*Designed for the maintenance of good nutrition of practically
all healthy people in the United States*

Water-Soluble Vitamins / Minerals

Vita-min C (mg)	Thia-min (mg)	Ribo-flavin (mg)	Niacin (mg NE)[f]	Vita-min B₆ (mg)	Fo-late (µg)	Vita-min B₁₂ (µg)	Cal-cium (mg)	Phos-phorus (mg)	Mag-nesium (mg)	Iron (mg)	Zinc (mg)	Iodine (µg)	Sele-nium (µg)
30	0.3	0.4	5	0.3	25	0.3	400	300	40	6	5	40	10
35	0.4	0.5	6	0.6	35	0.5	600	500	60	10	5	50	15
40	0.7	0.8	9	1.0	50	0.7	800	800	80	10	10	70	20
45	0.9	1.1	12	1.1	75	1.0	800	800	120	10	10	90	20
45	1.0	1.2	13	1.4	100	1.4	800	800	170	10	10	120	30
50	1.3	1.5	17	1.7	150	2.0	1,200	1,200	270	12	15	150	40
60	1.5	1.8	20	2.0	200	2.0	1,200	1,200	400	12	15	150	50
60	1.5	1.7	19	2.0	200	2.0	1,200	1,200	350	10	15	150	70
60	1.5	1.7	19	2.0	200	2.0	800	800	350	10	15	150	70
60	1.2	1.4	15	2.0	200	2.0	800	800	350	10	15	150	70
50	1.1	1.3	15	1.4	150	2.0	1,200	1,200	280	15	12	150	45
60	1.1	1.3	15	1.5	180	2.0	1,200	1,200	300	15	12	150	50
60	1.1	1.3	15	1.6	180	2.0	1,200	1,200	280	15	12	150	55
60	1.1	1.3	15	1.6	180	2.0	800	800	280	15	12	150	55
60	1.0	1.2	13	1.6	180	2.0	800	800	280	10	12	150	55
70	1.5	1.6	17	2.2	400	2.2	1,200	1,200	320	30	15	175	65
95	1.6	1.8	20	2.1	280	2.6	1,200	1,200	355	15	19	200	75
90	1.6	1.7	20	2.1	260	2.6	1,200	1,200	340	15	16	200	75

[c] Retinol equivalents. 1 retinol equivalent = 1 µg retinol or 6 µg β-carotene.

[d] As cholecalciferol. 10 µg cholecalciferol = 400 IU of vitamin D.

[e] α-Tocopherol equivalents. 1 mg d-α tocopherol = 1 α-TE.

[f] 1 NE (niacin equivalent) is equal to 1 mg of niacin or 60 mg of dietary tryptophan.

Estimated Safe and Adequate Daily Dietary Intakes of Selected Vitamins and Minerals[a]

Category	Age (years)	Vitamins	
		Biotin (µg)	Pantothenic Acid (mg)
Infants	0–0.5	10	2
	0.5–1	15	3
Children and adolescents	1–3	20	3
	4–6	25	3–1
	7–10	30	4–5
	11 +	30–100	4–7
Adults		30–100	4–7

Category	Age (years)	Trace Elements[b]				
		Copper (mg)	Man-ganese (mg)	Fluoride (mg)	Chromium (µg)	Molybdenum (µg)
Infants	0–0.5	0.4–0.6	0.3–0.6	0.1–0.5	10–40	15–30
	0.5–1	0.6–0.7	0.6–1.0	0.2–1.0	20–60	20–40
Children and adolescents	1–3	0.7–1.0	1.0–1.5	0.5–1.5	20–80	25–50
	4–6	1.0–1.5	1.5–2.0	1.0–2.5	30–120	30–75
	7–10	1.0–2.0	2.0–3.0	1.5–2.5	50–200	50–150
	11 +	1.5–2.5	2.0–5.0	1.5–2.5	50–200	75–250
Adults		1.5–3.0	2.0–5.0	1.5–4.0	50–200	75–250

[a] Because there is less information on which to base allowances, these figures are not given in the main table of RDA and are provided here in the form of ranges of recommended intakes.

[b] Since the toxic levels for many trace elements may be only several times usual intakes, the upper levels for the trace elements given in this table should not be habitually exceeded.

Basic Nutrition
and
Diet Therapy
Ninth Edition

Sue Rodwell Williams, Ph.D., M.P.H., R.D.
President, SRW Productions, Inc., and Director,
The Berkeley Nutrition Group,
Berkeley, California; Nutrition Consultant,
Kaiser-Permanente Northern California Regional
Newborn Screening and Metabolic Program,
Kaiser-Permanente Medical Center, Oakland

with 80 illustrations

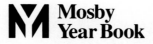
Mosby
Year Book

St. Louis   Baltimore   Boston   Chicago   London   Philadelphia   Sydney   Toronto

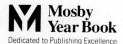
**Mosby
Year Book**
Dedicated to Publishing Excellence

Editor: Vicki Van Ry-Malinee
Editorial assistant: Francine Trtanj
Project manager: Peggy Fagen
Design: Jeanne Wolfgeher
Cover illustration: Barbara Maslen

Photo Credits
P. 146, Cathy Lander-Goldberg/Lander Photographics; p. 209, Judy Canty/Stock Boston; p. 230, Elizabeth Crews/Stock Boston; p. 250, Sue Klemens/Stock Boston; p. 255, Joel Gordon/Joel Gordon Photography © 1990.

Ninth edition

Printed in the United States of America

Mosby–Year Book, Inc.
11830 Westline Industrial Drive, St. Louis, MO 63146

International Standard Book Number 0-8016-5686-9

92 93 94 95 96   GW/DC   9 8 7 6 5 4 3 2 1

To my son, **JIM,** *with love —*
his expert work and personal support
have helped me shape this book —
he is a true "Renaissance man" — and friend

S.R.W.

PREFACE

For many years, through eight highly successful editions, this compact "little" book has provided a sound learning resource and a handy manual in basic nutrition for support personnel in health care. It has filled a practical need among various allied health workers and students for a realistic and easily comprehended reference. It has always maintained a person-centered approach to nutrional study and client/patient care. This new ninth edition continues this important central focus.

The field of nutrition is a dynamic *human* endeavor. It has been expanding and changing since publication of earlier editions. We want to capture the excitement of this current, constantly developing nutrition knowledge and its application to human needs in this new edition with its modern format and style.

Three main factors continue to expand and change this modern face of nutrition. First, the science of nutrition is growing more and more rapidly with basic research. New knowledge, as is true in all fields, always challenges some traditional ideas and develops new ones. This is especially true in applying current nutritional science to the modern movement in health promotion and disease prevention in health care for younger populations and to a preventive early risk-reduction approach to management of chronic disease in our aging population. Second, the rapidly increasing multiethnic diversity in the changing nature of the general population in the United States both enriches our food patterns and presents varying health care needs. Thrid, the overall general public is more aware and concerned about health promotion and the role of nutrition, largely through increasing attention of the media. General interest in nutrition has grown. Our clients and patients are raising more questions and seeking intelligent answers. They want sound information to deal with common misinformation and fads, as well as with legitimate controversy. They want to be more personally involved in their own health care. Nothing, perhaps, is more human a part of that care than food.

This new edition reflects these far-reaching changes. Its guiding principle continues to be my own commitment, along with that of my publisher, to the integrity of each previous edition. *Our expanded goal here is to produce a new book for today's needs, completely updated and rewritten, with new design and format and sound content to meet the expectations and changing needs of students, faculty, and practitioners in basic health care.*

OBJECTIVES OF THE BOOK

This text is designed primarily for students and health workers in beginning assistance level programs for practical or licensed vocational nurses (LPNs and LVNs), as well as for diet technicians or diet aides. As in previous editions, it assumes a limited background in nutrition-related basic sciences, so basic concepts are carefully explained when introduced. But with the changing public health awareness, it also assumes an expanded general base in nutrition and health. Thus, building on this interest, its general purpose is to introduce some basic principles of scientific nutrition and present their applications in *person-centered* care in health and disease. In addition, my personal concerns are ever present: (1) that this introduction to the science and practice I love will continue to lead students and readers to enjoy learning about human nutrition in the lives of people and stimulate further reading in personal interest areas; (2) that these caretakers will be alert to nutrition news and to questions raised by their increasingly diverse clients and patients; and (3) that contact and communication with professional nutrition resource persons will help build a strong team approach to clinical nutrition problems in all patient care.

MAJOR CHANGES IN THIS EDITION

In a real sense, this new edition of this classic basic text continues to be a new book for our new times and needs. To accommodate the demands of a rapidly developing science and society, yet retain a clearly understood writing style, I have rewritten a large portion of the text and made major changes to increase its usefulness.

1. New Chapter Materials. All chapters include new materials to help meet current practice needs: Chapter 1 provides a strengthened current focus on new directions in health care — health promotion, risk reduction for disease prevention, and new community health care delivery systems with emphasis on team care and the active role of clients in educated self-care. New research updates all of the basic nutrient-energy chapters in the remainder of Part I. In Part II, the separate life cycle Chapters 10, 11, and 12 reflect new material on human growth and development needs at each age. For example, the new Academy of Sciences guidelines for a more liberal positive weight gain to support the metabolic demands of pregnancy and lactation are presented and discussed. Positive growth support for infancy, childhood, and adolescence, as well as health-maintenance needs of adults throughout the aging process, focuses on the building of a healthy lifestyle to reduce disease risks. New community nutrition material in Chapter 13 highlights food-borne disease through bacterial contamination, environmental contaminants such as lead, and food labeling reform for the 1990s, and in Chapter 14 a reorganized and greatly expanded section on America's multiethnic cultural food patterns includes new descriptions of Moslem, Native American Navajo, African Americans, Cajun, and Southeast Asian patterns. Chapter 16 contains new material on athletics to clarify current practices of glycogen loading for endurance events, the proliferation of sports drinks, and the illegal use of steroids by athletes and body builders. Additional changes in each clinical nutrition chapter are described below.

2. New Book Format and Design. The chapter format enhances the book's appeal and encourages its use. Basic chapter concepts and overview, illustrations, tables, boxes, definitions, headings, and subheadings make it easier and more interesting to read.

3. New Learning Aids. Educational aids have been developed to assist both student and instructor in the teaching-learning process. These aids are described later in detail.

4. New Illustrations. A number of new illustrations, including artwork, graphs, charts, and photographs, help both students and practitioners better understand the concepts and clinical practices presented.

5. Enhanced Readability and Student Interest. This ninth edition is written in a style that not only continues its simple unfolding of the material, but also creates new interest and helps students understand basic concepts better by expanding explanations to "flesh out" the topics discussed.

ADDITIONAL CHANGES NEW TO THIS EDITION

I have developed and reorganized the text material to reflect both current nutrition knowledge and changes in health care practices.

Part One: Principles of Nutrition

Introductory chapter. Chapter 1 expands its focus on our changing health-care system and the expanded role of nutrition in health promotion as well as disease prevention.

Nutrients and energy. Each chapter on the various macronutrients that supply energy, as well as each of those describing the large number of micronutrients that supply special metabolic needs, has been updated to include current nutritional science material and its application to human health and health problems. For example, new material addresses such current nutrition concerns as complex carbohydrates, fats and cholesterol, fiber, vitamins and minerals, and the issue of nutrient supplements.

Part Two: Community Nutrition and the Life Cycle

Expanded age group needs. Three expanded separate chapters provide needed new material on: (1) early fetal growth and development during pregnancy with liberal guidelines for weight gain to support metabolic demands of both pregnancy and breast-feeding of the newborn; (2) continued rapid growth of infancy, erratic growth patterns through childhood, followed by the rapid growth surge and changing male and female bodies of maturing adolescents; and (3) the leveling off of physical growth in adulthood, but continued psychosocial development throughout life with its gradual decline in the extended aging process. There is new material, for example, on the eating disorders of adolescence, adolescent pregnancy, and on the aging process, as well as practical ways of meeting nutritional needs in each period of growth and development.

Weight management and physical fitness. These two updated chapters meet current needs for positive health approaches to maintaining ideal weight and developing habits of regular exercise, with expanded discussion of athletic practices both useful and harmful.

Community nutrition and changing American food patterns. Chapters 13 and 14 have been rewritten to include much practical material for working with families in the community. There is new background, as indicated above, on the relation of health to the community food supply, the significance of cultural food patterns in our increasingly multi-ethnic society, the many community factors that influence food habits, and the effects of our changing American food patterns.

Part Three: Clinical Nutrition

Introductory chapter. The chapter introducing clinical nutrition in various health problems focuses on the *process* of modern health care, here relating nutritional aspects of care to total medical-nursing nutrition team care of individual patients. This person-centered care *process* follows interrelated stages of assessment, intervention, and evaluation in many forms.

Clinical disease chapters. The remaining chapters on major health problems have all been reorganized and updated to provide current diet therapy procedures for each condition. For example, new material is provided on the underlying disease process of atherosclerosis and essential hypertension as a major risk factor is reflected in the chapter on heart disease, on nephrotic syndrome and kidney dialysis in renal disease, on tube feedings and total parenteral nutrition (TPN) in the chapters on surgery and cancer, on care of the patient with burns in the surgery chapter, and on nutrition and immunity in the cancer chapter.

LEARNING AIDS THROUGHOUT THE TEXT

As indicated, this new edition is especially significant in its use of many learning aids throughout the text.

Chapter openers. To immediately draw students into the topic for study, each chapter opens with a short list of the basic concepts involved, and a brief chapter overview leading into the topic to "set the stage."

Chapter headings. Throughout each chapter, the major headings and sub-headings in special type indicate the organization of the chapter material. This makes for easy reading and understanding of the key ideas. Main concepts and terms are also brought out with bold type and italics.

Boxed material. Additional boxed information has been expanded and numbered for easy reference. New Clinical Applications boxes go a step further on a given topic or present a case study for analysis. This enhances the understanding of concepts through further explanation or application.

Definitions of terms. Key terms important to the student's understanding and application of the material in patient care are presented in two ways. First, they are identified in the body of the text, often with interesting derivation and description of the words. Second, they are listed in a summary glossary at the back of the book for quick reference.

Illustrations. The expanded use of new illustrations throughout the text creates interest and helps the student better understand important concepts and applications.

Chapter summaries. Brief summary paragraphs review chapter highlights and help students see the "big picture." Then the student can return to any part of the material for repeated study and clarification of details as needed.

Review questions. To help the student understand key parts of the chapter or to apply it to patient care problems, questions are given after each chapter for review and analysis of the material presented.

Self-test questions. In addition, self-test items in both true-false and multiple choice forms are provided at the end of each chapter for students to check their basic knowledge at that point.

Suggestions for further study. Also, at the end of each chapter a variety of activities are suggested for better understanding and application of the text material. These suggestions include many projects, surveys, situational problems, and analysis of information gathered.

Case studies. In clinical care chapters, case studies have been highlighted in separate Boxes to focus the student's attention to related patient care problems. Each case is accompanied by questions for case analysis. Students can use these examples for similar patient care needs in their own clinical assignments.

Diet guides. In clinical chapters, various diet therapy guides provide practical help in patient care and education.

Cited references. Expanded use of background references throughout the text provide more resources for students who may want to "dig further" into a particular topic of interest.

Further annotated readings. To encourage further reading of useful materials for expanding knowledge of key concepts or applying the material in practical ways for patient care and education, a brief list of annotated resources is provided at the end of each chapter.

Appendixes. The Appendixes include a table of food values and several materials, such as food sources of cholesterol, dietary fiber, sodium and potassium, as well as the food exchange lists for meal-planning, for use as reference tools and guides in learning and practice. The newly revised standard Recommended Dietary Allowances (RDA) tables have been placed inside the book covers for easy quick reference.

A PERSONAL APPROACH

In the past, users of this basic text have responded very positively to the person-centered approach I have tried to develop. In this new edition I have sought to strengthen this approach in several ways.

Personal writing style. In this new edition, I have continued to use a personal writing style to reflect the very personal nature of human nutrition and health care, and to speak more directly to the reader. I wish to share my own self and feelings, born of many years of experience in clinical work and teaching. I want to create interest and involvement in our rapidly advancing knowledge of nutrition, the exciting process of learning, and in sound humanistic practice. In this manner, I want to express my concern for students and their learning, and for clients or patients and their needs.

Practical application. In most human endeavors, theory is useful only in its human application. So it is with nutritional care. Thus all of the chapters here supply expanded practical applications of current scientific knowledge in very realistic human terms. My goal is always to bring together science and human needs to make them "come alive" for students and in turn for their clients and patients. Often there are no single "pat" answers to many health care problems, and individual situations require individual solutions. But a basic understanding of the principles involved will make for better person-centered care in any case.

ACKNOWLEDGMENTS

A realistic and useful textbook is never the work of one person. It develops into the planned product through the committed hands and hearts of a number of persons. It would be impossible to name all the individuals involved here, but several groups deserve special recognition.

First, I am indebted to Mosby–Year Book Publishing and the many persons there, new and old friends, who have had a part in this project. Especially do I thank my publisher and editorial staff, including Ed Murphy, Vicki Van Ry-Malinee, Francine Trtanj, and Peggy Fagen, all of whom helped shape the manuscript and support my efforts and goals.

Second, I am grateful to the reviewers who gave their valuable time and skills to help strengthen the manuscript:

Elaine Hammes
Indian Hills Community College

Leona McCoy
Flint Hills Area Vocational School

Elaine Schmidt
Indiana Votech College

Diane Suchman
Sarasota County Vocational Technical School

Barbara Vredeveld
Iowa Western Community College

Third, I am grateful to my own production staff, especially to my expert business manager and systems analyst, Jim Williams, who has developed and set up my expanded computer system, a true joy to work with. And to Tony Rinella, friend and computer expert, who has responded with grace to my calls for help at all sorts of odd hours, I give special thanks for being there when I needed him.

Fourth, many students and interns, colleagues, clients, and patients over the years have enriched my life; their contributions are revealed in all my work. Each one has taught me something about human experience, and I am grateful for those opportunities for personal growth.

And finally, but most of all, I want to thank my family — my "home team." These beautiful people never cease to provide loving support for all my work, and to each one I am eternally grateful.

I hope that those who use this text will continue to give me feedback and suggestions for future editions. My constant purpose is to provide a useful and practical beginning text for students, one that can help them understand some of the elemental principles of nutritional science and apply them in personal patient care — and one that they can enjoy.

Sue Rodwell Williams

CONTENTS

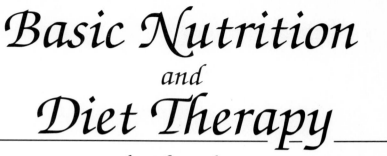

Basic Nutrition
and
Diet Therapy

Ninth Edition

❖

Food, nutrition, and health

K E Y   C O N C E P T S

An integral component of health promotion is optimal personal and community nutrition.

Certain nutrients in the food we eat are essential to our health and well-being.

Food and nutrient guides help us to plan a balanced diet according to individual needs and goals.

*W*e live in a world with rapidly changing elements — our environment, food supply, population, and scientific knowledge. Within individual environments, our physical bodies and our personalities change and with them our personal needs and goals. These *constant changes* of life must be in some kind of *positive balance* to produce healthy living. Thus within these life concepts of change and balance, to be realistic our study of food, nutrition, and health care must focus on **health promotion**. Although we may view and define health and disease in different ways, a primary basis for promoting health and preventing disease must always be good food and the sound nutrition it provides. This basic study of nutrition, then, has primary importance in two ways. First, of course, it is fundamental for our own health. But as health care workers, we also know that good nutrition is essential for the health and well-being of our patients and clients.

HEALTH PROMOTION

Basic definitions

Nutrition and dietetics. *Nutrition* concerns the food people eat and how their bodies use it. *Nutritional science* comprises the body of scientific knowledge governing the food requirements of humans for maintenance, growth, activity, reproduction, and lactation. *Dietetics* is the health profession responsible for the application of nutritional science to promote human health and treat disease. The *registered dietitian (RD)*, especially the *clinical nutrition specialist*, or the *public health nutritionist* in the community, is the nutrition authority on the health care team. These health care professionals carry the major responsibility for nutritional care of patients and clients.

Health and wellness. Good nutrition is essential to good health throughout life, beginning with prenatal life and extending through old age. In its simplest terms, *health* is defined as the absence of disease. But this is far too narrow a definition. Life experience shows that it is much more. It must include broader attention to the roots of health in meeting basic human needs—physical, mental, psychological, and social well-being.[1] This approach recognizes the individual as a whole person and relates health to both internal and external environments. The added positive concept of *wellness* carries this broader approach one step further. It seeks for all individuals full development of their potential, within whatever environment they may find themselves. It implies a balance among activities and goals: work versus leisure, life-style choices versus health risks, and personal needs versus expectations of others. Wellness implies a positive dynamic state motivating a person to seek a higher level of function.

Wellness movement and national health goals. The current wellness or fitness movement began in the 1970s in response to the medical care system's emphasis on illness and disease and the rising costs of medical care. Since then, "holistic" health and health promotion have focused on life-style and personal choice in helping individuals and families develop plans for wellness. During the past decade the U.S. national health goals have reflected this wellness philosophy. The current report of the U.S. Department of Health and Human Services, Public Health Service, *Healthy People 2000*, focuses on the nation's main objective of positive health promotion and disease prevention. It outlines specific objectives for meeting three broad public health goals over the next 10 years: an increase in the span of healthy life for Americans, reduction of health disparities among Americans, and access to preventative health care services for all Americans.[2] A major theme throughout the report is the encouragement of healthy choices in diet, weight control, and other risk factors for disease, especially in its 21 specific nutrition objectives. Community health agencies are implementing these goals and objectives in local and state public and private health programs.[3] All of these efforts recognize personal nutrition as an integral component of health and health care.

Traditional and preventive approaches to health. The *preventive* approach to health involves identifying risk factors that increase an individual's chances of developing a particular health problem.[4] Knowing these factors, individuals can then make behavior choices that will prevent or minimize their risks of disease. On the other hand, the *traditional* approach to health attempts change only when symptoms of illness or disease already exist. Then ill persons seek out a physician to diagnose, treat, and "cure" the condition. This approach has little value for lifelong positive health. Major chronic problems such as heart disease or cancer may be developing long before overt signs become apparent.

Importance of a balanced diet

Food and health. Food has always been one of the necessities of life. Many people, however, are concerned only with food that relieves their hunger or satisfies their appetites but are not concerned about whether it supplies their bodies with all the components of good nutrition. The health care team core practitioners—physician, clinical nutritionist, and nurse—are all aware of the important part that food plays in maintaining good health and recovery from illness. Chronic ill health in patients requires checking food habits as possible contributing factors. Thus assessing the patient's nutritional status and identifying nutritional needs are primary activities in planning care.

Signs of good nutrition. Evidence of good nutrition is a well-developed body, ideal weight for body composition (ratio of muscle mass to fat) and height, and good muscle development and tone. The skin is smooth and clear, the hair glossy, and the eyes clear and bright. Posture is good, and the facial expression alert. Appetite, digestion, and elimination are normal. Well-nourished persons are much more likely to be alert, both mentally and physically, and to have a positive outlook on life. They are also more able to resist infectious diseases than are undernourished people. Proper diet not only creates healthier persons but also extends the years of normal functioning.

FUNCTIONS OF NUTRIENTS IN FOOD

To sustain life, the nutrients in foods must perform three basic overall functions within the body: provide energy sources, build tissue, and regulate metabolic processes. *Metabolism* refers to the sum of all body processes that accomplish these three basic life-sustaining tasks.

An important nutritional-metabolic fact emerges in the following outline of these three basic nutrient functions. It is the fundamental principle of *nutrient interaction*. This means two things: individual nutrients have many specific metabolic functions, including primary and supporting roles, and no nutrient ever works alone. The human body is a fascinating whole made up of many parts and processes. Intimate metabolic relationships exist among all the basic nutrients and their metabolic products. This key principle of nutrient interaction will be demonstrated more clearly in the following chapters. Although the various nutrients may be separated for study purposes, remember that in the body they do not exist that way. They always interact as a dynamic whole to produce and maintain the human body.

Energy sources

Carbohydrates. Dietary carbohydrates—starches and sugars—provide the body's primary source of fuel for heat and energy. They also maintain the body's backup store of quick energy as *glycogen*, sometimes called "animal starch" (p. 17). Each gram of carbohydrate consumed yields 4 kilocalories (kcalories or kcal) of body energy. This number is called the "fuel factor" for carbohydrates. In a well-balanced diet, carbohydrates should provide about 55% to 60% of the total kcalories.

Fats. Dietary fats, from both animal and plant sources, provide the body's secondary, or storage, form of heat and energy. It is a more concentrated form of energy, yielding 9 kcal for each gram consumed. Thus its fuel factor is 9. In a well-balanced diet, fats should provide no more than 25% to 30% of the total kcalories, with the majority of this amount, approximately two thirds, being unsaturated fats from plant sources (p. 26).

Proteins. The body may draw on dietary or tissue protein to obtain needed energy when the supply of fuel from carbohydrates and fats is insufficient. When this occurs, protein can yield 4 kcal/g, making its fuel factor 4. In a well-balanced diet, quality protein should provide about 15% to 20% of the total kcalories. Thus, although protein's primary function is tissue building, some may be available for energy as needed.

Tissue building

Proteins. The primary function of protein is tissue building. Dietary protein provides *amino acids*, the building units, necessary for constructing and repairing body tissues. This is a constant process that ensures growth and maintenance of a strong body structure and vital substances for its tissue functions.

Other nutrients. Several other nutrients that contribute to building and maintaining tissues are described in the following paragraphs.

1. *Minerals.* Two major minerals, calcium and phosphorus, function in building and maintaining bone tissue. Iron contributes to building the oxygen carrier, hemoglobin.

2. *Vitamins.* An example of vitamins used in tissue building is that of vitamin C in developing the cementing intercellular ground substance. This substance helps build strong tissue and prevent tissue bleeding.

3. *Fatty acids.* Fatty acids derived from fat metabolism help build the central fat substance of cell walls, which promotes transport of fat-soluble materials across the cell wall.

Regulation and control

All of the multiple chemical processes in the body, required for providing energy and building tissue, must be carefully regulated and controlled to maintain a smooth, balanced operation. Otherwise there would be chaos within the body systems and death would result. Life and health result from a dynamic balance among all the body parts and processes. Nutrients that help regulate body processes are described in the following list.

1. *Vitamins.* Many vitamins function as coenzyme factors, components of cell enzymes, in governing chemical reactions in cell metabolism. This is true, for example, of most of the B-complex vitamins.

2. *Minerals.* Many minerals also serve as coenzyme factors with cell enzymes in cell metabolism. An interesting structural example is that of cobalt, which is a central constituent of vitamin B_{12} (cobalamin) and functions with this vitamin to combat pernicious anemia.

3. *Other nutrients.* Water and fiber also function as regulatory agents. In fact, water is *the* fundamental agent for life itself, providing the essential base for all metabolic processes. Dietary fiber helps regulate the passage of food material through the gastrointestinal tract and influences absorption of various nutrients.

GOOD NUTRITION
Optimal nutrition

Optimal or good nutrition, then, means that a person receives and uses substances that are obtained from a *varied* diet containing carbohydrates, fats, proteins, certain minerals, vitamins, water, and dietary fiber in optimal amounts. The optimal amounts of these nutrients should be greater than the minimum requirements, to cover variations in health and disease and provide reserves.

Undernutrition

Dietary surveys have shown that approximately one third of the U.S. population lives on diets below the optimal level. This does not necessarily mean that these Americans are undernourished. Some persons can maintain health with less than the optimal amounts of various nutrients in a state of borderline nutrition. On the average, however, a person receiving less than the desired amounts has a greater risk of physical illness than a person receiving the appropriate amounts. Such nutritionally deficient persons are limited in physical work capacity, immune system function, and mental activity.[5] They lack nutritional reserves to meet any added physiologic or metabolic demands from injury or illness, or to sustain fetal development during pregnancy or proper growth in childhood. This state may result from poor eating habits or an unrelieved continuous stressful environment with little or no income.

Malnutrition

Signs of more serious malnutrition appear when nutritional reserves are depleted and nutrient and energy intake is not sufficient to meet day-to-day needs or added metabolic stress. Many malnourished people live in conditions of poverty. These conditions influence the health of all persons involved, but especially the most vulnerable ones—pregnant women, infants, children, and elderly adults. Here in the United States, one of the wealthiest countries on earth, many studies document widespread hunger and malnutrition among the poor, indicating that food security problems involve urban development issues, economic policy and more general poverty issues.[6] The Physician Task Force on Hunger in America has found that in the United States alone at least 20 million persons suffer hunger some days each month.[7] Worldwide about 40,000 to 50,000 people die *each day* as a result of malnutrition, and an estimated 450 million to 1.3 billion people do not have enough to eat.[8]

Frank malnutrition also occurs in hospitals. For example, extended illness, especially among older persons with chronic disease, places added stress on the body, and the person's daily nutrient and energy intake is insufficient to meet needs.

Overnutrition

Some persons may be in a state of overnutrition that results from excess nutrient and energy intake over time. In a sense, overnutrition can be viewed as another form of malnutrition, especially when excess caloric intake produces gross harmful body weight—morbid obesity. Harmful overnutrition also occurs in persons who use excessive "megadose" amounts of nutrient supplements over time that produce damaging tissue effects (see p. 66).

NUTRIENT AND FOOD GUIDES FOR HEALTH PROMOTION
Nutrient standards

Most developed countries of the world have set up nutrition standards for the major nutrients to serve as guidelines for maintaining healthy populations. These standards are not intended to indicate individual requirements or therapeutic needs, but rather serve as a reference for levels of intake of the essential nutrients considered, on the basis of current scientific knowledge, to adequately meet the known nutritional needs of most healthy population groups. Although these standards are similar in different countries, they may vary somewhat according to the philosophy of scientists and practitioners in a particular country as to their purpose and use. In the United States these standards are called the *Recommended Dietary Allowances (RDAs)*.

U.S. standards: Recommended Dietary Allowances. The U.S. nutrient standard for population groups is outlined by age and sex. It is developed and maintained by a group of leading scientists and practitioners in the field of nutrition, working through the National Academy of Sciences in Washington, D.C. The Academy has numerous divisions of councils and is supported by the National Institutes of Health. The working group of nutrition scientists responsible for the RDAs make up the Food and Nutrition Board of the National Research Council.

The U.S. RDA standard was first published in 1943, during World War II, as a guide for planning and obtaining food supplies for national defense and providing average population standards as a goal for good nutrition. The RDAs have been revised and expanded over the years. A revision usually comes out every 4 or 5 years, with the current 10th edition in 1989, and reflects increasing scientific knowledge as well as expanding social concerns about nutrition and health.[9,10] (See the current U.S. RDA tables inside book covers.)

Other standards. Canadian and British standards are similar to the U.S. standard. In less developed countries where factors such as quality of protein foods available must be considered, workers look to standards such as those set by the Food and Agriculture Organization (FAO) of the World Health Organization (WHO). Nonetheless, all of these standards provide a guideline to help health workers in a variety of population groups promote good health through sound nutrition.

Food guides

To interpret and apply sound nutrient standards, health workers need practical food guides to use in nutrition education and food planning with individuals and families. Such tools include the long-used but limited basic four food groups, and the more recent U.S. dietary guidelines.

Basic food groups. Nutritionists have worked to clarify nutrition concepts so people can estimate whether their food choices supply enough of all essential nutrients. By the mid-1950s various food plans evolved into one, the four food groups: milk, meat, fruits and vegetables, and breads and cereals. In 1979 the names of the groups were revised by the U.S. Department of Agriculture, and a fifth group—fats, sweets, and alcoholic beverages—was added. This plan was designed to provide a minimum foundation for a diet, representing about 1200 to 1400 kcalories. In 1991 the USDA revised this guide to represent a *total* diet, not just a foundation (Table 1-1). The major changes include an increase in servings of fruits and vegetables (from 4 per day to 5 to 9), and bread and cereal (from 4 per day to 6 to 11). The goal of these changes is to provide the bulk of dietary energy intake from carbohydrate while limiting fat intake.

U.S. dietary guidelines. The U.S. dietary guidelines were issued as a result of growing public concern beginning in the 1960s and subsequent Senate investigations studying hunger and nutrition in the United States. They are based on our developing concern about chronic health problems in an aging population and a changing food environment. From the beginning, they have encountered controversy, centering mainly on the broad issue of the roles of government and science in maintaining health. The U.S. Departments of Agriculture and Health and Human Services reissued this food guide in 1980 under the new title "The Dietary Guidelines for Americans." These statements relate current scientific thinking to America's leading health problems. Recent review by expert committees have led to only minimal updating changes over the past decade. The current 1990 issue is titled "Nutrition and Your Health: Dietary Guidelines for Americans."[11-13] It reflects a comprehensive evaluation of the scientific evidence of a relationship between diet and health, based on the findings in two important reports: the Surgeon General's 1988 report *Nutrition and Health,* and the National Academy of Sciences 1989 report *Diet and Health: Implications for Reducing Chronic Disease.*[14,15] The seven statements in the current guidelines serve as a useful general guide for a concerned public (Box 1-1). Although no guidelines can guarantee health or well-being, and people differ widely in their food needs, these general statements can lead people to evaluate their food habits and move toward general improvements. Good food habits based on moderation and variety can help to build sound, healthy bodies.

Individual needs

Person-centered care. Regardless of the type of food guide used, health workers must remember that food patterns vary with individual needs, living situations, and energy demands. However, usually persons who eat nutritionally well-balanced meals spread fairly evenly throughout the day can work more efficiently and sustain a more even energy supply.

Changing food environment. In recent years our food environment has been rapidly changing. There are more processed food items of variable or unknown nutrient quality. American food habits may have deteriorated in some ways. Despite a plentiful food supply, surveys show evidence of malnutrition, even

❖ **TABLE 1-1**   *The guide to daily food choices—a summary*

Food group	Serving	Major contributions	Foods and serving sizes*
Milk, yogurt, and cheese	2 (adult‖) 3 (children, teens, young adults, and pregnant or lactating women)	Calcium Riboflavin Protein Potassium Zinc	1 cup milk 1½ oz cheese 2 oz processed cheese 1 cup yogurt 2 cups cottage cheese 1 cup custard/pudding 1½ cups ice cream
Meat, poultry, fish, dry beans, eggs, and nuts	2-3	Protein Niacin Iron Vitamin B-6 Zinc Thiamin Vitamin B-12†	2-3 oz cooked meat, poultry, fish 1-1½ cups cooked dry beans 4 T peanut butter 2 eggs ½-1 cup nuts
Fruits	2-4	Vitamin C Fiber	¼ cup dried fruit ½ cup cooked fruit ¾ cup juice 1 whole piece of fruit 1 melon wedge
Vegetables	3-5	Vitamin A Vitamin C Folate Magnesium Fiber	½ cup raw or cooked vegetables 1 cup raw leafy vegetables
Bread, cereals, rice, and pasta	6-11	Starch Thiamin Riboflavin§ Iron Niacin Folate Magnesium‡ Fiber‡ Zinc	1 slice of bread 1 oz ready-to-eat cereal ½-¾ cup cooked cereal, rice, or pasta
Fats, oils, and sweets	Foods from this group should not replace any from the other groups. Amounts consumed should be determined by individual energy needs.		

From Wardlaw G and Insel P; Contemporary nutrition, St. Louis, 1992, Mosby—Year Book, Inc.
* May be reduced for child servings.   § If enriched.
† Only in animal food choices.   ‖ ≥25 years of age.
‡ Whole grains especially.

among hospitalized patients. Nurses and other health workers have an important responsibility in observing patients' diets carefully. In general, however, it is encouraging to note that Americans are gradually learning that what they eat *does* influence their health. Even fast-food restaurants, where Americans

BOX 1-1

❖ ────────── CLINICAL APPLICATION ────────── ❖

Dietary Guidelines for Americans

Eat a variety of foods

About 40 different known nutrients, and probably additional as yet unknown factors, are needed to maintain health. No single food can supply all the essential nutrients in the amounts needed to maintain health. Thus the greater the variety of foods used, the less likely a person is to develop either a deficiency or an excess of any single nutrient. One way to ensure a varied balanced diet, is to select foods each day from all the major food groups.

Maintain healthy weight

Excessive fatness is associated with some chronic disorders such as hypertension and diabetes, which in turn relate to heart disease. The healthy body weight, however, must be determined individually because many factors are involved, such as body composition (muscle/fat ratio), body metabolism, genetics, and physical activity.

Choose a diet low in fat, saturated fat, and cholesterol

Americans have traditionally consumed a high-fat diet. In some persons, excess fat leads to high levels of blood fats and cholesterol. Elevated blood levels of these fats and cholesterol are associated with a higher risk of coronary heart disease. Thus it is wise to reduce intake of fats in general, using them only in moderation.

Choose a diet with plenty of vegetables, fruits, and grain products

Increasing use of these foods will help supply more of the needed starches (complex carbohydrates) for energy, many essential nutrients, and necessary dietary fiber. Research indicates that certain types of dietary fiber may help control chronic bowel diseases, contribute to improved blood glucose management for persons with diabetes mellitus, and bind dietary cholesterol.

Use sugars only in moderation

The major health hazard from eating too much sugar is tooth decay (dental caries). Contrary to popular opinion, however, too much sugar does not in itself cause diabetes. It can only contribute to poor control of diabetes in persons who have inherited the disease. Most Americans consume a relatively large amount of sugar, over 100 pounds per person per year, much of it in processed food products. Again, moderation is the key.

Use salt and sodium only in moderation

Our main source of dietary sodium is in ordinary table salt. Excessive salt is not healthy for anyone and certainly not for persons with hypertension. Many processed food products contain considerable amounts of salt and other sodium compounds, and many Americans use more salt in foods than they need. Thus it is wise to limit salt use in food preparation or at the table and to reduce the use of "salty" food products. This approach will lower individual salt tastes, which are learned habits and not biologic necessities. There is ample sodium as a natural mineral in foods to meet usual needs.

If you drink alcoholic beverages, do so in moderation

Alcoholic beverages tend to be high in kcalories and low in other nutrients. Limited food intake may accompany excessive alcohol intake. Heavy drinking also contributes to chronic liver disease and some neurologic disorders, as well as some throat and neck cancers. Moreover, it is a major factor in highway deaths. Thus, moderation is the key, if alcohol is used at all, and persons should *never* drink and drive.

eat one in 12 meals, are beginning to respond to their customers' desires for less fat in fast foods, although some nutritional concerns still exist.[16,17] More than ever, people are being more selective about what they eat.

SUMMARY

Good food and key nutrients are essential to life and health. In our changing world an emphasis on health promotion and disease prevention through reducing health risks has become our primary health goal. The importance of a balanced diet in meeting this health goal through the functioning of its component nutrients is fundamental. Food guides that help persons plan such a healthy diet include the recommended dietary allowances (RDAs), the basic four food groups, and the U.S. dietary guidelines.

❖ REVIEW QUESTIONS

1. What is the current U.S. national health goal? Define this goal in terms of health, wellness, and the differences between traditional and preventive approaches to health.
2. Why is a balanced diet important? List and describe some signs of good nutrition.
3. What are the three basic functions of foods and their nutrients? Describe the general roles of nutrients in relation to each function: (1) main nutrient(s) for that function, and (2) other nutrients contributing.
4. Compare a nutrient standard such as the RDAs with a food guide in purpose and use.
5. Plan a day's food pattern for a selected person using the basic four food group as a guide with modifications according to the Dietary Guidelines for Americans.

❖ SELF-TEST QUESTIONS

True-false
For each item you answer "false," write the correct statement.
1. The diet planning tool "Dietary Guidelines for Americans" stresses the two basic concepts of variety and moderation in food habits.
2. Food processing has little influence on food taste, appearance, safety, or nutrient values.
3. Certain foods are called "complete foods" because they contain all the nutrients essential for full growth and health and are therefore essential in everyone's diet.

Multiple choice
1. Nutrients are:
   a. Chemical elements or compounds in foods that have specific metabolic functions
   b. Foods that are necessary for good health
   c. Metabolic control substances such as enzymes
   d. Nourishing foods used to cure certain illnesses
2. All nutrients needed by the body:
   a. Must be obtained by specific food combinations
   b. Must be obtained by vitamin/mineral supplements
   c. Have a variety of functions and uses in the body
   d. Are supplied by a variety of foods in many different combinations
3. All persons throughout life, as indicated by the RDAs, need:
   a. The same nutrients but in varying amounts
   b. The same amount of nutrients in any state of health
   c. The same nutrients at any age in the same amounts
   d. Different nutrients in varying amounts

❖ SUGGESTIONS FOR ADDITIONAL STUDY

1. Keep a notebook throughout the course. Cut out any articles on nutrition that you find. Bring them to class for discussion and evaluation, then paste them in your notebook.
2. Make a list of your food intake for 3 days and analyze each day using: (1) the basic four food groups guide, and (2) the "Dietary Guidelines for Americans." Compare the two results. Which of the two food guides do you think is more useful? Why?
3. At some time during the first half of the course, give a special report on the phase of nutrition that interests you most. Present your report to the class, and then place it in your notebook.

References

1. Joseph MV and Conrad AP: Social work influence on interdisciplinary ethical decision making in health care settings, Health Soc Work 14:22, February 1989.
2. US Department of Health and Human Services, Public Health Service: Healthy people 2000: National health promotion and disease prevention objectives—Nutrition priority area, Nutr Today 25(6):29, 1990.
3. Report: For your information: Healthy people 2000, J Am Diet Assoc 90(9):1215, 1990.
4. Foege WH: Preventive medicine, JAMA 261:2879, May 26, 1989.
5. Buzina R and others: Workshop on functional significance of mild-to-moderate malnutrition, Am J Clin Nutr 50:172, July 1989.
6. Cohen BE: Food security and hunger policy for the 1990s, Nutr Today 25(4):23, 1990.
7. Physician Task Force on Hunger in America: The growing epidemic, Cambridge, Mass, 1985, Harvard University Press.
8. American Dietetic Association: Hunger—worldwide problem, J Am Diet Assoc 86(10):1414, 1986.
9. National Research Council, Food and Nutrition Board: Recommended Dietary Allowances, ed 10, Washington, DC, 1989, National Academy Press.
10. Guthrie HA: Recommended dietary allowances 1989: changes, consensus and challenges, Nutr Today 25(1):43, 1990.
11. Report: Dietary guidelines for Americans released, Nutr Today 25(6):44, 1990.
12. Peterkin BB: Dietary guidelines for Americans, 1990 edition, J Am Diet Assoc 90(12):1725, 1990.
13. US Department of Agriculture and US Department of Health and Human Services: Nutrition and your health: Dietary guidelines for Americans, ed 3, Home and Garden Bull No 232, Nov 1990.
14. US Department of Health and Human Services, Public Health Service: The surgeon general's report on nutrition and health, PHS88-50210, Washington, DC, 1988, Government Printing Office.
15. Committee on Diet and Health, National Research Council, Food and Nutrition Board: Diet and health: implications for reducing chronic disease risk, Washington, DC, 1989, National Academy Press.
16. Shields JE and Young E: Fat in fast foods—evolving changes, Nutr Today 25(2):32, 1990.
17. Marens CL and others: Fast-food fare, N Engl J Med 322:557, Feb. 22, 1990.

Annotated readings

Executive summary: National Nutrition Monitoring System: nutrition monitoring in the United States: an update report on nutrition monitoring, Nutr Today 25(1):33, 1990.

Just how well are we doing nutritionally as a nation? This report of surveys conducted by the U.S. Departments of Agriculture and Health and Human Services provides some answers. It evaluates the dietary and nutritional status of the U.S. population, as well as the factors that determine status. Overall it suggests that some changes are occurring in eating patterns consistent with recommended dietary guidelines for Americans to avoid too much fat, saturated fat, and cholesterol and to consume adequate amounts of starch and dietary fiber.

Food: Does your diet meet the current RDAs? Better Homes and Gardens 69(2):M4, 1991.

Just how well are *you* doing with your own diet? How does it compare with the new Recommended Dietary Allowances (RDAs)? If you can answer *yes* to the four questions asked in this concise, one-page review, you're probably doing very well. You'll find a lot of basic nutrition information packed into this review, with emphasis on key food sources for the main nutrients.

2

❖

Carbohydrates

K E Y   C O N C E P T S

Carbohydrate foods provide practical body fuel sources because of their availability, relatively low cost, and storage capacity.

Carbohydrate structure varies from simple to complex, so it can provide both quick and extended energy for the body.

An indigestible carbohydrate, dietary fiber, serves separately as a body regulatory agent.

*A*s discussed in Chapter 1, key nutrients in the foods we eat sustain life and promote health. This tremendous result is possible because of the human body's unique use of these nutrients to provide three essential life and health needs: (1) *energy* to do its work, (2) *building materials* to maintain its form and functions, and (3) *control agents* to regulate these processes efficiently.

These three basic life and health nutrient functions are closely related—no one nutrient ever works alone. For this study, as indicated in the previous chapter, we will look at each of the nutrients separately, aware that in our bodies they do not exist and work that way. In this chapter we consider the first of these life needs—*energy production*—and the body's primary fuel for its energy system—*carbohydrates*.

NATURE OF CARBOHYDRATES
Relation to energy

Basic fuel source. Energy is a necessity for life. It is the power an organism requires to do its work. Any energy system must first have a basic fuel supply. In the human energy system, this major basic fuel comes from carbohydrate foods, the starches and sugars we eat.

Energy production system. To produce energy from a basic fuel supply, a successful energy system must be able to do three things: (1) change the basic fuel to a refined fuel that the machine is designed to use, (2) carry this refined fuel to the places that need it, and (3) burn this refined fuel at these places in the special equipment set up there to do it. Far more efficient than any man-made machine, the body easily does these three things. It digests its basic fuel, carbohydrate, changing it to glucose. The body then absorbs and carries this refined fuel, through blood circulation to the cells that need the glucose. Glucose is burned in the cells in the highly specific and intricate equipment, releasing energy through its amazing process of cell metabolism. Thus, since the human body can rapidly break down the starches and sugars we eat to yield energy, carbohydrates are called "quick energy" foods. They are our major source of energy.

Practical dietary importance. There are also practical reasons for the large quantities of carbohydrates in diets all over the world. First, carbohydrates are widely available, easily grown in grains, legumes, other vegetables, and fruits. In some countries, carbohydrate foods make up almost the entire diet of the people. In the American diet about half of the total kcalories is in the form of carbohydrates. Second, carbohydrates are relatively low in cost as compared with many other food items. Third, carbohydrates may be easily stored. They can be kept in dry storage for relatively long periods without spoilage. Modern processing and packaging extend the shelf life of carbohydrate products almost indefinitely.

The Continuing Survey of Food Intakes by Individuals (CSFII) conducted by the U.S. Department of Agriculture (1988) has indicated that about half (47%) of the total kcalories in the American diet come from carbohydrates, with children consuming somewhat more carbohydrates than adults.[1,2] The Food and Drug Administration (FDA) estimates that daily intake of sugars by Americans accounts for 21% of total kcalories—half from added sugars and half naturally occurring sugars.[3] The remainder of the total carbohydrate kcalories come from starches.

Classes of carbohydrates

The name *carbohydrate* comes from its chemical nature. It is composed of carbon (C), hydrogen (H), and oxygen (O), with the hydrogen/oxygen ratio usually that of water—H_2O. Its abbreviated name often used in medical charts or various notations is CHO, from the chemical symbols of its three components. The term *saccharide* used as a carbohydrate class name comes from the Latin word *saccharum* meaning "sugar." Thus a saccharide unit is a single sugar unit. Carbohydrates are classified according to the number of sugar, or saccharide, units making up their structure: *mono*saccharides with one sugar unit, *di*saccharides with two sugar units, and *poly*saccharides with many sugar

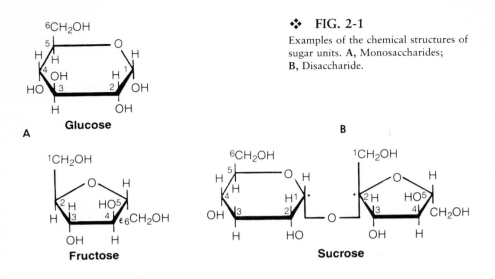

❖ **FIG. 2-1**

Examples of the chemical structures of sugar units. **A,** Monosaccharides; **B,** Disaccharide.

units. Monosaccharides and disaccharides are small, simple structures of only one and two sugar units, so they are called **simple carbohydrates**. Polysaccharides, on the other hand, are large complex compounds of many saccharide units in long chains, so they are called **complex carbohydrates**. For example, starch, the most significant polysaccharide in human nutrition, is made up of many coiled and branching chains in a "tree-like" structure. Each of the multiple branching chains is composed of 24 to 30 sugar units of glucose that are gradually split off in digestion to supply a steady source of energy over a period of time. A summary of the classes of carbohydrates is given in Table 2-1.

Monosaccharides. The three important simple single sugars in nutrition are glucose, fructose, and galactose.

1. Glucose. The basic single sugar in body metabolism is glucose. This is the form of sugar, sometimes called *dextrose*, circulating in the blood and supplying the primary fuel for the cells. It is not usually found as such in the diet, except for undiluted corn syrup or in processed food items. The body supply comes mainly from the digestion of starch. Glucose is a moderately sweet sugar.

2. Fructose. Fructose is found mainly in fruits, from which it gets its name, or in honey. Honey therefore is a form of sugar and cannot be used as a sugar substitute. The amount of fructose in fruits depends on the degree of ripeness. As the fruit ripens, some of the stored starch turns to sugar. High-fructose corn syrups are increasingly being used in processed food products. Fructose is the sweetest of the simple sugars.

3. Galactose. Galactose also is not usually found as such in the diet but comes mainly from the digestion of milk sugar, lactose.

All of these monosaccharides, or simple single sugars, require no digestion. They are quickly absorbed from the intestine into the bloodstream and carried to the liver. There they are converted by liver enzymes into glycogen, a constant backup energy supply, or used for immediate energy needs.

❖ **TABLE 2-1**   *Summary of carbohydrate classes*

Chemical class name	Class members	Sources

Polysaccharides
  Multiple sugars,
    complex car-
    bohydrates
	Starch	Grains and grain products
		    Cereal, bread, crackers, and other
		      baked goods
		    Pasta
		    Rice, corn, bulgur
		  Legumes
		  Potatoes and other vegetables

	Glycogen	Animal tissues, liver and muscle meats
	Dietary fiber	Whole grains Fruits Vegetables Seeds, nuts, skins

Disaccharides
  Double sugars,
    simple carbo-
    hydrates
	Sucrose	"Table" sugar: sugar cane, sugar beets
		Molasses

	Lactose	Milk
	Maltose	Starch digestion, intermediate Sweetener in food products Starch digestion, final

Monosaccharides
  Single sugars,
    simple carbo-
    hydrates
	Glucose (dextrose)	Corn syrup (large use in processed
		    foods)

	Fructose	Fruits, honey
	Galactose	Lactose (milk)

Disaccharides. Disaccharides are the simple double sugars, made up of two single sugar units linked together. The three disaccharides important in nutrition are sucrose, lactose, and maltose.

1. Sucrose. Sucrose is common table sugar. Its two single sugar units are glucose and fructose. It is used in the form of granulated, powdered, or brown sugar, and is made from sugar cane or sugar beets. Molasses, a by-product of sugar production, is also a form of sucrose. When people speak of "sugar" in the diet, usually they mean sucrose.

2. Lactose. The sugar in milk is lactose. Its two single sugar units are glucose and galactose. Lactose is the only common sugar not found in plants. It is less soluble and less sweet than sucrose. It remains in the intestine longer than other sugars and encourages the growth of certain useful bacteria. Lactose is formed in the mammary glands and comprises about 40% of the milk solids. Cow's milk contains 4.8% lactose and human milk has 7% lactose. Since lactose aids calcium and phosphorus absorption, the presence of all three nutrients in one natural "package" food is a fortunate circumstance.

3. Maltose. Maltose is not usually found as such in the diet. It is derived in the body from the intermediate digestive breakdown of starch. Because starch is made up entirely of many single glucose units, the two single sugar units that compose maltose are both glucose. Maltose is used as a sweetener in various processed foods.

Polysaccharides. Polysaccharides are complex carbohydrates composed of many single sugar units. The important polysaccharides in nutrition include starch, glycogen, and dietary fiber.

1. Starch. Starches, by far the most significant polysaccharides in the diet, are found in grains, in legumes and other vegetables, and in minute amounts in some fruits. Since starches are more complex than simple sugars, they break down more slowly and supply energy over a longer period of time. For starch to be used more promptly by the body, the outer membrane can be broken down by grinding or cooking. The cooking of starch not only improves its flavor but also softens and ruptures the starch cells, making digestion easier. Starch mixtures thicken when cooked because the portion that encases the starch granules has a gel-like quality, thickening the starch mixture in the same way that pectin causes jelly to set.

Starch is the most important dietary carbohydrate worldwide. Recently, the value of starch in human nutrition and health has received a great deal of recognition. The U.S. dietary guidelines (p. 9) recommend that about 50% to 55% of the total kcalories come from carbohydrates, with a greater portion of that intake coming from complex carbohydrate forms of starch. In many other countries where starch is a staple food, it makes up an even higher portion of the diet. The major food sources of starch (Fig. 2-2) include grains

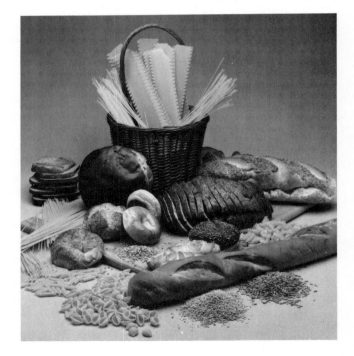

❖ **Fig. 2-2**
Complex carbohydrate foods.

in many forms such as cereals, pastas, crackers, breads, and other baked goods; legumes in many forms of dried beans, peas, lentils; potatoes, rice, corn, and bulgur; and other vegetables, especially root varieties.

2. *Glycogen*. Glycogen is similar in structure to starch and is therefore sometimes called *animal starch*. However, the animal body contains little glycogen, and that small amount drains away in meat preparation for market. Thus glycogen is not a significant carbohydrate in diets but is a tissue carbohydrate crucial to the body's metabolism and energy balance. It is found in the liver and muscles, where it is constantly being "recycled"—broken down to form glucose for immediate energy needs and resynthesized for liver and muscle storage. These small stores of glycogen help sustain normal blood sugar during fasting periods such as sleep hours and provide immediate fuel for muscle action.

3. *Dietary fiber*. Several types of dietary fiber are polysaccharides. Since humans lack the necessary enzymes to digest dietary fiber, these substances have no direct nutrient value as do other carbohydrates. However, their inability to be digested makes these materials important dietary assets. Through the observations of Burkitt, a British physician working in Africa, increasing attention has focused on the relation of fiber to health promotion and disease prevention, especially to gastrointestinal problems and management of diabetes.[4,5] The types of dietary fiber, important in human nutrition, are described below.

CELLULOSE. Cellulose is the chief part of the framework of plants. It remains undigested in the gastrointestinal tract and provides important bulk to the diet. This bulk helps move the food mass along, stimulates normal muscle action in the intestine, and forms the feces for elimination of waste products. The main sources of cellulose are stems and leaves of vegetables, and coverings of seeds and grains.

NONCELLULOSE POLYSACCHARIDES. Hemicellulose, pectins, gums and mucilages, and algal substances are noncellulose polysaccharides. They absorb water and swell to a larger bulk. Thus they slow the emptying of the food mass from the stomach, bind bile acids including cholesterol in the intestine, and prevent spastic colon pressure by providing bulk for normal muscle action. They also provide fermentation material for colon bacteria to work on.

LIGNIN. Lignin, the only noncarbohydrate type of dietary fiber, is a large compound forming the woody part of plants. It also combines with bile acids and cholesterol in the intestine, preventing their absorption.

A summary of these dietary fiber classes with their sources and functions is given in Table 2-2. Currently, as a method to simplify fiber for the public and practitioners alike, dietary fiber is being divided into two groups on the basis of solubility.[4,5] Cellulose, lignin, and most hemicelluloses are not soluble in water. The remainder, most pectins and other polysaccharides such as gums and mucilages, are water soluble. These two classes of dietary fiber are summarized in Table 2-3.

In general, the food groups providing needed dietary fiber include whole grains in their many food item forms, legumes, and vegetables and fruits with as much of their skins remaining as possible. Whole grains provide a special natural "package" of both the complex carbohydrate starch and the fiber in

❖ **TABLE 2-2** *Summary of dietary fiber classes*

	Source	Function
Cellulose	Main cell wall constituent of plants	Holds water; reduces elevated colonic intraluminal pressure; binds zinc
Noncellulose polysaccharides		Slows gastric emptying; provides fermentable material for colonic bacteria with production of gas and volatile fatty acids; binds bile acids and cholesterol
Gums	Secretions of plants	
Mucilages	Plant secretions and seeds	
	Algae, seaweeds	
Algal polysaccharides	Intercellular cement plant	
Pectin substances	material	
Hemicellulose	Cell wall plant material	Holds water and increases stool bulk; reduces elevated colonic pressure; binds bile acids
Lignin	Woody part of plants	Antioxidant; binds bile acids, cholesterol, and metals

❖ **TABLE 2-3** *Summary of soluble and insoluble fibers in total dietary fiber*

Insoluble	Soluble
Cellulose	Gums
Most hemicelluloses	Mucilages
Lignin	Algal polysaccharides
	Most pectins

the coating. In addition, whole grains contain an abundance of vitamins and minerals. In comparison, refined grains have no fiber left and only three B vitamins and iron restored in the enrichment process. The Nationwide Food Consumption Survey of the U.S. Department of Agriculture in its reports of the Continuing Survey of Food Intakes of Individuals estimates the dietary fiber intake of women to be approximately 11 g/day; men 17.5 g/day; and young children, 9.8 g/day.[1,5] Many health organizations have recommended increasing the intake of complex carbohydrates in general or dietary fiber in particular, and a range of dietary intakes has been suggested by study groups.[6-8]

There is no RDA standard for dietary fiber, but the committee does state that a desirable fiber intake should be achieved not by adding concentrated fiber supplements to the diet, but by eating a higher-fiber diet of whole grains, fruits, vegetables, and legumes, which also provide vitamins and minerals.[9] Although specific needs remain to be determined, a general daily increase to about 25 g/1000 kcal up to 40 g of total dietary fiber appears to be a reasonable goal. This intake would require consistent use of whole grains, legumes, vegetables, fruits, seeds, and nuts. A table of dietary fiber content of some commonly used foods is provided in the Appendix.

FUNCTIONS OF CARBOHYDRATES
Primary energy function
Basic fuel supply. The main function of carbohydrates is to provide the primary fuel for the body. To meet energy needs, carbohydrates burn in the body at the rate of 4 kcal/g. Thus the fuel factor for carbohydrate is 4. Carbohydrates furnish readily available energy that is needed not only for physical activities but also for all the work of the body cells. Fat is also a fuel, but the body needs only a small amount of dietary fat, mainly to supply the essential fatty acids (p. 29).

Reserve fuel supply. Glycogen reserves supply vital backup fuel. The total amount of carbohydrate in the body, including both glycogen and blood sugar, is relatively small (Table 2-4). However, without resupply this total amount of available glucose provides energy sufficient for only about a half day of moderate activity. Thus, to maintain a normal blood glucose level and to prevent a breakdown of fat and protein in tissue, people must eat carbohydrate foods regularly and at fairly frequent intervals to meet energy demands.

Special tissue functions
Carbohydrates also serve special functions in many body tissues, as part of their basic function as the body's main energy source.

Liver. Glycogen reserves in the liver and muscles provide a constant exchange with the body's overall energy balance system. These reserves, especially in the liver, protect cells from depressed metabolic function and resulting injury.

Protein and fat. Carbohydrates help regulate both protein and fat metabolism. If there is sufficient dietary carbohydrate to meet general body energy needs, protein will not have to be drained off to supply energy. Instead protein will be used for its main purpose of tissue building. This *protein-sparing action* of carbohydrate thus protects protein, allowing it to be used for its major role in tissue growth and maintenance. In a similar manner, with sufficient carbohydrate for energy, fat will not be used for large amounts for energy. Such a rapid breakdown of fat would produce excess materials called *ketones*, which result from incomplete fat oxidation in the cells. These ketones are strong acids, so this condition of acidosis, or *ketosis*, upsets the normal acid-base

❖ **TABLE 2-4**   *Postabsorptive carbohydrate storage in normal adult man**

	Glycogen (g)	Glucose (g)
Liver (weight 1800 g)	72	
Muscles (mass weight 35 kg)	245	
Extracellular fluids (10 L)		10
Component totals	317	10
TOTAL STORAGE	327	

* 70 kg (154 pounds)

balance of the body and can become serious. This protective action of carbohydrate is called its *antiketogenic* effect.

Heart. The constant action of the heart muscle sustains life. Although fatty acids are the preferred regular fuel for the heart muscle, glycogen is vital emergency fuel. In a damaged heart, low glycogen stores or inadequate carbohydrate intake may cause symptoms of cardiac disorder and angina.

Central nervous system. Constant carbohydrate intake and reserves are necessary for proper functioning of the central nervous system (CNS). The master center of the CNS, the brain, has no stored supply of glucose. It is especially dependent on a minute-to-minute supply of glucose from the blood. Sustained and profound shock from low blood sugar may cause brain damage.

FOOD SOURCES OF CARBOHYDRATES
Starches

As indicated earlier, starches provide fundamental complex carbohydrate foods for sustained primary energy sources. They are the central type of food for a balanced diet. In unrefined forms, they also provide important sources of fiber and other nutrients.

Sugars

Sugar as such is not the villain in the story of health. The problem lies in the large quantities of sugar many people consume, often to the exclusion of other important foods.[10] High-sugar diets do carry health risks, such as dental caries and obesity. The average American consumes about *one-third pound* a day, which may lead to problems. So, as with many things, *moderation* is the key.

BODY NEEDS FOR CARBOHYDRATES

Recommended dietary allowances. There is no recommended dietary allowance for carbohydrate as such in the RDAs. In this nutrient standard, energy needs are listed as total kcalories, which include caloric intake from fat and protein as well as from carbohydrate. Nor is there any specific RDA standard for dietary fiber beyond the general recommendation that a desirable fiber intake be achieved by consumption of whole-grain cereals, legumes, vegetables, and fruits, which also provide minerals and vitamins, rather than by adding fiber concentrates as supplements.[9]

U.S. dietary guidelines. The recommended relative amount of carbohydrate in the diet outlined in the U.S. dietary guidelines for health is given in terms of percent of total kcalories. To achieve a better balance, these guidelines recommend that 55% to 60% of the total kcalories in the diet come from carbohydrate foods, with the large majority as *complex* carbohydrates, or starches. This would mean a reduction in the amount of sugar and sweets consumed, a health habit improvement for many persons.

DIGESTION OF CARBOHYDRATES
Mouth

The digestion of carbohydrate foods, starches and sugars, begins in the mouth and progresses through the successive parts of the gastrointestinal tract, accomplished by two types of actions: (1) mechanical or muscle functions that break the food mass into smaller particles, and (2) chemical processes in which specific **enzymes** break down the food nutrients into still smaller usable metabolic products. In the mouth the chewing of the food, a process called *mastication*, breaks food into fine particles and mixes it with saliva. During this process, the salivary enzyme *ptyalin* is secreted by the *parotid* glands, which lie under each ear at the back of jaw. Ptyalin acts on starch to begin its breakdown into dextrins, intermediate starch products, and maltose.

Stomach

Wavelike contraction of the muscle fibers of the stomach wall continue the mechanical digestive process. This action is called *peristalsis*. It further mixes food particles with gastric secretions to allow chemical digestion to take place more easily. The gastric secretions contain no specific enzyme for the breakdown of carbohydrate. The hydrochloric acid in the stomach stops the action of the salivary ptyalin in the food mass from the mouth. But before the food mixes completely with the acid stomach secretions, as much as 20% to 30% of the starch may have been changed to maltose. Muscle action continues to mix the food mass and move it to the lower part of the stomach. Here the food mass is a thick creamy *chyme*, ready for its controlled emptying through the *pyloric valve* into the *duodenum*, the first portion of the small intestine.

Small intestine

Peristalsis continues to aid digestion in the small intestine by mixing and moving the chyme along the length of the tube. Chemical digestion of carbohydrate is completed in the small intestine by specific enzymes from both the pancreas and the intestine.

Pancreatic secretions. Secretions from the *pancreas* enter the duodenum through the common bile duct. These secretions contain a starch enzyme—*pancreatic amylase*—commonly called *amylopsin*. This enzyme continues the breakdown of starch to maltose.

Intestinal secretions. Secretions from small glands in the intestinal wall contain three disaccharidases—*sucrase, lactase*, and *maltase*. These specific enzymes act on their respective disaccharides to render the monosaccharides—glucose, galactose, and fructose—ready for absorption directly into the **portal** blood circulation.

A summary of the major aspects of carbohydrate digestion through the successive parts of the gastrointestinal tract is shown in Table 2-5.

❖ **TABLE 2-5** *Summary of carbohydrate digestion*

Organ	Enzyme	Action
Mouth	Ptyalin	Starch → Dextrins → Maltose
Stomach	None	(Above action continued to minor degree)
Small intestine	Pancreatic amylopsin	Starch → Dextrins → Maltose
	Intestinal:	
	Sucrase	Sucrose → Glucose + Fructose
	Lactase	Lactose → Glucose + Galactose
	Maltase	Maltose → Glucose + Glucose

SUMMARY

The primary source of energy for most of the world's populations is carbohydrate foods. These foods are from widely distributed plant sources, such as grains, legumes, vegetables, and fruits. For the most part, these food products store easily and are relatively low in cost.

Two basic types of carbohydrates supply energy: complex and simple. *Simple carbohydrates* are made up of single and double sugar units (monosaccharides and disaccharides). Since simple carbohydrates are easy to digest and absorb, they provide quick energy. *Complex carbohydrates*, or polysaccharides, are made up of many sugar units. They break down more slowly and thus provide sustained energy over a longer period of time.

Dietary fiber in most of its forms is complex carbohydrate that is not digestible. It occurs mainly as the structural parts of plants and provides important bulk in the diet, affects nutrient absorption, and benefits health.

Carbohydrate digestion starts briefly in the mouth with initial action of the salivary enzyme ptyalin to begin the breakdown of starch into maltose. There is no enzyme for starch breakdown in the stomach, but muscle action continues to mix the food mass and forward it to enter the small intestine. Final starch and disaccharide digestion occurs in the small intestine with action of specific enzymes—sucrase, lactase, and maltase—to produce single sugar units glucose, fructose, and galactose, which then are absorbed directly into the portal blood circulation to the liver.

❖ REVIEW QUESTIONS

1. Why is carbohydrate the predominant type of food in the world's diets? Give some basic examples of these carbohydrate foods.
2. What are the main classes of carbohydrates? Describe each in terms of general nature, functions, and main food sources.
3. Compare starches and sugars as a basic fuel. Why are complex carbohydrates a significant part of a healthy diet? What is the recommendation about the use of sugars in such a diet? Why?
4. Describe the types and functions of dietary fiber. What are the main food sources? Give the generally recommended amount of fiber for a healthy diet.
5. What is glycogen? Why is it a vital tissue carbohydrate?

❖ SELF-TEST QUESTIONS

True-false
For each item you answer "false," write the correct statement.
1. Carbohydrates are composed of carbon, hydrogen, oxygen, and nitrogen.
2. The main carbohydrate in our diet is starch.
3. Lactose is a very sweet, simple, single sugar found in a number of foods.
4. Glucose is the form of sugar circulating in the blood.
5. Glycogen is an important long-term storage form of energy because relatively large amounts are stored in the liver and muscles.
6. Modern food processing and refinement has reduced dietary fiber.

Multiple choice
1. Which of the following carbohydrate foods provides the *quickest* energy?
   a. Slice of bread
   b. Chocolate candy
   c. Milk
   d. Orange juice

2. A quickly available but limited form of energy is stored in the liver by conversion of glucose to:
   a. Glycerol
   b. Glycogen
   c. Protein
   d. Fat

❖ SUGGESTIONS FOR ADDITIONAL STUDY

1. Cut pictures from magazines illustrating carbohydrate foods. Put them in your notebook under two headings, simple and complex carbohydrates.
2. Compare the taste of a very ripe banana with that of a partially ripe one. Describe the difference in taste. Why are they different?
3. Check the carbohydrate and dietary fiber values on labels of six different food products.

References

1. US Department of Agriculture: Nationwide Food Consumption Survey, Continuing Survey of Food Intakes by Individuals: Low income women 19-50 years and their children 1-5 years, 4 days, 1985, Report No 85-5, Nutrition Monitoring Division, Human Nutrition Information Service, Hyattsville, MD, 1988, US Government Printing Office.
2. Executive summary, National Nutrition Monitoring in the United States: an update report on nutrition monitoring, Nutr Today 25(1):33, 1990.
3. Glinsmann WH and others: Evaluation of health aspects of sugar contained in carbohydrate sweeteners: FDA report of Sugar Task Force, 1986, J Nutr 116:S12-S216, 1986.
4. Slavin JL: Dietary fiber: mechanisms or magic on disease prevention? Nutr Today 25(6):6, 1990.
5. National Research Council, Food and Nutrition Board: Diet and health: implications for reducing chronic disease risk, Washington, DC, 1989, National Academy Press.
6. Lanza E and others: Dietary fiber intake in the U.S. population, Am J Clin Nutr 46:790, 1987.
7. Anderson JW and others: Dietary fiber content of a simulated American diet and selected research diets, Am J Clin Nutr 49:352, Feb 1989.
8. Report: Council on Scientific Affairs, American Medical Association: Dietary fiber and health, JAMA 262:542, July 28, 1989.
9. National Research Council, Food and Nutrition Board: Recommended dietary allowances, ed 10, Washington, DC, 1989, National Academy Press.
10. Campbell VS: Are children consuming too much sugar? Food Management 25:58, May 1990.

Further reading

Fletcher AM: The sweet truth: sugar myths vs. the facts, Better Homes and Gardens 69(2):124, 1991.

The author of this excellent, succinct two-page article, a registered dietitian and author, provides clear answers for seven common myths about sugar with the verdict of not guilty on the basis of both scientific wisdom and common sense. She also tells you how to "think smart" about sugar and be a sugar sleuth. For good measure, there is an eight-item multiple-choice quick quiz to test your sweetness IQ. This review is guaranteed to raise your own sugar IQ.

Owen AL: The impact of future foods on nutrition and health, J Am Diet Assoc 90(9):1217, 1990.

In this interesting current and future look at changing food trends and the forces driving them, the author provides a number of good reference charts of products being marketed or under preliminary testing for future release. Two of these charts list sweeteners and dietary fiber products and their uses in the diet.

3

❖

Fats

KEY CONCEPTS

*Fat in foods supplies essential diet and body tissue needs, both
as an energy fuel and a structural material.*

*Food from animal and plant sources supplies distinct forms
of fat that affect health in different ways.*

*Excess dietary fat, especially from animal
sources, is a health risk factor.*

$\mathcal{T}$raditionally, Americans and people in most other developed countries have eaten a relatively high-fat diet. In the United States we have maintained a rich food pattern with about 45% of our total caloric intake coming from fat. Now, however, we have justified health concerns and are beginning to eat less fat, especially animal fats.

In this chapter, we consider fat not only as an essential nutrient, a concentrated storage fuel, and tissue need, but also as a health hazard. We want to help achieve realistic balance in attitudes and habits about fat and health.

NATURE OF FATS
Fat as fuel

Fats supply a storage form of concentrated fuel for the human energy system. As such they back up carbohydrates as an available energy source. Food fats include materials such as solid fats, liquid oils, and related compounds such as cholesterol. Fats are not soluble in water and are greasy.

Classes of fats

Lipids. The overall chemical group name for all fats and fat-related compounds is **lipids.** This term comes from the Greek word *lipos*, meaning "fat." This group name lipid appears in combination words used for fat-related health problems. For example, the condition of an elevated level of blood fats is called *hyperlipidemia*.

Triglycerides. Fats are made up of the same basic chemical elements that make up carbohydrates—carbon, hydrogen, and oxygen. As a group, fats are called **glycerides** because they are composed of *glycerol* with *fatty acids* attached. Whether in food or in the body tissue, fatty acids combine with glycerol to form glycerides. Most natural fats, whether in animal or plant sources, have three fatty acids attached to their glycerol base; thus their chemical name is **triglyceride.** When you encounter "triglycerides" in your reading, just think of the term as the chemical name for fat.

Fatty acids. The main building blocks of fats are **fatty acids.** They have two significant characteristics, one relating to the concept of saturation and the other to essential fatty acids.

1. Saturated fatty acid. When a substance is described as **saturated**, it simply means that it contains all the material that it is capable of holding. For example, a sponge is saturated with water when it holds all the water that it is capable of holding. In the same manner, fatty acids are called "saturated" or "unsaturated" according to whether or not they are filled with hydrogen. Thus a saturated fatty acid is one whose structure is completely filled with all the hydrogen it can hold and as a result is heavier, more dense, and more solid. If most of the fatty acids making up a given fat are saturated, that fat is said to be a *saturated fat.* Naturally it would be a more solid fat, such as meat fats. Saturated fats are of animal origin (Fig. 3-1).

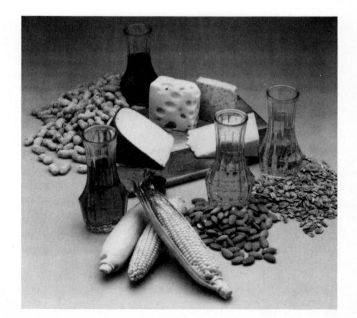

❖ **Fig. 3-1**
Food sources of fats.

2. Unsaturated fatty acid. A fatty acid that is not completely filled with all the hydrogen it can hold is unsaturated, and as a result is less heavy, less dense, such as a liquid oil. If most of the fatty acids making up a given fat are unsaturated, that fat is said to be an *unsaturated fat.* If the component fatty acids have *one* unfilled spot, the fat is called a *mono*unsaturated fat. Olives and olive oil, peanuts and peanut oil, canola oil (rapeseed), almonds, pecans, and avocados supply monounsaturated fats. If the component fatty acids have two or more unfilled spots, a fat is called a *poly*unsaturated fat. Examples of such fats, in order of their degree of unsaturation, are the vegetable oils: safflower, corn, cottonseed, and soybean. Fats from plant sources usually are unsaturated (Fig. 3-1). Notable exceptions are coconut oil, palm oil, and cocoa butter, which are saturated. Although world production of the saturated tropical oils (palm, palm kernel, and coconut) increased rapidly over the past two decades, use of these oils in the United States has not followed this world trend. Current surveys indicate that these saturated oils contribute less than 4% of Americans' total daily fat intake and about 8% of the daily saturated fat intake.[1]

3. Essential fatty acid. The term *essential* or *nonessential* is applied to a nutrient according to its relative necessity in the diet. The nutrient is essential if (1) its absence will create a specific deficiency disease, or (2) the body cannot manufacture it and must obtain it from the diet. A diet with 10% or less of its total kcalories from fat cannot supply adequate amounts of essential fatty acids. The only fatty acids known to be essential for complete human nutrition are linoleic, linolenic, and arachidonic. Actually, of these three, only **linoleic acid** is the true *dietary* essential fatty acid, since the body can synthesize the other two from it. All three of these fatty acids serve important functions related to tissue strength, cholesterol metabolism, muscle tone, blood clotting, and heart action. Linoleic acid is found primarily in polyunsaturated vegetable oils.

Cholesterol. Although cholesterol is often discussed in connection with dietary fat, it is not a fat itself. Many people confuse cholesterol with saturated fats. Actually, **cholesterol** belongs to a group of chemical substances called *sterols.* Its name comes from the material in which it was first identified— gallstones, hence "chole-" referring to bile or the gallbladder, and "-sterol" referring to its family group name. Cholesterol occurs naturally in all animal foods. Since it is synthesized in animal tissue, there is none in plant foods. Its main food sources are egg yolks and organ meats such as liver and kidney. (See Appendix.) Cholesterol has widespread functions essential to life and is found in practically all body tissues, especially brain and nerve tissue, bile, blood, and liver, where most cholesterol synthesis takes place.

Lipoproteins. The **lipoproteins** are combinations of fat (lipids) with protein (the protein part is called an *apoprotein*) and other fat-related substances that serve as the major vehicle for fat transport in the bloodstream. Since fat is insoluble in water and the blood is mainly water, fat cannot travel freely in the blood. It needs a water-soluble carrier. The body solves this problem by wrapping the small particles of fat with a covering of protein, which is soluble in water. These little packages of fat wrapped in water-soluble protein are then carried by the blood to and from the cells to supply needed nutrients. The lipoproteins contain triglycerides, cholesterol, and other materials such as fat-soluble vitamins. The lipoprotein's relative load of fat and protein determines its density. The higher the fat load, the lower its density.The groups of *low-density lipoproteins* (LDLs) carry fat and cholesterol to cells. The *high-density lipoproteins* (HDLs) carry free cholesterol from body tissue to the liver for breakdown and excretion. All the lipoproteins are closely associated with lipid disorders and the underlying blood vessel disease in heart attacks, *atherosclerosis*. These relationships are discussed in greater detail in Chapter 19.

FUNCTIONS OF FAT
Fat in foods

Energy. Fat serves as one of the body's fuels for energy production. Because carbohydrate can be easily converted to fat, fat is an important storage form of body fuel for energy reserves. It is a much more concentrated form of fuel, yielding 9 kcal/g when burned by the body, in comparison to carbohydrate, which yields 4 kcal/g.

Essential nutrients. Food fats supply the essential fatty acids, especially linoleic acid, and cholesterol to supplement the amount synthesized by the body. Also, food fats carry fat-soluble vitamins (p. 67) and aid in their absorption.

Flavor and satisfaction. Some fat in the diet adds flavor to foods and contributes to a feeling of *satiety* or satisfaction after a meal. Satiety is caused partly by the slower rate of digestion of fats in comparison to that of carbohydrate. Satiety is also the result of the fuller texture and body that fat gives to food mixtures and the slower stomach-emptying time it brings. The absence of satiation and hunger delay experienced by some persons using low-fat diets may contribute to client dissatisfaction and problems with needed food habit changes. Several new fat substitutes, compounds that are not absorbed and thus contribute few or no kcalories, are being marketed or tested to provide improved flavor and physical texture to low-fat foods and help reduce the total dietary fat.[2] Two examples of these fat substitutes are Simplesse, made by reshaping the protein of either milk whey or egg whites, and Olestra, a non-digestible form of sucrose.[3,4]

Fat in the body

Adipose tissue. Fat stored in various parts of the body is called **adipose** tissue, from the Latin word *adiposus* meaning "fatty." A weblike padding of this tissue supports and protects vital organs. A layer of fat directly under the skin is important in regulating body temperature. The fat covering also protects nerve fibers and helps relay the nerve impulses.

Cell membrane structure. Fat forms the fatty center of cell walls, helping to carry nutrient materials across cell membranes.

FOOD SOURCES OF FAT
Variety of sources

Animal fats. Animal sources supply saturated fats, as shown in Fig. 3-2. Food sources include meat fats, bacon and sausage, dairy fats, cream, butter, and cheese, as well as egg yolk. Traditionally the American diet has featured

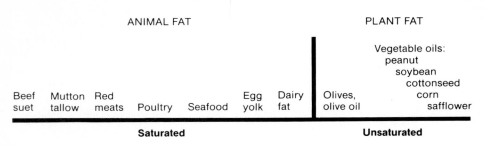

ANIMAL FAT   PLANT FAT

									Vegetable oils:
									  peanut
									  soybean
									  cottonseed

Beef suet	Mutton tallow	Red meats	Poultry	Seafood	Egg yolk	Dairy fat	Olives, olive oil		corn safflower

Saturated   **Unsaturated**

❖ **Fig. 3-2**

Spectrum of food fats according to degree of saturation of component fatty acid.

meats and other foods of animal origin. Current surveys show that animal products in particular—red meats (beef, veal, pork, lamb), poultry, fish and shellfish, separate animal fats (tallow and lard), milk and milk products, and eggs—contribute more than half of the total fat to U.S. diets, three fourths of the saturated fat, and all the cholesterol.[5,6]

Plant fats. Plant sources supply unsaturated fats. Food sources include the vegetable oils made from safflowers, corn, cottonseed, soybeans, peanuts, and olives (Fig. 3-2). Three plant fats, used mainly in food processing, are exceptions in that they yield saturated fats: coconut oil, palm oil, and cocoa butter.

Hydrogenated fat. Margarine and shortenings are made from vegetable oils by the introduction of hydrogen into the fat molecule. This process is called *hydrogenation*, a word that appears frequently on the labels of such commercial fat products. To make margarine a substitute for butter, the hydrogenated product may also be churned with cultured milk to give it a butter flavor and fortified with vitamins A and D. Fortified margarine is the nutritional equivalent of butter and has the same caloric value. Margarine, which is economical, tasteful, and lower in saturated fat, is 80% fat and fortified with 15,000 international units (IU) of vitamin A per pound.

Characteristics of sources

For practical purposes, food fats are sometimes classified as *visible* fats or *invisible* fats, to help persons become aware of all food sources of fat.

Visible fat. The obvious fats are plain to see. These include butter, margarine, separate cream, salad oils and dressings, lard, shortening, fat meat such as bacon, sausage, or salt pork, and the visible fat of any meat. It is easier to control visible fats in the diet than those that are less apparent.

Invisible fat. Some dietary fats are less visible, so a person who wants to control fat needs to be aware of these food sources also. Invisible fats include the cream portion of homogenized milk, cheese, egg yolk, nuts, seeds, olives, avocados, and lean meat. Even when all of the visible fat has been removed from meat, such as the skin on poultry and the obvious fat on the lean portions, about 6% of the total fat remains surrounding the muscle fibers.

Digestibility of fats

The digestibility of fats varies somewhat according to the food source and cooking method. Butter digests more completely than meat fat. Fried foods, especially those saturated with fat in the frying process, are digested more slowly than baked or broiled foods. Fried foods cooked at too high a temperature are more difficult to digest, and substances in the fat break down into irritating materials. Fried foods should be used sparingly, and the temperature of the fat should be controlled carefully. In general, the health goal is to reduce the amount of fat used in the diet.

BODY NEEDS FOR FAT
Dietary fat and health

American diet. The traditional American diet is high in fat. The average amount consumed per person, about 100 pounds per year, provides about 40% to 45% of the diet's total kcalories. This amount of fat exceeds that needed by the average person. Not more than 25% to 30% of the diet's total kcalories needs to come from fat. This amount would easily provide an adequate amount of the essential fatty acids, especially linoleic acid, to meet the physiologic needs of the body.

Health problems. If fat is vital to human health as indicated, what is the concern about fat in the diet? This is not a fully resolved question. However, current research does indicate that health problems with fat result from too much dietary fat and too much of that fat from animal food sources.

1. Amount of fat. Too much fat in the diet supplies more kcalories than required for immediate energy needs. The excess is stored as increasing body fat. Increased body fat and weight has been associated with risk factors in health problems such as diabetes, hypertension, and heart disease. Look for more details about these relationships in later chapters in the section on clinical

❖

BOX 3-1
How Much Fat Are You Eating?

- Keep an accurate record of everything you eat or drink for 1 day. Be sure to estimate and add amounts of all fat or other nutrient seasonings used with your foods. (If you want a more representative picture and have a computer available with nutrient analysis programming, keep a 1-week record and calculate an average of the 7 days.)
- Calculate the total kilocalories (kcal) and grams of each of the energy nutrients (carbohydrate, fat, and protein) in everything you eat. Multiply the total grams of each energy nutrient by its respective fuel value:

$$fat \underline{\hspace{1cm}} g \times 9 = \underline{\hspace{1cm}} kcal$$
$$protein \underline{\hspace{1cm}} g \times 4 = \underline{\hspace{1cm}} kcal$$
$$carbohydrate \underline{\hspace{1cm}} g \times 4 = \underline{\hspace{1cm}} kcal$$

- Calculate the percentage of each energy nutrient in your total diet:

$$\frac{Fat\ kcal}{Total\ kcal} \times 100 = \%\ fat\ kcal\ in\ diet$$

- Compare with fat in American diet (40% to 45%); with the U.S. dietary goals (25% to 30%).

nutrition. How much fat is in your own diet? You might try figuring it out for a day (Box 3-1).

2. Type of fat. An excess of cholesterol and saturated fat in the diet, which comes from animal food sources, has been associated as a specific risk factor with atherosclerosis, the underlying blood vessel disease that contributes to heart attacks and strokes. A decrease in dietary saturated fats, using polyunsaturated fats instead, has been shown to reduce serum total cholesterol. Recent studies indicate that monounsaturated fats, as in olive oil, when substituted for saturated fat in the diet, also reduced the LDL cholesterol—the main target for control.[7,8] The exact nature of these associations is not yet clear and is the focus of continuing research.

Health promotion. The current movement in American health care is toward health promotion and prevention of disease through reduction of identified risk factors related to chronic disease. Heart disease is the leading cause of death in developed countries such as the United States, and much attention is given to reducing the various risk factors leading to this disease process (Table 3-1). Excess dietary fat, particularly saturated fat and cholesterol, contributes to these risk factors, which include obesity, diabetes, elevated blood fats, and elevated blood pressure. Additional life-style factors include smoking, lack of exercise, and increased stress. Thus a middle-aged or older adult who is overweight and has a high level of blood cholesterol and blood pressure should reduce both weight and amount of dietary fat, especially animal fat. Children are beginning to learn in grade school and practice in their cafeterias healthier food habits with less fat.[9,10] This need is especially great for children in high-risk families (those families having identified lipid disorders and heart disease at young adult ages), who should develop moderation in fat use, as well as other aspects of a healthy life-style, at an early age.

Dietary fat requirements

Recommended dietary allowances. No fat requirement is stated in the RDA nutrient standard. As an energy source the fat allowance in the diet is included in the general kcalorie allowances. However, the study committee has issued general guidelines for dietary fat use. After comprehensive evaluation of the

❖ **TABLE 3-1**   *Multiple risk factors in cardiovascular disease*

Personal characteristics (no control)	Learned behaviors (intervene and change)	Background conditions (screen-treat)
Sex	Stress/coping	Hypertension
Age	Smoking cigarettes	Diabetes mellitus
Family history	Sedentary life	Hyperlipidemia (especially
	Obesity	hypercholesterolemia)
	Food habits	
	Excess fat	
	Excess sugar	
	Excess salt	

evidence, the National Research Council's Committee on Diet and Health has recommended that the fat content of the U.S. diet not exceed 30% of the total kcalories, that less than 10% of the kcalories should be provided from saturated fats, and that dietary cholesterol should be less than 300 mg/day.[6,11]

U.S. dietary guidelines. In line with the current national health goal of health promotion through disease prevention by reducing identified risks of chronic disease, the U.S. dietary guidelines recommend control of fat in the diet, especially saturated fat and cholesterol (pp. 25-26). The guidelines reflect the previously mentioned recommendations of the Diet and Health Committee. Several practical ways of lowering fat in the diet are listed below.

1. *Meat.* Use only lean cuts of all meats, and use more poultry and seafood. Remove skin from poultry and trim fat from all meats. Avoid added fat in cooking. Use smaller portions—2 to 4 oz.

2. *Eggs.* Limit intake of eggs to approximately two or three a week. Cook and serve without added fat.

3. *Milk and milk products.* Use low-fat or fat-free milk and milk products. Use cheeses with lower fat content.

4. *Food preparation.* Avoid fat as much as possible in food preparation and cooking. Use alternate seasonings such as herbs, spices, lemon juice, onion, garlic, fat-free broth, and wine.

DIGESTION OF FATS
Mouth

The various animal and plant fats (triglycerides) that naturally occur in foods are taken into the body with the diet. Then the task is to change these basic fuel fats into a refined fuel form of fat that the cells can burn for energy. This key refined fuel form is the individual *fatty acid*. The body accomplishes this task through the process of fat digestion. When fat foods are eaten no chemical fat breakdown takes place in the mouth. In this first portion of the gastrointestinal tract, fat is simply broken into smaller particles through chewing and moistened with saliva for passage into the stomach with the food mass.

Stomach

Little if any chemical fat digestion occurs in the stomach. General muscle action continues to mix the fat with the stomach contents. No significant amount of enzymes specific for fats is present in the gastric secretions except a *gastric lipase* (tributyrinase), which acts on emulsified butterfat. As the main gastric enzymes act on other specific nutrients in the food mix, fat is separated from them and made ready for its own specific chemical breakdown in the small intestine.

Small intestine

Not until fat reaches the small intestine do the chemical changes necessary for fat digestion occur. The specific digestive agents come from three major sources—a preparation agent from the gallbladder and specific enzymes from the pancreas and the small intestine itself.

1. *Bile from the gallbladder.* The fat coming into the duodenum, the first section of the small intestine, stimulates the secretion of *cholecystokinin*, a

local hormone from glands in the intestinal walls. In turn, cholecystokinin causes contraction of the gallbladder, relaxation of its opening muscle, and subsequent secretion of **bile** into the intestine by way of the common bile duct. The liver first produces the bile in large dilute amounts, then sends it to the gallbladder for concentration and storage, ready for use with fat as needed. Bile functions as an **emulsifier**. *Emulsification* is not a chemical digestive process itself, but is an important first preparation of fat for chemical digestion by its specific enzymes. This preparation process accomplishes two important tasks: (1) it breaks the fat into small particles, which greatly enlarges the total surface area available for action of the enzyme, and (2) it lowers the surface tension of the finely dispersed and suspended fat particles, which allows the enzymes to penetrate more easily. This process is similar to the wetting action of detergents. The bile also provides an alkaline medium necessary for the action of the fat enzyme lipase.

2. Enzymes from the pancreas. Pancreatic juice contains an enzyme for fat and another one for cholesterol. First, *pancreatic* **lipase**, a powerful fat enzyme, breaks off one fatty acid at a time from the glycerol base of fats (triglycerides). One fatty acid plus a diglyceride, then another fatty acid plus a monoglyceride, are produced in turn. Each succeeding step of this breakdown occurs with increasing difficulty. In fact, separation of the final fatty acid from the remaining monoglyceride is such a slow process that less than a third of the total fat present actually reaches complete breakdown. The final products of fat digestion to be absorbed are fatty acids, diglycerides, monoglycerides, and glycerol. Some remaining fat may pass into the large intestine for fecal elimination. Second, the enzyme *cholesterol enterase* acts on free cholesterol to form a combination of cholesterol and fatty acids in preparation for absorption, first into the lymph vessels and finally into the bloodstream (see Chapter 9).

3. Enzyme from the small intestine. The small intestine secretes an enzyme in the intestinal juice called *lecithinase*. As its name indicates, it acts on lecithin, another lipid compound, to break it down into its components for absorption.

A summary of fat digestion in the successive parts of the gastrointestinal tract is given in Table 3-2.

❖ **TABLE 3-2**   *Summary of fat digestion*

Organ	Enzyme	Activity
Mouth	None	Mechanical, mastication
Stomach	No major enzyme	Mechanical separation of fats as protein and starch digested out
	Small amount of gastric lipase tributyrinase	Tributyrin (butterfat) to fatty acids and glycerol
Small intestine	Gallbladder bile salts (emulsifier)	Emulsifies fats
	Pancreatic lipase (steapsin)	Triglycerides to diglycerides and monoglycerides in turn, then fatty acids and glycerol

---

SUMMARY

Fat is an essential body nutrient. It serves important body needs as a backup storage fuel, secondary to carbohydrate, for energy. Fat also supplies important tissue needs as a structural material for cell walls, protective padding for vital organs, insulation to maintain body temperature, and covering for nerve fibers.

Food fats have different forms and body uses. Saturated fats come from animal food sources and carry health risks for the body. Unsaturated fats come from plant food sources and reduce health risks. Cholesterol is a fat-related substance that in excess amounts also contributes to health risks.

In general, Americans consume more fat than they need or is healthy. For health promotion, a reduction of fat and cholesterol in the diet is recommended. When various foods containing fat and cholesterol are eaten, specific digestive agents including bile and the enzyme pancreatic lipase prepare and break down the fats (triglycerides) into fatty acids and glycerides for absorption via the lymphatic system into the blood circulation.

❖ REVIEW QUESTIONS

1. Compare fat to carbohydrate as fuel sources in the body's energy system. Name several other important functions of fat in human nutrition and health.
2. Define the terms lipids, triglycerides, fatty acids, cholesterol, and lipoproteins. Distinguish between saturated and unsaturated fats, giving food sources for each type.
3. Why is a controlled amount of dietary fat recommended for health promotion? What amount of fat should a healthy diet contain?

❖ SELF-TEST QUESTIONS

True-false
For each item you answer "false," write the correct statement.
1. Fat has the same energy value as carbohydrate.
2. Fat is composed of the same basic chemical elements as carbohydrate.
3. Corn oil is a saturated fat.
4. Polyunsaturated fats usually come from animal food sources.
5. Lipoproteins, produced mainly in the liver, carry fat in the blood.

Multiple choice
1. The fuel form of fat found in food sources is:
   - a. Triglyceride
   - b. Fatty acid
   - c. Glycerol
   - d. Lipoprotein
2. Which of the following statements are correct concerning the saturation of fats?
   - (1) The degree of saturation depends on the relative amount of hydrogen in the fatty acids that make up the fat.
   - (2) The more unsaturated fats come from animal food sources.
   - (3) The more saturated the fat, the softer it tends to be.
   - (4) Fats composed of fatty acids with two or more "unfilled" spaces in their structure are called *polyunsaturated*.
     - a. 1 and 2
     - b. 3 and 4
     - c. 1 and 4
     - d. 2 and 4
3. If a person used a low saturated—fat diet to lower his risk of heart disease, which of the following foods would he use frequently?
   - a. Whole milk
   - b. Oil-vinegar salad dressing
   - c. Butter
   - d. Cheddar cheese

❖ SUGGESTIONS FOR ADDITIONAL STUDY

1. Visit a community food market and survey the fats and fat-related foods. Read the labels carefully. Look for the words *imitation, hydrogenated, fortified, hardened, saturated, polyunsaturated,* and *P/S (polyunsaturated/saturated) ratio.* Include foods such as margarines, shortenings, oils, frozen desserts, whipped toppings, cream substitutes, nondairy creamers, milks, egg and cheese foods, egg substitutes, and special low-fat cheeses. Make a list of the terms you found on labels of the fat-related food products you located and describe the product involved. What does each term mean? How has the product been processed? Prepare a report of your survey for your notebook.

2. Plan your meals for 1 day using as little fat as possible. Describe how you would prepare and serve the food to avoid fat.

References

1. Park YK and Yetley EA: Trend changes in use and current intakes of tropical oils in the United States, Am J Clin Nutr 51:738, May 1990.
2. Dziezak JD: Fats, oils, and fat substitutes, Food Technology 43:65, July 1989.
3. Lynch PM: Sugar and fat substitutes: the challenge for today and tommorow, Diabetes Educator 16:101, Mar/Apr 1990.
4. Owen AL: The impact of future foods on nutrition and health, J Am Diet Assoc 90(9):1217, 1990.
5. National Research Council, Board on Agriculture: Designing foods: animal product options in the marketplace, Washington, DC, 1988, National Academy Press.
6. National Research Council, Food and Nutrition Board, Committee on Diet and Health: Diet and health, implications for reducing chronic disease risk, Washington, DC, 1989, National Academy Press.
7. Grundy SM: Monounsaturated fatty acids and cholesterol metabolism, implications for dietary recommendations, J Nutr 119:529, Apr 1989.
8. Trevisan M and others: Consumption of olive oil, butter, and vegetable oils and coronary heart disease risk factors, JAMA 263:688, Feb 2, 1990.
9. Frank GC and others: Cardiovascular health promotion for school children, the Heart Smart Nutrition Intervention, School Food Service Research Review 13:130, Fall 1989.
10. Resnicow J and others: Plasma cholesterol levels of 6,585 children in the United States: results of the Know Your Body screening in five states, Pediatrics 84:969, Dec 1989.
11. National Research Council, Food and Nutrition Board: Recommended dietary allowances, ed 10, Washington, DC, 1989, National Academy Press.

Further reading

Krance N: A dietary olive branch, Am Health 9(3):64, 1990.

Chalkley, G: Mediterranean feasts, Am Health 9(3):72, Apr 1990.

These two articles provide a feast for food and thought for including monounsaturated olive oil in your diet as part of your serum cholesterol control efforts. Both a sound review of the background and a mouth-watering set of recipes from the Mediterranean to tempt your taste are included.

Raeburn P: The great cholesterol debate: Is it a myth—or a killer, Am Health 9(1):79, 1990.

The author tackles head-on perhaps the hottest nutrition controversy around: Is cholesterol really life-threatening or does it just have a bad reputation? To find some answers, a science writer interviews an investigative reporter, whose new book, *Heart Failure* (Random House), sparked the controversy, and two leading lipid researchers from Johns Hopkins Hospital and the University of Texas Southwestern Medical School. Also included are sidebars for a layman's glossary of terms, the bigger picture of the heart's other risk factors, and why cholesterol could be more dangerous than previously thought.

Stoy DB: Controlling cholesterol with diet, Am J Nurs 89:1625, Dec 1989.

This article provides an overview of the rationale and guidelines for reducing dietary fat and cholesterol, many practical suggestions for implementing such a diet, a "patient-friendly" primer of dietary fat, and a color graphic of major sources of dietary fats. Other companion articles in this issue's focus include a continuing education credit study of cholesterol, interpreting the new guidelines, and controlling cholesterol with drugs.

4

❖

Proteins

KEY CONCEPTS

*Food proteins provide the amino acids necessary
for building and maintaining body tissue.*

*Protein balance, both within the body and in
the diet, is essential to life and health.*

*The value of foods for meeting body protein needs is determined
by their composition of essential amino acids.*

*M*any different proteins in the body make human life possible. Each one of these thousands upon thousands of specific body proteins has a unique structure designed to perform an assigned task.

The essential building units for constructing our bodies are the amino acids. They are the building blocks of all protein. We obtain amino acids from the variety of food proteins we eat every day.

In this chapter we look at the specific nature of proteins, both in our food and in our bodies. We see why protein balance is essential to life and health and how we maintain that balance.

NATURE OF PROTEINS
Amino acids: basic building material

Role as building units. All protein, whether in our bodies or in the food we eat, is made up of building units or compounds known as **amino acids.** These amino acids are joined in unique chain sequence to form specific proteins. When we eat protein foods, the protein (for example, casein in milk and cheese, albumin in egg white, or gluten in wheat products) is broken down into amino acids in the digestive process. Amino acids are then reassembled in the body in the proper *specific* order to form *specific* tissue proteins (for example, collagen in connective tissue, myosin in muscle tissue, hemoglobin in red blood cells [Fig. 4-1], cell enzymes, or insulin) that are needed by the body.

Role as nitrogen supplier. Amino acids are named for their chemical nature. The word *amino* refers to compounds containing nitrogen. Like carbohydrates and fats, proteins have a basic structure of carbon, hydrogen, and oxygen. But unlike carbohydrates and fats, which contain no nitrogen, protein is about 16% nitrogen. In addition, some proteins contain small but valuable amounts of sulfur, phosphorus, iron, and iodine.

Classes of amino acids

There are 22 common amino acids, all of which are vital to human life and health. However, they are classified as essential or nonessential *in the diet* according to whether or not the body can make them.

Essential amino acids. Nine amino acids are classed as essential amino acids because the body cannot manufacture them. Thus *essential* means that they are necessary in the diet. Histidine was previously known as essential for infants, but was not demonstrated to be required by adults until recently.[1,2]

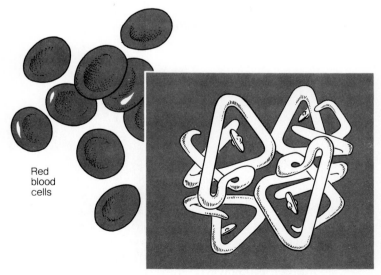

Red
blood
cells

Hemoglobin molecule

❖ **FIG. 4-1**
Hemoglobin is an oxygen-carrying protein of red blood cells.

❖ TABLE 4-1   *Amino acids required in human nutrition, grouped according to nutritional (dietary) essentiality*

Essential amino acids	Semiessential amino acid*	Nonessential amino acids
Histidine	Arginine	Alanine
Isoleucine		Aspargine
Leucine		Aspartic acid
Lysine		Cystine (cysteine)
Methionine		Glutamic acid
Phyenylalanine		Glutamine
Threonine		Glycine
Tryptophan		Hydroxyproline
Valine		Hydroxylysine
		Proline
		Serine
		Tyrosine

* Considered semiessential because the rate of synthesis in the body is inadequate to support growth; therefore essential for children.

The nine essential amino acids are histidine, isoleucine, leucine, lysine, methionine, phenylalanine, threonine, tryptophan, and valine (Table 4-1). During the growth years, arginine is also essential to meet normal childhood growth demands. Although arginine is synthesized by the body, it may not be made in sufficient amounts to meet the rapid growth of infants (especially premature infants) and young children.[2]

Nonessential amino acids. In this instance, the word *nonessential* is misleading, since amino acids have essential tissue-building and metabolic functions in the body. However, as used here, the term refers to the remaining 12 amino acids that the body can synthesize, so they are not essential in the diet.

Balance

The term *balance* refers to the relative intake and output of substances in the body to maintain the normal levels of these substances needed for health in various circumstances during life. We can apply this concept of balance to life-sustaining protein and the nitrogen it supplies.

Protein balance. The body's tissue proteins are constantly being broken down into amino acids, a process called *catabolism*, and then resynthesized into tissue proteins as needed, a process called *anabolism*. To maintain nitrogen balance, the nitrogen-containing amino part of the amino acid may be removed by a process called *deamination*, converted to ammonia (NH_3), and the nitrogen excreted as urea in the urine. The remaining non-nitrogen residue can be used to make carbohydrate or fat, or reattach to make another amino acid according to need. The rate of this protein and nitrogen turnover varies in different tissues, according to their degree of metabolic activity. It is always a continuous process, reshaping and rebuilding, and adjusting as needed to maintain overall protein balance within the body. Also, the body maintains a balance between tissue protein and plasma protein. Then, in turn, these two body protein stores are further balanced with dietary protein intake. With this finely balanced

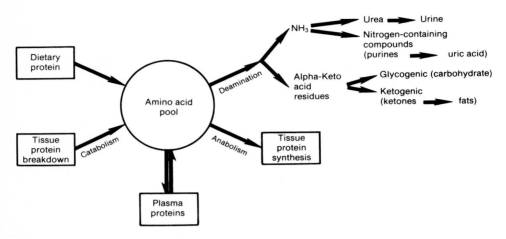

❖ **Fig. 4-2**

Balance between protein compartments and amino acid pool.

system, a "pool" of amino acids from both tissue protein and dietary protein is always available to meet construction needs (Fig. 4-2).

Nitrogen balance. The body's nitrogen balance indicates how well its tissues are being maintained. The intake and use of dietary protein is measured by the amount of nitrogen intake in the food protein and the amount of nitrogen excreted in the urine. For example, 1 g of urinary nitrogen results from the digestion and metabolism of 6.25 g of protein. Therefore, if for every 6.25 g of protein consumed, 1 g of nitrogen is excreted in the urine, the body is said to be in nitrogen balance. This is the normal pattern in adult health, but at different times of life, or in states of malnutrition or illness, this balance may be either positive or negative.

1. Positive nitrogen balance. A positive nitrogen balance exists when the body takes in more nitrogen than it excretes. This means that the body is storing nitrogen by building more tissue than it is breaking down. This situation occurs normally during periods of rapid growth such as infancy, childhood, adolescence, and during pregnancy and lactation. It also occurs in persons who have been ill or malnourished and are being "built back up" with increased nourishment. In such cases protein is being stored to meet increased needs for tissue building and associated metabolic activity.

2. Negative nitrogen balance. A negative nitrogen balance exists when the body takes in less nitrogen than it excretes. This means that the body has an inadequate protein intake and is losing nitrogen by breaking down more tissue than it is building up. This situation occurs in states of malnutrition and illness. For example, this nitrogen imbalance is seen in America in cases in which specific protein deficiency, even when kcalories from carbohydrate and fat may be adequate, causes the classic protein deficiency disease kwashiorkor.[3] Failure to maintain nitrogen balance may not become apparent for some time, but it will eventually cause loss of muscle tissue, impairment of body organs and functions, and increased susceptibility to infection. In children, negative nitrogen balance will cause growth retardation.

FUNCTIONS OF PROTEIN
Primary tissue building

Protein is the fundamental structural material of every cell in the body. In fact the largest portion of the body, excluding the water content, is made up of protein. Body protein, mainly the lean body mass of muscles, accounts for about three fourths of the dry matter in most tissues other than bone and adipose fat.[4] Protein not only makes up the bulk of the muscles, internal organs, brain, nerves, skin, hair, and nails, but also is a vital part of regulatory substances such as enzymes, hormones, and blood plasma. All of these tissues must be constantly repaired and replaced. The primary functions of protein are to repair worn-out, wasted, or damaged tissue and to build up new tissue. Thus protein meets growth needs and maintains tissue health during adult years.

Additional body functions

In addition to its basic tissue-building function, protein has other body functions. These functions relate to energy, water balance, metabolism, and the body defense system.

Energy system. As described in previous chapters, carbohydrate is the primary fuel source in the body's energy system, assisted by fat as a stored fuel. However, in times of need protein may furnish additional body fuel to sustain body heat and energy. This is a less efficient back up source for use only when there is an insufficient supply of carbohydrate and fat. The available fuel factor of protein is 4 kcal/g.

Water balance. Plasma protein, especially albumin, helps to control water balance throughout the body by exerting osmotic pressure to maintain normal circulation of tissue fluids and capillary blood flow.

Metabolism. Protein aids metabolic functions by: (1) combining with iron to form hemoglobin, the vital oxygen-carrier in the red blood cells (Fig. 4-1) and (2) manufacturing agents that control metabolic processes, such as digestive and cell enzymes, as well as hormones.

Body defense system. Protein is used to build special white blood cells (lymphocytes) and antibodies as part of the body's immune system to help defend against disease and infection.

FOOD SOURCES OF PROTEIN
Types of food proteins

Fortunately, most foods contain a mixture of proteins that complete one another. In a mixed diet, animal and plant foods provide a wide variety of many nutrients as well as proteins that supplement each other. Thus the key to a balanced diet is *variety*. Food proteins are classified as complete or incomplete proteins, depending on their amino acid composition (Fig. 4-3).

Complete proteins. Protein foods that contain all of the nine essential amino acids (p. 37) in sufficient quantity and ratio to meet the body's needs are called *complete proteins*. In general, these proteins are of animal origin: egg, milk, cheese, and meat. A notable exception is gelatin. Although this protein food is an animal product, it is a relatively worthless protein, for it lacks three essential amino acids—tryptophan, valine, and isoleucine—and has only small amounts of another—leucine.

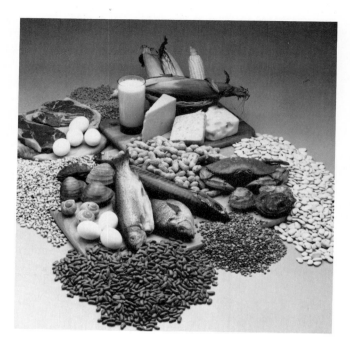

❖ **FIG. 4-3**
Complete and incomplete
protein foods.

Incomplete proteins. Protein foods that are deficient in one or more of the nine essential amino acids are called *incomplete proteins*. These proteins are of plant origin: grains, legumes, nuts, seeds, vegetables, and fruits. However, these foods make valuable contributions to the total dietary protein.

Vegetarian diets

Complementary protein. The principle of complementary protein foods to provide adequate amounts of essential amino acids is the base for planning vegetarian diets. However, current knowledge of protein metabolism and the "pooling" of amino acid reserves (Fig. 4-2) indicates that careful meal-by-meal balance of complementary amino acids is not as necessary as previously thought. A normal eating pattern through the day, together with the body's reserve supply, usually ensures that complementary amino acid balance. The underlying requirement for vegetarians, as for all people, is to eat a sufficient amount of varied foods to meet caloric or energy needs (Box 4-1).

Types of vegetarian diets. Vegetarian diets differ according to the beliefs of persons following these food patterns. In general, there are three basic types of vegetarians.

1. Lacto-ovo vegetarians. Lacto-ovo vegetarians follow a food pattern that allows dairy products and eggs. Some may even accept fish and perhaps occasional poultry. Their mixed diet of both plant and animal food sources, excluding only meat, especially red meats, poses no nutritional problems.

BOX 4-1

❖ ——————— CLINICAL APPLICATION ——————— ❖

Essential Amino Acids—Nine or Eleven?—and Their Complementary Food Proteins

All of the nine essential amino acids must be supplied by the diet. But two of them, phenylalanine and methionine, have helpers as interactive backup. The body makes the amino acid tyrosine, which can spare some of the phenylalanine, and cystine which can interact with methionine. Thus, although there are only nine essential amino acids because the body can't make them, some may speak of eleven when they add the two helpers tyrosine and cystine.

The real life concern in a vegetarian diet is to obtain a balanced amount of the essential amino acids to complement one another and make complete food combinations. Only three of these nine essential amino acids are critical, however; if persons eat foods to supply enough of these three in a combined pattern, they will get sufficient amounts of the others, too. These three amino acids are thus called the *limiting amino acids*—lysine, methionine, and tryptophan. Of these three, lysine is the most limiting one.

The answer to balancing the vegetarian diet lies in mixing families of foods like grains, legumes, and milk products to make complementary food combinations to balance these needed amino acids. For example, grains are low in lysine and high in methionine, whereas legumes are just the opposite—low in methionine and high in lysine. So basically, grains and legumes will always balance one another, and additions of milk products and eggs will enhance their adequacy. Here are a few sample food combination dishes to illustrate:

Rice + black-eyed peas—a Southern U. S. dish called "hopping John"

Whole wheat or bulgur + soybeans + sesame seeds—protein enhanced by the addition of yogurt

Cornmeal + kidney beans—a combination in many Mexican dishes, protein enhanced by the addition of cheese

Soybeans + peanuts + brown rice + bulgur wheat—an excellent sauce dish served over the rice and wheat

Prepared with a variety of herbs and spices, onions, and garlic, to suit your taste, such dishes can supply needed nutrients and good eating.

2. Lacto-vegetarians. Lacto-vegetarians accept only dairy products from animal sources to complement their basic diet of plant foods. The use of milk and milk products such as cheese with a varied mixed diet of grains, legumes, nuts, seeds, fruits, and vegetables in sufficient quantities to meet energy needs provides a balanced intake.

3. Vegans. Vegans follow a strictly vegetarian diet and use no animal foods. Their food pattern is composed entirely of plant foods—grains, legumes, nuts, seeds, fruits, and vegetables. Careful planning and sufficient intake is necessary for adequate nutrition (Box 4-2).

BOX 4-2

❖ ———————— **CLINICAL APPLICATION** ———————— ❖

Case Study: A Vegan Child and Her Family

A vegan couple decided to raise their 2-year-old daughter according to their strict vegetarian diet. Often the child did not finish her meals and ate snacks of fruits and biscuits. Eventually the parents began to notice that she was not growing at the same rate as the other children and was becoming thin.

Questions for Analysis

1. What food patterns would you expect in this family? What dietary factor may have been involved in the child's poor growth?
2. What advice would you offer these parents to improve their child's nutritional status?
3. Plan one day's food for this family that would meet their nutritional needs within their vegetarian pattern. Indicate any added foods to meet the child's needs.
4. Would nutrient supplementation be indicated for this family, especially for the child? Why or why not? What would you suggest to them?

BODY NEEDS FOR PROTEIN
Influencing factors

Three main factors influence our requirement for protein: (1) tissue growth needs, (2) quality of the dietary protein, and (3) added needs from illness or disease.

Tissue growth. During the rapid growth periods of the human life cycle, more protein per unit of body size is required to build new tissue as well as maintain present tissues. Human growth is most rapid during three periods: fetal growth during the mother's pregnancy, infant growth during the first year of life plus lactation needs of a breast-feeding mother, and adolescent growth and development into adulthood. The period of young childhood is a sustained time of continued growth but at a somewhat slower rate. For adults protein requirements level off to meet tissue maintenance needs, but individual needs vary.

Dietary protein quality. The nature of the protein foods used and their pattern of amino acids significantly influence the quality of the dietary protein. Also, sufficient kcalories or energy intake, especially from nonprotein foods, is necessary to conserve protein for tissue building. Finally, the digestion and absorption of the protein consumed is affected by the comparative complexity of its structure as well as its preparation and cooking. The comparative quality of protein foods has been determined by the four basic measures below.

1. Chemical score (CS). is a value derived from the amino acid pattern of the food. Using a high-quality protein food such as egg and giving it a value of 100, other foods are compared according to their amino acid ratios.

2. Biologic value (BV). is based on nitrogen balance.

3. Net protein utilization (NPU). is based on biologic value and degree of the food protein's digestibility.

4. Protein efficiency ratio (PER). is based on weight gain of a growing test animal in relation to its protein intake.

❖ **TABLE 4-2**   *Comparative protein quality of selected foods*

Food	Chemical score*	BV†	NPU‡	PER§
Egg	100	100	94	3.92
Cow's milk	95	93	82	3.09
Fish	71	76	—	3.55
Beef	69	74	67	2.30
Unpolished rice	67	86	59	—
Peanuts	65	55	55	1.65
Oats	57	65	—	2.19
Polished rice	57	64	57	2.18
Whole wheat	53	65	49	1.53
Corn	49	72	36	—
Soybeans	47	73	61	2.32
Sesame seeds	42	62	53	1.77
Peas	37	64	55	1.57

Data adapted from Guthrie H: Introductory nutrition, ed 6, St. Louis, 1986, Times Mirror/
Mosby College Publishing; and Food and Nutrition Board: Recommended dietary allowances,
ed 9, Washington, DC, 1980, National Academy of Sciences.
* Amino acid   ‡ Net protein utilization
† Biologic value   § Protein efficiency ratio

A comparison of various protein food scores based on these measures of
protein quality is shown in Table 4-2. As shown, egg and milk proteins lead
all the lists. A sound diet is the best way for a healthy person to obtain quality
protein without need for amino acid supplements.

Illness or disease. An illness or disease, especially when accompanied by
fever and increased tissue breakdown (catabolism), increases the need for protein and kcalories to meet the demands of increased metabolic rate and for
rebuilding tissue. Traumatic injury requires extensive tissue rebuilding. After
surgery extra protein is needed for wound healing and restoring losses. Extensive tissue destruction as in massive burns requires a large protein increase
for the healing and grafting processes.

Dietary guides

Recommended dietary allowances. The RDA standards are based on age
and sex of the "average" person. For example, the reference man used for
these determinations weighs 70 kg (154 lbs), and the reference woman 55 kg
(120 lbs). They were assumed to be in good health and doing moderate activity.
The present RDA standard for adults is based on 0.8 g/kg of protein per day.[2]
Of course, individual needs vary at all ages. Thus this standard refers mainly
to population groups, not to specific individuals.

U.S. dietary guidelines. The dietary guidelines for Americans indicate that
about 15% to 20% of the diet's total kcalories should come from protein.
However, because there are no known benefits and possibly some risks in
consuming diets with a high animal protein content, the Diet and Health
Committee recommends that adult protein intake be maintained at moderate
levels, meeting the RDA standard of 0.8 g/kg of desirable body weight per
day but holding any increase to less than twice the RDA, that is, less than 1.6
g/kg.[4] In general Americans eat more protein than necessary, especially in the

❖ **TABLE 4-3** *Foods high in protein*

Food	Approximate amount	Protein (g)
Beef, chuck roast	3 oz cooked	23.4
Beef, hamburger	3 oz cooked	20.5
Beef, round	3 oz cooked	24.7
Beef, club steak	4 oz cooked	27.6
Lamb leg	3 oz cooked	21.6
Liver (beef, calf, and pork)	3 oz cooked	20.4
Pork loin	3 oz cooked	20.7
Ham	3 oz cooked	20.7
Veal, leg or shoulder	3 oz cooked	25.2
Chicken	¼ broiler	22.4
Chicken, fryer	½ breast (4 oz raw)	26.9
Chicken, hen, stewed	1 thigh or ½ breast	26.5
Duck, roasted	3 slices (3½ × 2¾ × ¼)	20.6
Goose, roasted	3 slices (3½ × 2¾ × ¼)	25.3
Turkey	3 slices (3½ × 2¾ × ¼)	27.8
Haddock	3 oz cooked	20.2
Halibut	3 oz cooked	21.0
Oysters	6 medium	15.1
Salmon	⅔ cup	20.5
Scallops	5-6 medium	23.8
Tuna	½ cup	15.9
Peanut butter	4 tbs	15.9
Milk	1 cup	8.5
Cottage cheese	5-6 tbs	19.5
American cheddar cheese	1 oz	7.0
Egg	1 medium	7.0

form of meat, which carries considerable animal fat. Consuming leaner, more moderate portions of meat would also bring the health benefits of reducing saturated animal fat intake. A comparison of protein food portions is shown in Table 4-3.

DIGESTION OF PROTEINS
Mouth

After the food protein is secured, it must be changed into the needed ready-to-use building units, the amino acids. This work is done through the successive parts of the gastrointestinal tract by the mechanical and chemical processes of digestion. In the mouth only the mechanical breaking up of the protein foods by chewing occurs. The food particles are mixed with saliva and passed on as a semisolid mass into the stomach.

Stomach

Because proteins are such large complex structures, a series of enzymes is necessary to finally break them down to produce the amino acids. These chemical changes begin in the stomach. In fact, the stomach's chief digestive function in relation to all foods is the initial partial enzymatic breakdown of protein.

Three agents in the gastric secretions help with this task: pepsin, hydrochloric acid, and rennin.

1. Pepsin. Pepsin is the main gastric enzyme, specific for proteins. It is first produced as an inactive **proenzyme,** *pepsinogen,* by a single layer of cells (the chief cells) in the stomach wall. Pepsinogen is then activated by the hydrochloric acid in the gastric juices to the enzyme pepsin. The active **pepsin** begins splitting the linkages between the protein's amino acids, changing the large amino acid chains that make up the protein into smaller parts called *peptides.* If the protein were held in the stomach longer, pepsin could continue the breakdown until individual amino acids resulted. But with normal gastric emptying time, only the beginning stage is completed by the action of pepsin.

2. Hydrochloric acid. Hydrochloric acid provides the acid medium necessary to convert pepsinogen to active pepsin.

3. Rennin. The gastric enzyme **rennin** is present only in infancy and childhood and disappears in adulthood. It is especially important in the infant's digestion of milk. Rennin and calcium act on the casein of milk to produce a curd. By coagulating milk, rennin prevents too rapid a passage of the food from the child's stomach into the small intestine.

Small intestine

Protein digestion begins in the acid medium of the stomach and is completed in the alkaline medium of the small intestine. A number of enzymes from secretions of both the pancreas and the intestine take part in protein digestion.

1. Pancreatic secretions. Three enzymes produced by the pancreas continue breaking down proteins into simpler and simpler substances. (1) **Trypsin,** secreted first as inactive trypsinogen, is activitated by a local hormone from glands in the wall of the duodenum, the first part of the small intestine. Then the active enzyme works on protein and large polypeptide fragments carried from the stomach, producing small polypeptides and dipeptides.(2) **Chymotrypsin,** secreted first as inactive chymotrypsinogen, is activated by the trypsin already present. Then the active enzyme continues the same protein-splitting action of trypsin. (3) **Carboxypeptidase** attacks the acid (carboxyl) end of the peptide chains and produces in turn smaller peptides and some free amino acids.

2. Intestinal secretions. Glands in the intestinal wall produce two more protein-splitting enzymes to complete the breakdown and free the remaining amino acids. (1) **Aminopeptidase** releases amino acids one at a time from the nitrogen-containing amino end of the peptide chain, producing peptides and free amino acids. (2) **Dipeptidase,** the final enzyme in the protein-splitting system, completes the large task by breaking the remaining dipeptides into their two, now free, amino acids.

This team system of protein-splitting enzymes breaks down the large complex proteins into progressively smaller peptide chains and finally frees each individual amino acid—a tremendous overall task. Now the free amino acids are ready to be absorbed directly into the portal blood circulation for use in building body tissues. A summary of this remarkable system of protein digestion is given in Table 4-4.

❖ **TABLE 4-4** *Summary of protein digestion*

Organ	Inactive precursor	Enzyme		Digestive action
		Activator	Active enzyme	
Mouth			None	Mechanical only
Stomach (acid)	Pepsinogen	Hydrochloric acid	Pepsin	Protein → polypeptides
			Rennin (infants) (calcium necessary for activity)	Casein → coagulated curd
Intestine (alkaline)				
Pancreas	Trypsinogen	Enterokinase	Trypsin	Protein, polypeptides → polypeptides, dipepetides
	Chymotrypsinogen	Active trypsin	Chymotrypsin	Protein, polypeptides → polypeptides, dipeptides
			Carboxypeptidase	Polypeptides → simpler peptides, dipeptides, amino acids
Intestine			Aminopeptidase	Polypeptides → peptides, dipeptides, amino acids
			Dipeptidase	Dipeptides → amino acids

SUMMARY

Proteins provide the human body with its primary tissue-building units, the amino acids. Of the 22 known amino acids, nine are essential in the diet because the body cannot manufacture them as it can the remaining ones. Foods that supply all the essential amino acids are called complete proteins. These foods are of animal origin—egg, milk, cheese, and meat. Plant protein foods are called incomplete because they lack one or more of the essential amino acids. Plant sources are grains, legumes, nuts, seeds, vegetables, and fruits. Strict vegetarian diets use only these plant proteins; other may use milk and egg and eliminate only meat. Carefully planned combinations of foods with complementary amino acid contents can provide adequate dietary protein quality.

Constant tissue protein turnover occurs between tissue building (anabolism) and tissue breakdown (catabolism). Adequate dietary protein and a body reserve "pool" of amino acids help to maintain overall protein balance. Nitrogen balance is a measure of this overall balance. A mixed diet of a variety of foods, together with sufficient nonprotein kcalories from the primary fuel foods, supplies a balance of protein and other nutrients. Only strict vegetarians—vegans—risk protein imbalance and other nutritional deficiencies in iron, zinc, calcium, and vitamin B_{12}.

Protein requirements are influenced mainly by growth needs and the nature of the diet in terms of protein quality and energy intake. Clinical influences on protein needs include fever, disease, surgery, or other trauma to body tissues. After protein foods are eaten, a powerful digestive team of six protein-splitting enzymes frees individual unique amino acids for their vital tissue-building tasks.

❖ REVIEW QUESTIONS

1. What is the difference between an *essential* and a *nonessential* amino acid? Why is this difference important?
2. Compare *complete* and *incomplete* protein foods. Give examples of each type.
3. Describe the factors that influence protein requirements.
4. Describe the different types of vegetarian diets. Compare each one in terms of protein quality and risk of nutrient deficiencies.

❖ SELF-TEST QUESTIONS

True-false

For each item you answer "false," write the correct statement.

1. Complete proteins of high biologic value are found in whole grains, dried beans and peas, and nuts.
2. The primary function of dietary protein is to supply the necessary amino acids to build and repair body tissue.
3. Protein provides a main source of body heat and muscle energy.
4. The average American diet is relatively moderate in protein.
5. Because they are smaller, infants and young children need less protein per unit of body weight than adults require.
6. In old age the protein requirement decreases because of lessened physical activity.
7. Healthy adults are in a state of nitrogen balance.
8. Positive nitrogen balance exists during periods of rapid growth, such as in infancy and adolescence.
9. When negative nitrogen balance exists, the person is less able to resist infections and general health deteriorates.
10. Wheat and rice are complete protein foods of high biologic value.
11. Egg protein has a higher biologic value than meat protein.

Multiple choice

1. Nine of the 22 amino acids are called "essential," meaning that:
   a. The body cannot make these nine and must get them in the diet.
   b. These nine are essential in body processes and the rest are not.
   c. The body makes these nine because they are the life-essential ones.
   d. After making these nine, the body uses them for essential growth.
2. A complete protein food of high biologic value would be one that contains:
   a. All 22 of the amino acids in sufficient amounts to meet human requirements.
   b. The nine essential amino acids in any proportion, since the body can always fill in the differences needed.
   c. All of the 22 amino acids from which the body can make additional amounts of the nine essential ones as needed.
   d. All nine essential amino acids in correct proportion to meet human needs.
3. A state of negative nitrogen balance occurs during periods of:
   a. Pregnancy
   b. Adolescence
   c. Injury or surgery
   d. Infancy

❖ SUGGESTIONS FOR ADDITIONAL STUDY

1. Collect illustrations of complete and incomplete protein foods for your notebook.
2. List the protein food combinations you usually have at daily meals.
3. Keep a record of everything you eat or drink for one day. Calculate your protein intake and compare it with your need according to the RDAs guideline. Identify your complete and incomplete protein food sources. How would you rate the protein quality of your diet?

References

1. Cho ES and others: Long-term effects of low histidine intake on men, J Nutr 114:369, 1984.
2. National Research Council, Food and Nutrition Board: Recommended dietary allowances, ed 10, Washington, DC, 1989, National Academy press.
3. Rossouw JE: Kwashiorkor in North America, Am J Clin Nutr 49:588, Apr 1989.
4. National Research Council, Food and Nutrition Board, Committee on Diet and Health: Diet and Health, implications for reducing chronic disease, Washington, DC, 1989, National Academy Press.

Further reading

Lappe FM: Diet for a small planet, New York, 1982, Ballantine Books.

This little book is still a classic, filled with information about combining plant protein foods to achieve complementary amino acid combinations and giving many vegetarian recipes for good cooking.

Madison D and Brown E: The Greens cookbook, New York, 1987, Bantam Books.

This cookbook provides a wide selection of gourmet vegetarian recipes from dishes made famous by Greens' Restaurant in San Francisco. The recipe collection is drawn from a wide variety of traditions—Mediterranean cooking of southern France, Italy, and Greece, foods of Asia, Mexico, and the American Southwest.

Robertson L, Flinders C, and Godfrey B: Laurel's kitchen, a handbook for vegetarian cookery and nutrition, Petaluma, California, 1981, Nilgiri Press.

As the subtitle indicates, this excellent book combines much sound nutrition with a variety of cooking suggestions and recipes for a "good-to-eat" vegetarian diet. Its pages are permeated by the warmth of its authors and their many practical guides along the way.

5

❖

Energy balance

KEY CONCEPTS

*Food energy is changed into body energy and cycled
throughout the body to do its work.*

*The body uses the major portion of its energy
intake for basal metabolic work needs.*

*A balance between food energy intake and body work
energy output maintains life and health.*

*States of underweight and overweight reflect
degrees of body energy imbalance.*

*O*ur efficient bodies constantly change the stored fuel energy in our food into the energy we use at work and play as well as at rest. Overall energy metabolism deals with *change* and *balance*, the constant facts of life.

Many constant changes and balances in our food and the nutrients it delivers to our body cells produce our needed energy. Fuel is "burned" and stored as needed to provide a continuous flow of energy for our body's work.

In this chapter we look at the "big picture" of energy balance among all the energy nutrients. We see how this energy intake is measured, cycled, and used to meet all our energy needs.

HUMAN ENERGY SYSTEM
Basic energy needs

The body needs constant energy to do the work required to maintain life and health. The actions involved are both voluntary and involuntary.

Voluntary work and exercise. Voluntary body work includes all the physical actions related to a person's usual activities, as well as any added physical exercise. Although this visible, conscious action would seem to require the major portion of our energy output, this is usually not true.

Involuntary body work. The greatest energy output is the result of involuntary body work, which includes all the activities in the body that are not consciously performed. These activities include such vital processes as circulation, respiration, digestion, absorption, and a multitude of other internal activities that maintain life.

Sources of fuel. The energy needed for voluntary and involuntary body work requires fuel, provided in the form of nutrients. As presented in the previous chapters, the only three "energy nutrients" are carbohydrate, fat, and protein. Carbohydrate is the body's primary fuel, with fat assisting as a storage fuel. Protein is occasionally a backup fuel, actually an inefficient one, available as needed. The body must have a supply of the food fuels to provide energy for work and to keep the body warm. If sufficient primary fuel, carbohydrate, is not consumed to supply these body energy needs, the body will burn more fat. The average daily food energy intake should equal the daily body energy needs to maintain health.

Measurement of energy

Unit of measure: kilocalorie. In common usage the word **calorie** refers to the amount of energy in foods or expended in physical actions. In human nutrition, however, the term **kilocalorie** (1000 calories) is used to designate the large calorie unit used in nutritional science to avoid dealing with such large numbers. These units of measure relate to heat production. A kilocalorie, abbreviated as *kcalorie* or *kcal*, is the amount of heat required to raise 1 kg of water 1° centigrade (C). Sometime in your reading you may see the international unit of measure for energy, *joule (J)*, usually expressed as *megajoule (MJ)*, which equals 239 kcal.

Food energy: fuel factors. As previously discussed, the three energy nutrients, carbohydrate and fat, with protein as a backup, have basic fuel factors. Beverage alcohol, from fermented grains and fruits, also adds fuel. These factors reflect their relative fuel densities: (1) carbohydrate, 4 kcal/g; (2) fat, 9 kcal/g; (3) protein, 4 kcal/g; and (4) alcohol, 7 kcal/g.

Caloric and nutrient density. The term *density* refers to the degree of concentration of material in a given substance. More material in a smaller amount of substance gives that substance a greater density. Thus the concept of *caloric density* means a higher concentration of energy (kcalories) in a smaller amount of food. Of the three energy nutrients, fat or foods high in fat would have the highest caloric density. In a similar manner, foods may be evaluated in terms of their relative *nutrient density*. High nutrient density refers to a relatively high concentration of nutrients, from all nutrient groups, in smaller amounts of a given food. A number of food guides base their listed "food scores" on the concentration of nutrients in given foods, compared to kcalorie values, in relation to health goals.

ENERGY BALANCE

Energy, like matter, cannot be "created." When we speak of energy as being "produced," what we really mean is that it is being transformed—changed in form and cycled throughout a system. Consider our human energy system as part of the total energy system on earth. In this sense, two energy systems support our lives: the one within us and the much larger one surrounding us.

1. *External energy cycle.* In our external environment, the ultimate source of energy in our world is the sun and its vast nuclear reactions. Growing plants, using water and carbon dioxide as raw materials, transform the sun's radiation into stored chemical energy, mainly carbohydrate and some fat. The food chain continues as animals eat the plants and transform the plant energy into animal food energy.

2. *Internal energy cycle.* As we eat the plant and animal foods, we change the stored energy into our own body fuels, glucose and fatty acids, and cycle them into various other energy forms to serve our body needs. These forms include: (1) chemical energy in the many new metabolic products made, (2) electrical energy in brain and nerve tissue, (3) mechanical energy in muscle contraction, and (4) thermal energy in the heat to keep our bodies warm. As this internal energy cycle continues, we excrete water, exhale carbon dioxide, and radiate heat, returning these end-products to the external environment. The overall energy cycle repeats constantly, sustaining our lives.

Energy intake

The total overall energy balance within the body depends on the measure of energy intake in relation to the energy output. The main source of energy for all body work is food, backed up by stored energy in body tissues.

Sources of food energy. The three energy nutrients in the food we eat keep our bodies supplied with fuel. You can easily estimate your own energy intake by recording a day's actual food consumption, using a form such as the one given in Box 5-1, and calculating its energy value (see Appendix).

Sources of stored energy. When food is not available, as in the short hours of sleep, longer periods of fasting, or the extreme stress of starvation, the body draws on its stores for energy.

1. *Glycogen.* A 12- to 48-hour reserve of glycogen exists in liver and muscles and is quickly depleted if not replenished by food. Glycogen stores, for example, maintain normal blood glucose levels for body functions during sleep hours. Our first meal, breakfast, so named because it "breaks the fast," is a significant function for energy intake.

2. *Adipose tissue.* Although fat storage is larger than glycogen, the supply varies from person to person, and a balanced amount needs to be maintained as an added energy resource.

3. *Muscle mass.* Energy stored as protein exists in limited amounts in muscle mass, but this lean muscle mass needs to be maintained for health. Only in longer periods of fasting or starvation does the body turn to these tissues for energy.

❖❖❖

BOX 5–1
Record of Food Energy Intake

List all meals and snacks for 1 day:

Food (description and amount)	Carbohydrates (g)	Fat (g)	Protein (g)	Kcalories
Breakfast				
Lunch				
Snacks				
Dinner				
Snacks				
TOTAL				

Energy output

The energy from our food and body reserves is spent in necessary activities of the various organs of the body, such as body function work, regulation of body temperature, and the processes of tissue growth and repair. The total chemical changes that occur during all of these body activities are called *metabolism*. This exchange of energy in overall balance is usually expressed in kcalories. The energy output of the body is based on three demands for energy: basal metabolism, physical activity, and eating.

Basal metabolism. The term **basal metabolism** refers to the sum of all internal working activities of the body at rest. In general use, interchangeable terms are **basal energy expenditure (BEE)**, **resting energy expenditure (REE)**, or **resting metabolic rate (RMR)**.[1,2] This is a vast amount of physiologic work, and the large majority of the body's energy is spent to maintain these metabolic functions. Most of this amount is used by small but highly active tissues—

liver, brain, heart, kidney, and gastrointestinal tract—which together amount to less than 5% of the total body weight. Yet these tissues contribute about 60% of the total basal metabolism needs. Although resting muscle and adipose fat are far larger in mass, they contribute much less to the body's basal metabolic rate.

1. *Measuring basal metabolic rate.* Formerly, in clinical practice, an involved basal metabolic rate (BMR) test was done with an instrument that measured the normal exchange of oxygen and carbon dioxide in regular breathing. Then the amount of energy was calculated as the amount of body heat produced. This test is now used only in research. Newer, more efficient tests are currently used in practice. These tests measure activity of the thyroid gland and blood levels of its hormone *thyroxine.* Two thyroid hormone compounds are measured: T_3 (the prethyroxine hormone), and T_4 (thyroxine). Then a measure called the *free thyroxine index* (FTI) is calculated as the product of these two hormones ($T_3 \times T_4$). Since these thyroid hormones control the body's overall BMR, these blood measures provide a much more easily determined test for basal metabolism. Also, since the thyroid gland uses iodine to make its hormone, two other tests may be performed: serum levels of protein-bound iodine (PBI), and radioactive iodine uptake tests. A general formula for calculating basal energy needs is: 1 kcal/kg body weight (weight in pounds divided by 2.2) per hour per day. Thus with this method the daily basal metabolic needs are calculated as:

$$1 \text{ kcal} \times \text{kg body weight} \times 24 \text{ hrs}$$

For adult hospitalized patients an alternate method of estimating the basal or resting energy expenditure is by the classic Harris-Benedict equations (also see p. 60, Further Reading reference):

Women: BEE = 655 + 9.56 × weight (kg) + 1.85 × height (cm) − 4.68 × age
Men: BEE = 66.5 + 13.8 × weight (kg) + 5 × height (cm) - 6.76 × age

2. *Factors influencing BMR.* Several factors influence BMR and should be remembered when reading related test results. The major factor affecting BMR is the leanness of the body.[1,2] This is due to the greater metabolic activity in lean tissues compared with fat and bones. The BMR is higher in lean bodies, thus requiring more energy. It is lower in fat bodies, thus requiring less energy. Other factors such as surface area, sex, and age only influence BMR as they relate to the lean body mass.[2]

During growth periods, the growth hormone stimulates cell metabolism and raises BMR 15% to 20%. Thus the BMR slowly rises during the first 5 years of life, levels off somewhat, rises again just before and during puberty, and then gradually declines into old age. During pregnancy, a rapid growth period, the BMR rises 20% to 25% due to the accelerated tissue growth and the increased work of heart and lungs. During the following period of lactation, the breast-feeding mother's BMR increases still further and she needs extra kcalories to cover this added metabolic process.

Fever increases BMR approximately 7% for each 0.83° C (1° F) rise. Diseases involving increased cell activity, such as cancer, cardiac failure, and respiratory problems (for example, emphysema) usually increase the BMR. In the abnormal states of starvation and malnutrition, the BMR is lowered, since the lean body mass is decreased.

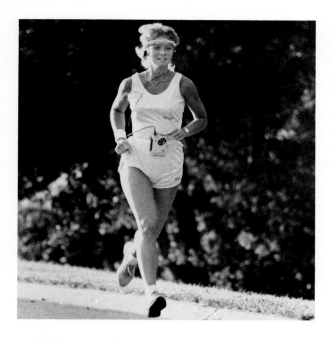

❖ **Fig. 5-1**
Energy output in exercise.

BMR rises in lower temperature to generate more body heat to maintain normal body temperature.

Physical activity. Exercise involved in work or recreation (Fig. 5-1) accounts for wide individual variations in energy output. (See Chapter 16.) Some representative kcalorie expenditures in different types of work and recreation are given in Table 5-1. Mental work or study does not itself require added kcalories. The feeling of fatigue is caused by muscle tension or moving about. Also, emotional states alone do not increase kcalorie needs, but may require energy intake to compensate for muscle tension, restlessness, and agitated movements.

Effect of eating. After we eat, the food stimulates our metabolism and requires extra energy for digestion, absorption, and transport of the nutrients to the cells. This overall stimulating effect of food is called its *specific dynamic action (SDA)* or more recently *dietary thermogenesis* ("heat generating"). About 5% to 10% of the body's total energy needs for metabolism is related to the handling of the food we eat.[2]

Total energy requirement. The basal energy requirement, individual physical activities, and the energy need involved with eating make up the person's overall total energy requirement. To maintain daily energy balance, food energy intake must match body energy output. An energy imbalance of an excess of food energy intake needed for body energy output causes obesity. Treatment should include a decrease in food kcalories and an increase in physical activity. Extreme weight loss as in anorexia nervosa results from an energy imbalance of deficient food energy intake to match body energy requirements. Treatment should include a gradual increase in food kcalories along with moderate activity and rest. A discussion of weight management is given in Chapter 15.

Where do you stand in your own energy balance? You can estimate your energy needs by using the steps in Box 5-2.

❖ TABLE 5-1   *Energy expenditure/hour during various activities**

Light activities: 120-150 kcal/hr	Light-moderate activities: 150-300 kcal/hr	Moderate activities: 300-420 kcal/hr	Heavy activities: 420-600 kcal/hr
Personal care	Domestic	Yard work	Yard work
Dressing	work	Digging	Chopping
Washing	Making	Mowing lawn	wood
Shaving	beds	(not motor-	Digging holes
Sitting	Sweeping	ized)	Shoveling snow
Rocking	floors	Pulling weeds	Walking
Typing	Ironing	Walking	5 mph
Writing	Washing	3½-4 mph on	Upstairs
Playing cards	clothes	level surface	Up hills
Peeling potatoes	Yard work	Up and down	Climbing
Sewing	Light gar-	small hills	Recreation
Playing piano	dening	Recreation	Bicycling 11-12
Standing or	Mowing	Badminton	mph or up
slowly moving	lawn	Calisthenics	and down
around	(power	Ballet exer-	hills
Billiards	mower)	cises	Cross-country
	Light work	Canoeing 4	skiing
	Auto repair	mph	Jogging 5 mph
	Painting	Dancing	Swimming
	Shoe repair	(waltz,	Tennis (singles)
	Store clerk	square)	Water-skiing
	Washing car	Golf (no cart)	
	Walking	Ping-Pong	
	2-3 mph on	Tennis (dou-	
	level sur-	bles)	
	face or	Volleyball	
	down		
	stairs		
	Recreation		
	Archery		
	Bicycling		
	5½ mph		
	on level		
	surface		
	Bowling		
	Canoeing		
	2½-3 mph		

*Energy expenditure will depend on the physical fitness (that is, amount of lean body mass) of the individual and continuity of exercise. Note that some of these activities can be used as aerobic activities to promote cardiovascular fitness. For more information, see Chapter 16.

❖

BOX 5-2
Estimate Your Own Daily Energy Requirement

- **Basal metabolism (BMR)**

Use general formula: Women—0.9 kcal/kg body weight/hr
                     Men—1.0 kcal/kg body weight/hr
Convert weight (pounds) to kg: 1 kg = 2.2 pounds
Multiply according to formula: 1 (or 0.9) × (hours in day)
- **Physical activity**

Estimate your general average level of physical (muscular) activity. Find energy cost of activity (% of BMR) and add it to BMR.

Average activity level	Energy cost: % of BMR
Sedentary	20%
Very light	30%
Moderate	40%
Heavy	50%

For example, if you are sedentary (mostly sitting): BMR (step 1) + (.20 × BMR).
- **Specific dynamic action (SDA) of food**

Record food intake for day and calculate approximate energy (kcal) value.
Find energy cost of food effect (10% of kcal in food consumed).
- **Total energy output**

BMR + physical activity + SDA

ENERGY REQUIREMENTS
General life cycle

Growth periods. During periods of rapid growth extra energy per unit of body weight is required to build new tissue. In childhood the most rapid growth occurs during infancy and adolescence, with continuous but slower growth in between (Table 5-2). The rapid growth of the fetus, placenta, and other maternal tissues makes increased energy intake during pregnancy and lactation a vital concern.

Adulthood. With full adult growth achieved, energy needs of young adults level off, meeting requirements for tissue maintenance and usual physical activities. As the aging process continues, the gradual decline in BMR and physical activity decreases the energy requirement (Table 5-3). This means that food choices should reflect a decline in caloric density but give greater attention to increased nutrient density.

Guidelines for health

Recommended dietary allowances. The RDA standard for energy needs at all ages is given in Table 5-4. As indicated earlier, these allowances are estimates of population needs, and individual needs within age groups may vary widely. The varying individual needs are indicated by the ranges given in the full RDA tables inside the book covers.

U.S. dietary guidelines. Energy needs are indicated by two recommendations in the U.S. dietary guidelines for healthy Americans: (1) maintain healthy weight, and (2) choose a diet low in fat, saturated fat, and cholesterol.[1] Fats, the most concentrated fuel source, have the highest caloric density, and most

❖ TABLE 5-2   *Approximate caloric allowances for ages 1 month to 19 years*

Age	Kcalories per pound	Age	Kcalories per pound
Infants		Boys	
1-3 mo	54.3	13-15 yr	30.0
4-9 mo	49.5	16-19 yr	25.5
10-12 mo	45.5	Girls	
Children		13-15 yr	24.3
1-3 yr	45.0	16-19 yr	20.0
4-6 yr	40.0		
7-9 yr	40.0		
10-12 yr	32.0		

❖ TABLE 5-3   *Gradual reduction of kcalorie needs during adulthood*

Age	Kcalorie reduction (%) for maintenance of ideal weight*
30-40	3.0
40-50	3.0
50-60	7.5
60-70	7.5
70-80	10.0

* Added percent decreases for each decade past the age of 25.

Americans eat too much fat. Following the guideline statements to use sugars only in moderation and to choose a diet with plenty of vegetables, fruits, and grain products (p. 9) also contributes to a healthier energy balance.

SUMMARY

Energy is the force or power to do work. In the human energy system, energy intake is provided by food. This energy is measured in the "large calorie" (1000 calories), or *kilocalorie (kcalorie* or *kcal)*. Energy from food is cycled through our internal energy system in balance with the external environment's energy system, powered by the sun.

Metabolism is the sum of the body processes that change our food energy from the three energy nutrients—mainly carbohydrate, some fat, and protein backup—into various forms of energy. These forms include *chemical* energy in many metabolic products, *electrical* energy in brain and nerve activities, *mechanical* energy in muscle contraction, and *thermal* (heat) energy to keep us warm. Throughout this cycling of our body energy, metabolism is balanced by two types of metabolic actions: (1) *anabolism*, which builds tissue and stores energy; and (2) *catabolism*, which breaks down tissue and releases energy. When food is not available the body draws on its stored energy: glycogen, fat, and tissue protein.

❖ **TABLE 5-4** *Median heights and weights and recommended energy intake**

Category	Age (years) or condition	Weight (kg)	Weight (lb)	Height (cm)	Height (in)	REE[a] (kcal/day)	Multiples of REE	Average energy allowance (kcal)[b] Per kg	Per day[c]
Infants	0.0-0.5	6	13	60	24	320		108	650
	0.5-1.0	9	20	71	28	500		98	850
Children	1-3	13	29	90	35	740		102	1,300
	4-6	20	44	112	44	950		90	1,800
	7-10	28	62	132	52	1,130		70	2,000
Males	11-14	45	99	157	62	1,440	1.70	55	2,500
	15-18	66	145	176	69	1,760	1.67	45	3,000
	19-24	72	160	177	70	1,780	1.67	40	2,900
	25-50	79	174	176	70	1,800	1.60	37	2,900
	51+	77	170	173	68	1,530	1.50	30	2,300
Females	11-14	46	101	157	62	1,310	1.67	47	2,200
	15-18	55	120	163	64	1,370	1.60	40	2,200
	19-24	58	128	164	65	1,350	1.60	38	2,200
	25-50	63	138	163	64	1,380	1.55	36	2,200
	51+	65	143	160	63	1,280	1.50	30	1,900
Pregnant	1st trimester								+0
	2nd trimester								+300
	3rd trimester								+300
Lactating	1st 6 months								+500
	2nd 6 months								+500

*National Research Council Recommended dietary allowances, ed 10, Washington DC, 1989, National Academy Press.
[a]Resting energy expenditure (REE). Calculation based on FAO equations (Table 3-1), then rounded.
[b]In the range of light to moderate activity, the coefficient of variation is ± 20%.
[c]Figure is rounded.

Total body energy requirements are based on: (1) basal (maintenance) metabolism needs, measured by basal metabolic rate (BMR) and making up the largest portion of our energy needs, and (2) energy for physical activities, digesting food, and absorbing and transporting nutrients.

❖ REVIEW QUESTIONS

1. What are the fuel factors of the three energy nutrients? Of alcohol? What do these figures mean? What is our primary energy nutrient? Why?
2. Define *basal metabolism*. What body tissues contribute most to our basal metabolic needs? Why? What factors influence basal energy needs (BMR)? Why?
3. What factors influence nonbasal energy needs?

❖ SELF-TEST QUESTIONS

True-false
For each item you answer "false," write the correct statement.
1. Kilocalories are nutrients in foods.
2. Glycogen stores provide a long-lasting energy reserve to maintain blood sugar levels.
3. Thyroid hormone controls the rate of overall body metabolism.
4. Energy requirements for children are less per kg (lb) of body weight than for adults because they are smaller.
5. The process of catabolism builds new tissues.
6. Different persons doing the same amount of physical activity will require the same amount of energy in kcalories.

Multiple choice
1. In human nutrition the kilocalorie is used to:
   a. Provide nutrients
   b. Measure body heat energy
   c. Control energy reactions
   d. Measure electrical energy
2. In this family of four, who has the highest energy needs per unit of body weight?
   a. 32-year-old mother
   b. 35-year-old father
   c. 2-month-old son
   d. 70-year-old grandmother
3. An overactive thyroid causes:
   a. Decreased energy need
   b. No effect on energy need
   c. Increased energy need
   d. Obesity due to lower BMR
4. Which of the following persons is using the most energy:
   a. Woman walking uphill
   b. Student studying for final examinations
   c. Teenager playing basketball
   d. Man driving a car
5. Which of these foods has the highest energy value per unit of weight?
   a. Bread
   b. Meat
   c. Potato
   d. Butter

6. A slice of bread contains 2 g of protein and 15 g of carbohydrate in the form of starch. What is its kcalorie value?
   a. 17 kcal
   b. 42 kcal
   c. 68 kcal
   d. 92 kcal

❖ SUGGESTIONS FOR ADDITIONAL STUDY

1. Calculate your own energy balance for 1 day, based on your energy intake (food) and your energy output (basal metabolism, physical activities according to Table 5-1, and energy needed to handle your food after eating meals or snacks). Describe your energy balance in terms of your body weight.
2. Calculate the energy value (kcalories) of the following foods:

Food	Carbohydrate (g)	Fat (g)	Protein (g)	Kcalories
1 cup milk	12	10	8	
½ cup ice cream	15	9	3	
½ cup cooked carrots	7	0	2	
½ grapefruit	10	0	0	

3. List 10 of your favorite foods. Check the kcalorie value of your usual portion of each one, using the Appendix. Do any of these energy values surprise you?

References

1. National Research Council, Food and Nutrition Board: Diet and health, implications for reducing chronic disease risk, Washington, DC, 1989, National Academy Press.

2. National Research Council, Food and Nutrition Board: Recommended dietary allowances, ed 10, 1989, National Academy Press.

Further readings

Havala T and Shronts E: Managing the complications associated with refeeding, Nutr Clin Prac 5(1):23, 1990.

The two nurse-authors provide helpful guidance for managing a gradual refeeding process for patients with protein-energy malnutrition. This energy imbalance problem of malnutrition has been shown to exist in 44% to 50% of hospitalized patients. Any health worker caring for chronically malnourished persons will find this article of practical assistance.

Harris TG: How to manage your energy, Am Health 6(2):115, 1987.

This conversation with well-known author/manager Peter Drucker, who has many demands on his energy, shows us some ways we can better manage our own energy and be our own best bosses.

Perry P: Are we having fun yet? Am Health 6(2):58, 1987.

This helpful article shows us that exercise to balance our energy and keep us fit should also be fun. A good chart of kcalories spent in various activities is included.

Mifflin MD and others: A new predictive equation for resting energy expenditure in healthy individuals, Am J Clin Nutr 51:241, Feb 1990.

This group of investigators has provided new simplified formulas for estimating resting energy expenditure (REE) for men and women. Since the widely used Harris-Benedict equations were developed some 70 years ago, these new formulas may apply more accurately to our modern population with obvious differences in body size and composition, levels of physical activity, and diet. These simplified formulas are:

Women: REE = 10 × weight (kg) + 6.25 × height (cm) − 5 × age − 161

Men: REE = 10 × weight (kg) + 6.25 × height (cm) − 5 × age + 5

6

❖

Vitamins

K E Y   C O N C E P T S

Vitamins are noncaloric essential nutrients, necessary for specific metabolic control and disease prevention.

Certain health problems are related to inadequate or excessive vitamin intake.

Vitamins occur in a wide variety of foods, packaged with the energy and tissue building macronutrients (carbohydrate, fat, protein) on which they work as specific catalysts.

Vitamin supplementation needs are individual and specific.

$\mathcal{V}$itamins, more than any other group of nutrients, have captured public interest and concern. Attitudes toward them have varied from wise attention to diet and specific functional use to wild claims, counterclaims, and abuse.

Clearly vitamins are essential nutrients. But just what do they do, how much do we need, and where can we get them? Are they better in food or in pills? Do we need more than nutrient guides indicate? Can large amounts hurt us? From their constant attention in the public press, and the billion-dollar industry supporting this attention, we know that vitamins *are* a general concern of many people, and we need sound answers, not biased blasts.

In this chapter we look at vitamins as a group and as specific nutrients. They are as diverse in nature as are individual members of any other nutrient group and need to be viewed as such. We explore our general and specific needs and how to approach vitamin use in a reasonable and realistic manner.

NATURE OF VITAMINS
Discovery
Early observations. Discoveries of vitamins were largely related to work on cures for classic diseases that early observers believed were associated in some way with deficiencies in the diet. For example, as early as 1753, a British naval surgeon, Dr. James Lind, observed that on long voyages when sailors were forced to live on very limited rations because no fresh foods were available, many of the men became ill and died. When he took some easier-to-store fresh lemons and limes on a later voyage, he learned that when he gave these fruits to the sailors, no one became ill. Thus originated the nickname of "limeys" for British sailors. This vital clue then led to the discovery that *scurvy*, the curse of sailors, was caused by some dietary deficiency and was cured by adding certain fresh fruits to the diet.

Early animal experiments. In 1906, Dr. Frederich Hopkins, working at Cambridge University in England, performed an experiment in which he fed a group of white rats a diet of a synthetic mixture of protein, fat, carbohydrate, mineral salts, and water. As a result, the animals all became ill and died. When he added milk to the purified ration, all the rats grew normally. This important discovery, that there are accessory food factors present in *natural* foods that are essential to life, reinforced the necessary foundation for the individual vitamin discoveries that followed.

Era of vitamin discovery. During the first half of the 1900s, the discoveries of our known vitamins occurred. The remarkable nature of these vital agents became increasingly more evident. The name *vitamin* developed during the first part of these research years when Casimir Funk, a Polish chemist working at the Lister Institute in London, discovered in 1911 a nitrogen-containing substance called an *amine*, which he thought was the chemical nature of these vital agents. So he called it *vitamine* ("vital-amine"). Later the final "e" was dropped when other similarly vital substances turned out to be a variety of organic compounds. The name *vitamin* has been retained to designate compounds of this class of essential substances. At first alphabet letter names were given to individual vitamins discovered. But as the number increased rapidly, this practice became confusing. So in recent years more specific names based on the vitamins' chemical structure or body function have been developed. Today these scientific names are preferred and commonly used, so they should be learned.

Definition
As the vitamins were discovered one by one during the first half of the 1900s and the list of them grew, two characteristics clearly emerged to define a compound as a vitamin.
1. It must be a vital organic dietary substance that is not a carbohydrate, fat, protein, or mineral and is necessary in only very *small* amounts to perform a specific metabolic function or to prevent an associated deficiency disease.

2. It cannot be manufactured by the body and therefore must be supplied by the diet.

On the basis of both of these characteristics, vitamins are essential to life and health. The amount of these substances needed by the body is very small, as indicated (hence the designation "micronutrients"), unless some special state or condition creates an increased need in a particular individual. Normally the total volume of vitamins a healthy person requires would barely fill a teaspoon. However, all are essential to existence.

Classes of vitamins

Vitamins are usually classified on the basis of their solubility as either *fat soluble* or *water soluble*. Although this is a somewhat arbitrary grouping with little real significance, it is traditional and is used here. The fat-soluble vitamins are A, D, E, and K. The water-soluble vitamins are C and all of the B vitamins.

Functions of vitamins

Although each vitamin has its specific metabolic task, two general functions that may be ascribed to vitamins as a group are (1) control agents in cell metabolism and (2) components of body tissue construction. A third function, preventing specific nutritional deficiency disease, may be considered a result of the primary role in cell metabolism.

1. Control agent: coenzyme partner. Specific enzymes and coenzymes control specific chemical reactions by acting as necessary *catalysts.* This term comes from the Greek word *katalysis*, meaning "to dissolve." In chemical usage, it refers to substances such as enzymes that are necessary control agents for breaking down compounds but are not themselves consumed in the process. In many of the cell reactions a particular vitamin is required as a specific coenzyme partner with the regular cell enzyme. Together these two substances allow the reaction to proceed. Without the vitamin the reaction cannot occur and the metabolic process involved cannot function. For example, several of the B vitamins—thiamin, niacin, and riboflavin—are essential components of the cell enzyme systems that metabolize glucose to produce energy.

2. Tissue structure. Some of the vitamins also act as tissue-building components. For example, vitamin C helps to deposit a cementlike substance in the spaces between cells to produce strong tissue. This material is called "ground substance" and is similar to collagen. In fact, the word *collagen* comes from a Greek word meaning "glue."

3. Deficiency disease prevention. If a vitamin deficiency becomes severe, a nutritional deficiency disease associated with the specific function of that vitamin becomes apparent. For example, the classic vitamin deficiency disease scurvy, a hemorrhagic disease with bleeding into the joints and other internal tissues from fragile capillaries breaking down under simple blood pressure, is caused by a lack of vitamin C. Without the vitamin to produce strong capillary walls, vital internal membranes finally disintegrate and death occurs, as with British sailors 200 years ago. The name given the vitamin—*ascorbic acid*—comes from the Latin word *scorbutus*, which means "scurvy," so the term *ascorbic* means "without scurvy." Today, in developed countries, we do not often see frank scurvy, but we *do* see it, even here in America, together with other forms and degrees of malnutrition among low-income and poverty-stricken population groups.

ISSUE OF SUPPLEMENTATION
Ongoing debate

The debate between vitamin supplement users and those who think they have no place in health maintenance continues, fueled by extremists on both sides. On one hand, conservative health workers dismiss anyone who suggests a need for vitamin supplements. On the other hand, self-proclaimed nutrition experts push megadoses of everything from A to Z to cure anything. Who is right? Probably someone with sound knowledge and something more—*wisdom*—who suggests a course between these two extreme views. Some people think that everybody should meet the precise RDA standards for all essential nutrients. Others take a more individual approach. Furthermore, not all ideas expressed are equal or have scientific basis. The RDAs are based on the average needs of a healthy population, not on individual needs, which can vary widely. But extremists can take these concepts too far. Extreme "traditionalists" try to apply these standards rigidly to every individual. "Pill-pushers" recommend megadoses of everything "to cover all the bases"—or to increase profits.

Concept of biochemical individuality

The term *biochemical individuality* means that the body's chemical composition is not precisely the same for every individual, and that this pattern changes within a given person at different times under various circumstances. This concept cannot be overlooked when assessing individual nutritional needs, because it is influenced by such things as age, personal habits, and health status. We shall consider some of these factors here.

Life cycle needs. At different ages and situations through the life cycle, additional vitamins are needed.

1. Pregnancy and lactation. The RDA standard takes into account increased nutrient requirements for pregnancy and lactation. In fact, to prevent two forms of damaging anemia during pregnancy, the RDA recommends a daily increment of 15 mg of the trace mineral iron, making the total need 30 mg, and a daily increase of 220 μg of folate (folic acid), making the total need 400 μg.[1,2] Women find meeting the increased nutrient needs of pregnancy by diet alone difficult because of marginal diets, food availability, tolerances, or food preferences. Supplements then become a necessary way of ensuring an adequate intake to meet the increased nutrient demands.

2. Infancy. Supplements for breast-feeding infants are recommended by the American Academy of Pediatrics to prevent certain clinical problems. The supplements include vitamins K and D and the trace minerals iron and fluoride. These nutrients are included in the composition of commercial formulas for bottle-fed babies. (See Table 11-2.)

3. Aging. The aging process may increase the need for some nutrients because of decreased food intake and impaired nutrient absorption, storage, and usage. Marginal or so-called subclinical deficiencies of ascorbic acid, thiamin, riboflavin, and pyridoxine have occurred in the elderly, even among individuals using supplements.

Life-style. Personal life-style choices and habits may also influence individual needs for nutrient supplementation.

1. Oral contraceptive use. Women choosing oral contraceptive agents (the "pill") as a means of family planning find that this practice lowers serum levels of several B vitamins, including pyridoxine and niacin, as well as vitamin C. If general nutrient intake levels are marginal, some supplements may be needed. Of course, poor diets need improvement.

2. Restricted diets. Persons who are eternally dieting may find it difficult to meet many of the nutrient standards, particularly if their meals provide less than 1200 kcal/day. Very strict diets are not recommended, anyway. A wise weight reduction program should meet all nutrient needs. Persons who follow strict vegetarian diets will need supplements of vitamin B_{12}, since the vitamin's food source is animal proteins.

3. Exercise programs. Women in extensive exercise programs increase their requirement for riboflavin.[3] The combination of a reducing diet and exercise increases this need even more. This combination may indicate the need for a B-complex supplement, especially in women who do not tolerate milk, the major food source of riboflavin.

4. Smoking. This unhealthy addictive habit can reduce vitamin C levels by as much as 30%.[4] If dietary intake is marginal, a small supplement (for example, 100 mg/day) may compensate. Of course, stopping this unhealthy, expensive addiction would be preferable. The U.S. Surgeon General has indicated from current evidence that even nonsmokers are placed at risk for loss of vitamin C by breathing tobacco smoke around them, and the number of laws limiting smoking in public places is increasing.

5. Alcohol. Chronic or abusive use of alcohol can interfere with absorption and use of B-complex vitamins, especially thiamin, and even destroy folate. Again, multivitamin supplements rich in B vitamins will help. However, a change in alcohol use must accompany this nutritional therapy to prevent recurrence of deficiency effects.

6. Caffeine. In large quantities, the amount in four to six cups of coffee a day, caffeine will flush water-soluble vitamins out of the body faster than usual. Small supplements of B vitamins and ascorbic acid may help, but reduced caffeine intake is recommended.

Disease. In states of disease, malnutrition, debilitation, or hypermetabolic demand, each patient requires careful nutrition assessment. In cases of need, nutritional support including therapeutic supplementation as indicated becomes part of the total medical therapy. Diet and supplementation needs for nutritional therapy are planned to meet individual clinical requirements. The increased nutrient needs are particularly evident in long-term illness.

Megadoses

Persons taking megadoses of vitamins are using them as drugs. At these high pharmacologic levels, vitamins no longer operate as normal nutritional agents. The body uses both nutrients and drugs in specific amounts to: (1) control or improve a physiologic condition or illness, (2) prevent a disease, or (3) relieve symptoms. But the similarity ends there for many people. They realize that too much of any drug can be harmful, sometimes fatal, and so take care to avoid overdoses. But they do not apply this same logic to nutrients. As a result, they learn the dangers of vitamin megadosing the hard way.

  1. Toxic effects. Because fat-soluble vitamins—especially vitamin A—can be stored in large amounts in the liver, the potential toxicity of megadoses, including liver and brain damage in extreme cases, is well known. Many people take physician- or self-prescribed megadoses of water-soluble vitamins, believing them to be safe because they are not stored in the body. However, toxic effects of at least two of these is now known. Gynecologist-prescribed pyridoxine at 1000 to 2700 times its RDA level, used to treat menstrual edema and discomfort, has instead caused severe nerve damage and provided no relief for the original discomfort.[5] Megadoses of ascorbic acid (vitamin C), 1 to 2 g/day, have caused gastrointestinal pain, raised the risk of forming kidney stones, and reduced action of leukocytes, special white blood cells, against bacteria.[6] Meanwhile, they have failed to cure colds, lower cholesterol, or lower cancer risk—reasons for which persons initially used these large amounts.

  2. "Artificially induced" deficiencies. When blood levels of one nutrient being taken in megadoses rise above normal, increased need for other nutrients with which it works in the body create deficiency symptoms. Deficiencies also occur when a person suddenly stops taking the large amounts and a "rebound effect" results. For example, infants born to mothers who took megadoses of ascorbic acid (vitamin C) during pregnancy have developed scurvy when their high nutrient supply was cut off at birth.

Supplementation Principles

To summarize, the following basic principles may help guide nutrient supplementation decisions.

  1. Vitamins, like drugs, can be harmful in large amounts. The only time larger doses may be helpful is when the body already has a severe deficiency or is unable to absorb or metabolize the nutrient efficiently.

  2. Identified individual needs govern specific supplement use. Each person's need should be the basis for determining which nutrients and amounts are used. This helps prevent problems of excess, which may increase with a cumulative effect over time. The "blanket insurance" approach puts more money in the multi-package manufacturer's pocket, not health in the buyer's body.

  3. All nutrients work together to promote good health. Adding large amounts of one vitamin only makes the body believe it is not getting enough of the others and increases the risk of developing deficiency symptoms.

  4. Food remains the best source of nutrients. Most foods are the best "package deal" in nutrition. They provide a wide variety of nutrients in every bite, as opposed to the dozen or so found in a vitamin bottle. And *by itself* a vitamin can do nothing. Its action is catalytic, and so it must have its substrate material to work on—carbohydrate, protein, fat, and their metabolites. With careful selection of a wide variety of foods and wise storage, meal planning and preparation, most people can secure an ample amount of essential nutrients. Then specific supplements for certain individuals in specific circumstances will have far more meaning.

Fat-soluble vitamins

Vitamin A

Functions. Vitamin A performs the following functions in the body.

1. Vision. Vitamin A is an essential part of a pigment in the eye, *rhodopsin*, commonly known as *visual purple*. This light-sensitive substance enables the eye to adjust to different amounts of available light. A mild deficiency of the vitamin causes night blindness, slow adaptation to darkness, or glare blindness.

2. Tissue strength. Vitamin A maintains healthy *epithelial* tissue: the vital protective tissue covering the body—skin—and the inner mucous membranes in the nose, throat, eyes, gastrointestinal tract, and genitourinary tract. These tissues provide our primary barrier to infection.

3. Growth. Vitamin A is essential to growth of skeletal and soft tissues. It influences stability of cell membranes and protein synthesis.

4. Deficiency disease. Adequate intake of vitamin A prevents two eye conditions: (1) *xerosis*—itching and burning, red inflamed lids and (2) *xerophthalmia*—blindness from severe deficiency.

Requirements. Vitamin A requirements are influenced by factors related to its two basic forms in food sources and its use in the body.

1. Food forms and units of measure. Vitamin A occurs in two forms: (1) **retinol**—the fully preformed vitamin A, named because of its function in the retina of the eye, and (2) **carotene**—the "provitamin A," a pigment in yellow and green plants that the body converts to the vitamin. Since vitamin A comes in these two food forms and the greater amount of our intake is usually as beta-carotene, the current unit of measure for vitamin A is *retinol equivalents* (RE). The former measure for vitamin A was International Units (IU). (One IU equals 0.3 µg retinol or 0.6 µg beta-carotene.)

2. Hypervitaminosis A. Because the liver can store large amounts of vitamin A and many persons take megadose supplements, it is possible to take in a potentially toxic quantity. *Hypervitaminosis A* symptoms include joint pain, thickening of long bones, loss of hair, and jaundice. Excessive vitamin A may also cause liver injury with two results: (1) portal hypertension—elevated blood pressure in the blood system going directly to the liver from the gastrointestinal tract, which carries absorbed nutrient loads following intake, and (2) ascites—fluid accumulation in the abdominal cavity.

3. Recommended dietary allowances. The RDA standard for adults is 800 µg RE for women and 1000 µg for men. The full standard is given in the tables inside book covers.

Food sources. Fish-liver oils, liver, egg yolk, butter, and cream are among the best sources of preformed natural vitamin A. Fat-soluble vitamin A occurs naturally only in the fat part of milk. Whole milk, low-fat and nonfat milks, and the butter substitute margarine are good sources of vitamin A only because they are enriched or fortified with added vitamin A. Some good sources of carotene are green leafy vegetables such as swiss chard, turnip greens, kale, spinach; and yellow vegetables and fruits such as carrots, sweet potatoes or yams, yellow corn, yellow squash, apricots, and peaches. Both carotene and preformed vitamin A require the presence of bile salts for proper absorption from the intestine. Bile acts as an antioxidant to protect and stabilize the easily oxidized vitamin and transports it through the intestinal wall.

Stability. Vitamin A is unstable in heat in contact with air. Cooking vegetables in an uncovered pot destroys much of their vitamin content. Quicker cooking with little water helps to preserve the vitamin. If fats are rancid or the vegetables are wilted, most of the vitamin A is destroyed.

Vitamin D

Functions. Vitamin D performs the following functions in the body.

1. Absorption of calcium and phosphorus. Vitamin D, actually a hormone in its body-activated form, *calcitriol*, acts with two other hormones, the *parathyroid hormone* and the thyroid hormone *calcitonin*. In balance with these two hormones, calcitriol stimulates the absorption of calcium and phosphorus in the small intestine.

2. Bone mineralization. Calcitriol works with calcium and phosphorus to form bone tissue. It directly regulates the rate of deposit and resorption of these minerals in bone. This balancing process builds and maintains bone tissue. Thus the vitamin D hormone has been used clinically in the treatment of *osteoporosis*, a bone loss in older women that leads to fractures.

3. Rickets. A deficiency of the vitamin D hormone causes *rickets*, a condition characterized by malformation of skeletal tissue in growing children (Fig. 6-1).

Requirements. A number of factors influence the requirements for vitamin D, and excessive intake is possible, especially in young infants.

1. Influencing factors. It is difficult to set requirements for this nutrient because of its unique hormonelike nature, its synthesis in the skin by the sun's irradiation of cholesterol there, and its limited number of food sources. The amount needed may vary between winter and summer, and with individual exposure to sunlight. Also, growth demands in childhood and in pregnancy and lactation make increased intake necessary.

2. Hypervitaminosis D. Excess intake of vitamin D, especially in infant feeding, can be toxic. Prolonged intakes of the main form of vitamin D in human nutrition, D_3 or **cholecalciferol**, above 50 μg/day (2000 IU)— five times the RDA—can produce elevated blood levels of calcium in infants and calcium deposits in kidney nephrons in both infants and adults. Infant feeding may bring more excess when fortified milk, fortified cereal, plus variable vitamin supplements are used. The infant needs 10 μg (400 IU) daily, but the amount of all the above items can total 100 μg (4000 IU) or more. The symptoms of vitamin D toxicity are calcification of soft tissues, such as lungs and kidneys, as well as fragile bones. Kidney tissue is particularly prone to calcify, affecting overall function.

3. RDA standard. The RDA standard is 10 μg of cholecalciferol (400 IU) daily for children and for women during pregnancy and lactation. The daily allowance for young adults is 10 μg and for older adults 5.0 μg.

Food sources. Few natural food sources of vitamin D exist—only yeast and fish-liver oils. The main food sources are those to which vitamin D has been added. Milk, because it is a common food and also contains calcium and phosphorus, has proved to be the most practical carrier. The standard com-

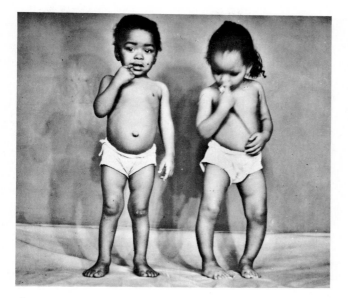

❖ **Fig. 6-1**

Rachitic children. Note knock-knees of child on left and bowlegs of child on right. (Therapeutic notes, Parke, Davis & Co., Detroit; courtesy Dr. Tom Spies and Dr. Orson D. Bird.)

mercial practice is to add 10 μg (400 IU)/quart. Butter substitutes such as margarines are also fortified. Children on vitamin D deficient diets, such as a rigid macrobiotic pattern with no milk products, are especially vulnerable to damaged bone development and rickets.[7]

Stability. Vitamin D is very stable to heat, aging, and storage.

Vitamin E

Functions. The single vital function of vitamin E relates to its action in many tissues as an antioxidant, an agent that prevents tissue breakdown by oxygen, the process of oxidation.

1. Antioxidant function. Vitamin E acts as nature's most potent fat-soluble antioxidant. The polyunsaturated fatty acids (p. 26) in lipid membranes of body tissues are particularly easy for oxygen to break down. Vitamin E, *tocopherol*, can interrupt this oxidation process, protecting the cell membrane fatty acids from damage. For example, vitamin E can protect fragile red blood cell walls in premature infants from breaking down and causing anemia (Box 6-1). Vitamin E helps protect both red blood cells and muscle tissue.

2. Selenium metabolism. Selenium is a trace mineral that works as a partner with vitamin E as an antioxidant. A selenium-containing enzyme is a second line of defense in preventing oxidative damage to cell membranes. So selenium spares vitamin E by reducing its requirement, as vitamin E does for selenium.

Requirements. Vitamin E requirements are expressed in terms of *alpha-*

BOX 6-1

❖ ——————————— CLINICAL APPLICATION ——————————— ❖

Vitamin E and Premature Infants

A medical problem found in infants, especially premature ones, has responded positively to vitamin E therapy. This problem is *hemolytic anemia.*

Anemia is a blood condition characterized by loss of mature functioning red blood cells. Different types of anemia are usually named according to cause, or to the nature of an abnormal nonfunctioning cell produced instead of the normal cell. In this case the name comes from the cause. The word *hemolysis* comes from two roots, *hemo-* referring to blood, and *lysis,* meaning dissolving or breaking. Thus hemolysis means the bursting or dissolving of red blood cells, and the resulting condition is a hemolytic anemia. Vitamin E can help prevent this destruction of red blood cells and the loss of their vital oxygen-carrying hemoglobin. It can do this important task because it is one of the body's foremost antioxidants.

An oxidant is a compound, or oxygen itself, that oxidizes other compounds and in the process breaks them down or changes them. Vitamin E is readily oxidized. When there is plenty of vitamin E among other compounds exposed to an oxidant, by its nature it can take on the oxidative attack and thus protect the others. Vitamin E is fat soluble so it is found in fat-rich tissues of the body among the polyunsaturated fatty acids that make up the core of the cell membranes. The cell membranes of red blood cells are particularly rich in these polyunsaturated lipids, and they are exposed to concentrated oxygen because they constantly circulate through the lungs. This would be a destructive situation were it not for the vitamin E present. It takes the oxygen itself, protecting the polyunsatured fatty acids, and preserving the red blood cells intact to continue their life-sustaining journey throughout the body. Thus vitamin E acts as nature's most potent fat-soluble antioxidant. It interrupts the oxidative breakdown by free radicals (parts of compounds broken off by cell metabolism) in the cell, protecting the cell membrane fatty acids from the oxidative damage.

Hemolytic anemia may develop in infants fed formulas rich in polyunsaturated fatty acids and supplemented with iron (an oxidant) as the fragile red blood cell membranes break down because of the high cell oxidative process and the induced deficiency of vitamin E. This protective need for increased vitamin E is especially great with small, premature infants who are fed formulas containing iron, which acts as an oxidant, and high concentrations of polyunsaturated fatty acids, which are vulnerable to oxidative breakdown. To avoid this problem and comply with American Academy of Pediatrics recommendations, manufacturers have increased the levels of vitamin E and lowered the iron content in formulas for premature infants. The improved formula ratio of vitamin E, polyunsaturated fatty acids, and iron no longer makes additional supplement necessary to prevent hemolytic anemia.

References
Bieri, JG, and others: Medical uses of vitamin E, N Engl J Med 308(18):1063, 1983.
National Research Council, Food and Nutrition Board, Recommended dietary allowances, ed 10, Washington, DC, 1989, National Academy Press.

tocopherol equivalents (α-TE). The RDA standard for adults is 10 mg for men and 8 mg for women. Needs during childhood growth years range from 3 to 10 mg. As you would expect from vitamin E's basic function, its requirement varies with the amount of polyunsaturated fat in the diet.

Food sources. The richest sources of vitamin E are the vegetable oils. It is interesting that vegetable oils are also the richest sources of polyunsaturated fatty acids, which vitamin E protects. Other food sources include milk, eggs, muscle meats, fish, cereals, and leafy vegetables.

Stability. Vitamin E is stable to heat and acids, but not to alkalis.

Vitamin K

Function. The major form of vitamin K found in plants has been named **phylloquinone** for its chemical structure. This is our dietary form. The single basic function of vitamin K is in the blood-clotting process. It is essential for the formation of *prothrombin*, a major clotting agent in the blood. Thus vitamin K can serve as an antidote for excess effects of anticoagulant drugs. It is often used in the control and prevention of certain types of hemorrhages. Since this fat-soluble vitamin is absorbed more completely if bile is present, conditions that hinder bile flow to the small intestine reduce blood-clotting ability. If bile salts are given with vitamin K concentrate, the blood-clotting time becomes normal.

Requirements. Since intestinal bacteria synthesize a form of vitamin K, a constant supply is normally available to support dietary sources. The current RDA standard for men is 80 μg/day and for women it is 65 μg. In the absence of specific information about the vitamin K requirements of children, RDA values for them are set at about 1 μg/kg body weight.[1] A deficiency is unlikely except in clinical conditions related to blood-clotting, malabsorption, or lack of intestinal bacteria for synthesis of the vitamin. For example, since the intestinal tract of a newborn is sterile, vitamin K is given routinely to prevent hemorrhage when the cord is cut. Also, patients treated with antibiotics that kill intestinal bacteria and who then have poor diets after surgery are susceptible to vitamin K deficiency, with resulting blood loss and poor wound healing.[8]

Food sources. Green leafy vegetables, which provide 50 to 800 μg of vitamin K per 100 g of food, are clearly the best dietary sources.[1] Small but significant amounts are contributed by milk and dairy products, meats, eggs, cereals, fruits, and vegetables.

Stability. Vitamin K is fairly stable, although sensitive to light and irradiation. Thus clinical preparations are kept in dark bottles.

A summary of the fat-soluble vitamins is given in Table 6-1.

WATER-SOLUBLE VITAMINS
Vitamin C

Functions. The basic function of vitamin C is related to tissue building. In this role it serves body metabolism.

1. Cement substance between cells. Vitamin C is necessary to build and maintain strong tissues in general, especially connective tissue such as bone, cartilage, dentin, collagen, and capillary walls. It acts like cement between cells to hold them together strongly. When vitamin C is absent, the important

❖ TABLE 6-1   *A summary of fat-soluble vitamins*

Vitamin	Functions	Results of deficiency	Food sources
A (retinol); provitamin A (carotene)	Vision cycle—adaption to light and dark; tissue growth, especially skin and mucuous membranes; toxic in large amounts	Night blindness, xerophthalmia, susceptibility to epithelial infection, changes in skin and membranes	Retinol (animal foods): liver, egg yolk, cream, butter or fortified margarine, fortified milk; carotene (plant foods): green and yellow vegetables, fruits
D (cholecalciferol)	Absorption of calcium and phosphorus, calcification of bones; toxic in large amounts	Rickets, faulty bone growth	Fortified or irradiated milk, fish oils
E (tocopherol)	Antioxidant—protection of materials that oxidize easily; normal growth	Breakdown of red blood cells, anemia	Vegetable oils, vegetable greens, milk, eggs, meat, cereals
K (phylboquinone)	Normal blood clotting	Bleeding tendencies, hemorrhagic disease	Green leafy vegetables, milk and dairy products, meats, eggs, cereals, fruits, vegetables

ground substance that builds the cementing material does not develop into collagen. When vitamin C is adequate, this special connecting substance develops quickly. Blood vessel tissue particularly depends on vitamin C to supply the cementing substance for strong capillary walls. Thus vitamin C deficiency causes signs of tissue bleeding: easy bruising, pinpoint skin hemorrhages, bone and joint bleeding, easy bone fracture, poor wound healing, and soft bleeding gums with loosened teeth. Extreme deficiency produces the disease *scurvy* (p. 62).

2. *General body metabolism.* The more metabolically active body tissues such as adrenal glands, brain, kidney, liver, pancreas, thymus, and spleen have greater concentrations of vitamin C. There is more of the vitamin in a child's actively growing tissue than in adult tissue. Vitamin C is an essential partner of protein for tissue building. It helps absorb iron and make it available for producing hemoglobin, thus helping prevent anemia. General clinical needs relate to wound healing, fevers and infections, and growth periods.

Requirements. Difficulties in setting requirements for vitamin C involve questions about individual tissue needs and whether minimum or optimum

❖ **TABLE 6-2**   *A summary of vitamin C (ascorbic acid)*

Functions	Clinical applications	Food sources
Intercellular cement substance; firm capillary walls and collagen formation	Scurvy (deficiency disease)	Citrus fruits, tomatoes, cabbage, leafy vegetables, potatoes, strawberries, melons, chili peppers, broccoli, chard, turnip greens, green peppers, other green and yellow vegetables
	Sore gums	
	Hemorrhages, especially around bones and joints	
Helps prepare iron for absorption and release to tissues for red blood cell formation	Tendency to bruise easily	
	Stress reactions	
	Growth periods	
	Fevers and infections	
	Wound healing, tissue formation	
	Anemia	

intakes are desired. The current RDA standard for the average healthy adult is 60 mg/day, with increases for women during pregnancy and lactation. Other age needs are given in the full RDA tables inside book covers.

Food sources. The best food sources of vitamin C are citrus fruits. Additional sources include tomatoes, cabbage and other leafy vegetables, berries, melons, peppers, broccoli, potatoes (white and sweet), and other green and yellow vegetables in general.

Stability. Vitamin C oxidizes easily on exposure to air and heat. Thus care must be taken in handling its food sources. It is not stable to alkaline substances, so soda should not be added to food being cooked. Acid fruits and vegetables retain their vitamin C content better than do nonacid ones. The vitamin is also very soluble in water, so only small amounts of water should be used for cooking.

A summary of the uses and sources of vitamin C is given in Table 6-2.

B-COMPLEX VITAMINS

Each of the eight "B vitamins" is a separate vitamin in name, structure, and function. The earliest discoveries were related to classic diseases. The general role of B-complex vitamins is that of coenzyme factor in various body metabolism tasks (p. 63). For general discussion here, we group them according to function as (1) classic deficiency disease factors: thiamin, riboflavin, and niacin; (2) more recently discovered coenzyme factors: pyridoxine (B_6), pantothenic acid, and biotin; and (3) cell growth and blood-forming factors: folate and cobalamin (B_{12}).

Thiamin

Functions. Thiamin was first discovered as the control agent relating to the deficiency disease *beriberi*, a paralyzing disease prevalent among the Asian countries for centuries. The name describes the disease well. It is Singhalese for "I can't, I can't," because the person was always too ill to do anything. The vitamin name *thiamin* comes from its chemical ringlike structure. Its basic function as a coenzyme factor relates to production of energy from glucose and storage of energy as fat, making energy available to support normal growth. Thiamin is especially necessary for maintaining good function of three body systems.

1. *Gastrointestinal system.* Lack of thiamin causes poor appetite, indigestion, constipation and poor stomach action from lack of muscle tone, and deficient gastric hydrochloric acid secretion. The cells of smooth muscles and secretory glands must have available energy to do their work; thiamin is a necessary agent for producing that energy.

2. *Nervous system.* The central nervous system depends on glucose for energy to do its work. Without sufficient thiamin, this energy is not produced and the nerves cannot do their work. Alertness and reflex responses decrease; apathy, fatigue, and irritability result. If the thiamin deficit continues, nerve tissue damage causes nerve irritation, pain, prickly or deadening sensations, and finally paralysis.

3. *Cardiovascular system.* Without constant energy, the heart muscle weakens and heart failure results. Also blood circulation becomes involved when muscles in vessel walls also weaken. This causes the vessels to dilate, which leads to fluid accumulation in the lower part of the legs.

Requirements. Since thiamin is directly related to energy and carbohydrate metabolism needs, the general thiamin requirement is stated in terms of caloric intake. Daily needs for healthy adults range from 0.23 to 0.5 mg/1000 kcal. The RDA adult standard is 0.5 mg/1000 kcal with a minimum of 1 mg for any intake between 1000 to 2000 kcal/day. Increased amounts are needed for childhood growth, during pregnancy and lactation, and for infectious diseases and alcoholism.

Food sources. Thiamin is widespread in almost all plant and animal tissues, but its content is usually small. Thus deficiency of thiamin is a distinct possibility when kcalories are markedly curtailed, as in alcoholism, or when a person is following some highly inadequate diet. Good food sources include lean pork, beef, liver, whole or enriched grains (flour, bread, cereals), and legumes. Eggs, fish, and a few vegetables are fair sources.

Stability. Thiamin is a fairly stable vitamin, but is destroyed by alkalis and prolonged heat at high temperatures. Since it is water soluble, little cooking water should be used. When cooking water is retained in the dish being prepared, the vitamin is preserved.

Riboflavin

Functions. The name *riboflavin* comes from its chemical nature. It is a yellow-green fluorescent pigment—the Latin word *flavus* means "yellow"—containing a sugar named *ribose*, hence the name "riboflavin." A deficiency of riboflavin has been given the general name "ariboflavinosis." Its symptoms relate to tissue inflammation and breakdown and poor wound healing. Even minor injuries easily become aggravated and do not heal well. Riboflavin operates as a vital coenzyme factor in both energy production and tissue protein building. Hence it is essential to tissue health and growth. Signs of riboflavin deficiency include cracked lips and mouth corners; swollen red tongue; eyes burning or itching and tearing from extra blood vessels in the cornea; and a scaly greasy dermatitis in skin folds. Since nutritional deficiencies are usually multiple rather than single, riboflavin deficiencies seldom occur alone. They are most likely to occur with deficiencies of other B vitamins and protein.

Requirements. Riboflavin needs are related to total energy requirements, level of exercise, body size, metabolic rate, and rate of growth. For practical purposes the general RDA standard is based on 0.6 mg/1000 kcal for all ages. The recommended daily intake of riboflavin for all ages is given in the RDA tables inside book covers. Requirements may increase for persons at risk: persons living in poverty or following bizarre diets, those with gastrointestinal disease or chronic illness where appetite and absorption are decreased, persons with poor wound healing, growing children and women during pregnancy and lactation.

Food sources. The most important food source of riboflavin is milk. One of the pigments in milk, *lactoflavin*, is the milk form of riboflavin. Each quart of milk contains 2 g of riboflavin, which is more than the daily requirement. Other good sources include animal protein sources such as meats, poultry, and fish. Enriched grains are also good sources of riboflavin. Green vegetables such as broccoli, spinach, asparagus, and turnip greens are good natural sources.

Stability. Riboflavin is destroyed by light, so milk is now sold and stored in cartons, not glass containers. Riboflavin is water soluble.

Niacin

Functions. Niacin's coenzyme role is that of a partner with riboflavin and thiamin in the cell metabolism system that produces energy. General niacin deficiency brings weakness, poor appetite, indigestion, and various disorders of the skin and nervous system. Skin areas exposed to sunlight develop a dark scaly dermatitis. Continuing deficiency causes central nervous system damage with resulting confusion, apathy, disorientation, and neuritis. The deficiency disease associated with niacin is *pellagra*, which is characterized by dermatitis, diarrhea, dementia, weakness, vertigo, and anorexia. When therapeutic doses of niacin are given, pellagra symptoms resolve.

Requirements. Factors such as age, growth periods, pregnancy and lactation, illness, tissue trauma, body size, and physical activity—all of which require more energy—influence niacin requirement. Since the body can make some of its niacin from the essential amino acid *tryptophan*, the total niacin requirement is stated in terms of "niacin equivalents" to account for both sources. About 60 mg of tryptophan can produce 1 mg of niacin, so this amount is designated as a *niacin equivalent* (NE). The RDA standard for adults is 6.6 mg NE/1000 kcal and not less than 13 niacin equivalents at intakes of less than 2000 kcal. The needs for different ages are given in the RDA tables inside book covers.

Food sources. Meat is a major source of niacin. Good sources include peanuts, legumes, and enriched grains. Fruits and vegetables are relatively poor sources.

Stability. Niacin is stable to acid and heat, but lost in excess-water cooking, unless cooking water is retained.

Pyridoxine (vitamin B₆)

Functions. The name *pyridoxine* comes from the vitamin's ringlike chemical structure called a "pyridine ring." Its basic coenzyme role is related to protein metabolism. Pyridoxine functions in many cell reactions involving amino acids. It aids neurotransmitter synthesis for brain activity and normal function of the central nervous system (CNS). Thus a deficiency would cause abnormal CNS function with hyperirritability, neuritis, and possible convulsions. Pyridoxine also participates in amino acid absorption, energy production, synthesis of the heme portion of hemoglobin, and niacin formation from tryptophan. In its coenzyme role niacin is also active in carbohydrate and fat metabolism.

Requirements. A deficiency of pyridoxine is unlikely because the amounts present in the general diet are large relative to the requirement. Since pyridoxine is involved in amino acid metabolism, its need varies directly with protein intake. The RDA standard for healthy adults is 2 mg/day. More is needed during pregnancy and by women using oral contraceptive pills. Pyridoxine abuse, in megadoses up to 5 g/day, has been reported, with severe nerve damage causing multiple symptoms.[5]

Food sources. Pyridoxine is widespread in foods, but many sources provide only very small amounts. Good sources include grains, seeds, liver and kidney, and other meats. There are limited amounts in milk, eggs, and vegetables.

Stability. Pyridoxine is stable to heat but sensitive to light and alkalis.

Pantothenic acid

Functions. The name *pantothenic acid* refers to the vitamin's widespread body function and food sources. It is based on the Greek word *pantothen*, which means "from every side." Pantothenic acid is present in all forms of living things. In its coenzyme role it is an essential part of the body's key activating agent, *coenzyme A*, which controls many metabolic reactions involving fat and cholesterol, heme formation, and amino acid activation.

Requirements. Deficiency of this widespread vitamin is unknown, so a specific requirement has not been established. The RDA's general "safe and adequate" range for adults is 4 to 7 mg/day. The daily intake in an average American diet of 2500 to 3000 kcal is about 10 to 20 mg. A deficiency is unlikely because of its widespread occurrence in food.

Food sources. Pantothenic acid occurs as widely in foods as in body tissues. It is especially abundant in animal tissues, whole-grain cereals, and legumes. Smaller amounts are found in milk, vegetables, and fruits.

Stability. Pantothenic acid is stable to acid and heat, but is sensitive to alkalis and is water soluble.

Biotin

Functions. The minute traces of biotin in the body perform multiple metabolic tasks. In its coenzyme role biotin serves as a partner with coenzyme A, of which pantothenic acid is an essential part. It is also involved in the synthesis of fatty acids, amino acids, and purines.

Requirements. Since the potency of biotin is great, even in its minute body amounts, a natural deficiency is unknown. The only induced deficiencies have occurred in patients receiving long-term total parenteral nutrition (TPN). There is no known toxicity. The amount needed for metabolism is so small that human requirement for biotin has not been established in specific terms. The RDA estimate for a "safe and adequate" adult intake is 100 to 200 μg/day. Most of the body's requirement is supplied from intestinal bacteria synthesis.

Food sources. Biotin is widely distributed in natural foods but is not equally available in various foods. For example, the biotin of corn and soy meals is completely available, but that of wheat is almost completely unavailable to the body. The best food sources are liver, egg yolk, soy flour, cereals (except bound forms in wheat), other meats, tomatoes, and yeast.

Stability. Biotin is a stable vitamin but is water soluble.

Folate

Functions. The name "folic acid" comes from the Latin word *folium*, which means "leaf," and was used because a major source of its original discovery was in dark green leafy vegetables. Several compounds have been found to share similar structures and nutritional functions to those of folic acid. The term *folate* is now used as the common generic name for this group of substances with similar vitamin activity. In its basic coenzyme role, folate is essential for forming all body cells, because it is part of DNA, the important cell nucleus material that transmits genetic characteristics. It is also essential for forming hemoglobin. A deficiency of folate causes a special type of anemia— *megaloblastic anemia*. This is a particular risk during pregnancy because of increased fetal growth demands. Rapidly growing adolescents, especially ones with poor diets, develop low folate blood levels and risk anemia.[9]

Requirements. The average American diet contains about 0.6 mg of folate. The RDA standard for healthy adults is 200 μg/day for men and 180 μg for women. The need for pregnant women is increased to 400 μg/day to meet the increased requirements for fetal growth. The standard for all ages is given in the RDA tables inside book covers.

Food sources. Folate is widely distributed in foods. Rich sources include green leafy vegetables, liver, yeast, and legumes.

Stability. Folate is a relatively stable vitamin, but storage and cooking losses can be high, especially in excess-water cooking. As much as 50% of food folate may be destroyed during household preparation, food processing, and storage.[1]

Cobalamin (vitamin B₁₂)

Functions. Vitamin B_{12} was named **cobalamin** because of its unique structure with a single red atom of the trace element cobalt at its center. In its coenzyme role, cobalamin is essential to the synthesis of the nonprotein *heme* portion of hemoglobin. A component of the gastric secretions called "intrinsic factor" is necessary for the absorption of vitamin B_{12}. When this factor is missing, the vitamin cannot be absorbed to do its job in making hemoglobin, and a special anemia—*pernicious anemia*—results. In such cases the vitamin must be given by injection to bypass the absorption defect.

Requirements. The amount of dietary vitamin B_{12} needed for normal human metabolism is very small. Reported requirements range from 0.6 to 2.8 μg/ day for adults. The usual mixed diet easily provides this much and more. The only reported deficiencies have been among strict vegans, because the major food sources are of animal origin. The RDA standard for adults is 2 μg/day, with an increase to 2.6 μg for pregnant and lactating women. Other age group needs are given in the RDA tables inside book covers.

Food sources. Since vitamin B_{12} occurs as a protein complex in foods, its food sources are mostly from animals. The initial source, however, is synthesizing bacteria in the gastrointestinal tract of herbivorous animals. Some synthesis is done by human intestinal bacteria, but our major source of vitamin

❖ **TABLE 6-3**   *A summary of B-complex vitamins*

Vitamin	Functions	Results of deficiency*	Food sources
Thiamin	Normal growth; coenzyme in carbohydrate metabolism; normal function of heart, nerves, and muscle	Beriberi; GI: loss of appetite, gastric distress, indigestion, deficient hydrochloric acid; CNS: fatigue, nerve damage, paralysis; CV: heart failure, edema of legs especially	Pork, beef, liver, whole or enriched grains, legumes
Riboflavin	Normal growth and vigor; coenzyme in protein and energy metabolism	Ariboflavinosis; wound aggravation, cracks at corners of mouth, swollen red tongue, eye irritation, skin eruptions	Milk, meats, enriched cereals, green vegetables
Niacin (precursor: tryptophan)	Coenzyme in energy production; normal growth, health of skin, normal activity of stomach, intestines, and nervous system	Pellagra; weakness, lack of energy, and loss of appetite; skin: scaly dermatitis; CNS: neuritis, confusion	Meat, peanuts, legumes, enriched grains
Pyridoxine (B₆)	Coenzyme in amino acid metabolism: protein synthesis, heme formation, brain activity; carrier for amino acid absorption	Anemia: CNS: hyperirritability, convulsions, neuritis	Grains, seeds, liver and kidney, meats; milk, eggs, vegetables
Pantothenic acid	Coenzyme in formation of coenzyme A: fat, cholesterol, and heme formation and amino acid activation	Unlikely because of widespread occurrence	Meats, cereals, legumes; milk, vegetables, fruits
Biotin	Coenzyme A partner; synthesis of fatty acids, amino acids, purines	Natural deficiency unknown	Liver, egg yolk, soy flour, cereals (except bound form in wheat), tomatoes, yeast
Folic acid	Part of DNA, growth and development of red blood cells	Certain type of anemia: megaloblastic (large, immature red blood cells)	Liver, green leafy vegetables, legumes, yeast

* Key: GI, gastrointestinal; CNS, central nervous system; CV, cardiovascular.

❖ TABLE 6-3   *A summary of B-complex vitamins—cont'd*

Vitamin	Functions	Results of deficiency*	Food sources
Cobalamin (B$_{12}$)	Coenzyme in synthesis of heme for hemoglobin, normal red blood cell formation;	Pernicious anemia (B$_{12}$ is necessary extrinsic factor that combines with intrinsic factor of gastric secretions for absorption)	Liver, kidney, lean meats, milk, eggs, cheese

B$_{12}$ is animal foods. The richest sources are liver and kidney, lean meat, milk, eggs, and cheese. Natural dietary deficiency in a mixed diet is unknown. The only reported cases have been in some groups of strict vegetarians—vegans (p. 40), for whom B$_{12}$ supplements are recommended to prevent such deficiency. The general symptoms of such a deficiency include nervous disorders, sore mouth and tongue, amenorrhea, and neuritis.

Stability. Vitamin B$_{12}$ is stable in ordinary cooking processes.

•   •   •

A summary of the eight B vitamins is given in Table 6-3.

SUMMARY

Vitamins are organic, noncaloric food substances that are required in very small amounts for certain metabolic tasks. They cannot be made by the body. A balanced diet usually supplies sufficient vitamin intake. However, in individually identified situations, a designated supplement amount may be needed. Megadoses carry significant risk and are on the level of drug abuse.

The fat-soluble vitamins are A, D, E, and K. Their metabolic tasks are mainly structural in nature. The water-soluble vitamins are vitamin C and the eight B vitamins. Their major metabolic tasks relate to their roles as coenzyme factors, except for vitamin C, which helps protein build strong tissue. Little toxicity has been associated with these vitamins because they are water soluble and excess is excreted in the urine. However, megadose habits with two water-soluble vitamins have produced drug-level abuse results: (1) large amounts of pyridoxine (B$_6$) have caused severe nerve damage; and (2) large amounts of vitamin C have been associated with gastrointestinal problems and kidney stones. The possibility of toxicity is increased for fat-soluble vitamins because the body can store them. Such toxicity is no longer so rare, because of the current popularity of large vitamin A supplements.

All water-soluble vitamins, especially vitamin C, are easily oxidized, so care must be taken in food storage and preparation.

❖ REVIEW QUESTIONS

1. What is a vitamin? Describe three general functions of vitamins and give examples of each function.
2. How would you advise a friend who was taking "self-prescribed" vitamin supplements? Give reasons and examples to support your answer.

3. Describe the effects of three vitamins that some persons take in large amounts. What are the risks involved in such megadoses?
4. Describe four situations in which vitamin supplements should be used. Give reasons and examples in each case.
5. List four principles to guide a person's decisions about vitamin supplements and explain the basis for each one.

❖ SELF-TEST QUESTIONS

True-false
For each item you answer "false," write the correct statement.
1. A coenzyme acts alone to control a number of different types of reactions.
2. Carotene is preformed vitamin A found in animal food sources.
3. Exposure to sunlight produces vitamin D from cholesterol in the skin.
4. Extra vitamin C is stored in the liver to meet tissue infection demands.
5. Vitamin D and sufficient calcium and phosphorus can prevent rickets.
6. Vitamin K is found in meat, especially liver, and in leafy vegetables.

Multiple choice
1. Vitamin A is fat soluble, produced by humans from carotene in plant foods or consumed as the fully formed vitamin in animal foods. Hence the main sources of this vitamin would include:
   (1) Nonfat milk
   (2) Green leafy vegetables
   (3) Carrots
   (4) Oranges
   (5) Butter
   (6) Tomatoes
       a. 1, 2, and 4
       b. 2, 3, and 5
       c. 1, 3, and 6
       d. 3, 4, and 5
2. If you wanted to increase the vitamin C content of your diet, which of the following foods would you choose in larger amounts?
   a. Liver, other organ meats, and seafood
   b. Potatoes, enriched cereals, and fortified margarine
   c. Green peppers, tomatoes, and oranges
   d. Milk, cheese, and eggs
3. Which of the following statements are true about the sources of vitamin K?
   a. Vitamin K is found in a wide variety of foods so no deficiency occurs.
   b. Vitamin K is easily absorbed without assistance so we can get all we absorb into our systems.
   c. Vitamin K is rarely found in foods so a natural deficiency can occur.
   d. Most of our vitamin K for metabolic needs is produced by interstinal bacteria.

❖ SUGGESTIONS FOR ADDITIONAL STUDY

1. Use the following activities to survey the marketing and use of vitamins:
   a. Interview six persons to determine how many are buying and using vitamin pills, and if so, which ones, in what amounts, and for what reasons.
   b. Interview several clerks in pharmacies concerning any increase in sales of vitamin pills, and if so, why they think this may be happening.
   c. Visit a health food store, posing as a potential customer. Ask about taking vitamin pills, which ones to take, and possible benefits. Look over the stock carefully, reading labels and advertisements. Ask for any literature to take with you (booklets, leaflets, ads) to help you decide which ones to buy and to give to friends.

  d. Survey and evaluate vitamin advertisements in magazines, newspapers, and television.
Evaluate all of your survey information and prepare a report of your results for class discussion.
2. Analyze your dietary intake of vitamin A and vitamin C by recording all your food intake for one day and checking the total amount of each vitamin. Compare your totals to the RDA standard. Where do you stand? What foods could you add to increase your intake of each vitamin?

References

1. National Research Council, Food and Nutrition Board: Recommended dietary allowances, ed 10, Washington, DC, 1989, National Academy Press.
2. National Research Council, Food and Nutrition Board: Diet and health, implications for reducing chronic disease risk, Washington, DC, 1989, National Academy Press.
3. Belko AZ and others: Effects of exercise on riboflavin requirements of young women, Am J Clin Nutr 35:509, Apr 1983.
4. Schectman G and others: The influence of smoking on vitamin C status in adults, Am J Pub Health 79:158, Feb 1989.
5. Schaumburg H and others: Sensory neuropathy from pyridoxine abuse, N Engl J Med 309:445, 1983.
6. Rudman D: Megadose vitamins: use and abuse, N Engl J Med 309:489, 1983.
7. Dagnelie PC and others: High prevalence of rickets in infants on macrobiotic diets, Am J Clin Nutr 51:202, Feb 1990.
8. Usui Y and others: Vitamin K concentrations in the plasma and liver of surgical patients, Am J Clin Nutr 51:846, May 1990.
9. Tsui JC and Nordstrom JW: Folate status of adolescents: effects of folic acid supplementation, J Am Diet Assoc 90(11):1551, 1990.

Further reading

Bailey LB: The role of folate in human nutrition, Nutr Today 25(5):12, 1990.

Ross AC: Vitamin A—current understanding of the mechanisms of action, Nutr Today 26(1):6, 1991.

Song WO: Pantothenic acid—How much do we know about this B-complex vitamin? Nutr Today 25(2):19, 1990.

  These three articles from recent issues of this excellent journal provide expanded information about the vitamins folate, A, and pantothenic acid for persons who want to know more. As is the standard for this popular publication, each article has numerous displays in diagrams and tables to aid the reader's understanding and answer questions raised about the nature, functions, and current applications of each vitamin in nutrition and health.

7

❖

Minerals

KEY CONCEPTS

The human body requires a variety of minerals in different amounts to do numerous metabolic tasks.

A mixed diet of varied foods and adequate energy value provides our best source of needed minerals for health, with individual supplements according to specific age and growth needs or clinical requirements.

Of the total amount of mineral a person consumes, only a relatively limited amount of it is available to the body.

*D*uring the eons in which the earth was forming, shifting oceans and mountains deposited a large number of minerals into earth materials. Over time these minerals have moved from rocks to soil, then to plants, to animals, and to humans. As a result, the mineral content of the human body is quite similar to that of the earth. Our lives now depend on a number of these basic elements.

In comparison with the vitamins, which are large complex organic compounds, minerals — single inert elements — may seem very simple. However, these micronutrients perform a wide fascinating variety of metabolic tasks essential to our lives.

In this chapter we look at this array of minerals to see how they differ from vitamins in the variety of their tasks and in the amounts, relatively large to exceedingly small, needed to do these jobs. Elements for which our bodies require more than 100 mg/day are called **major minerals**. Those we need in much smaller amounts are called **trace elements**.

NATURE OF BODY MINERALS

Minerals are single inorganic elements that are widely distributed in nature. Of the 54 known earth elements in the periodic table of elements, 25 have been shown to be essential to human life. These 25 elements perform a variety of metabolic functions with a widely varying amount of each element needed in the body to do these tasks.

Variety of functions

These seemingly simple, single elements, in comparison with the much larger complex organic structure of vitamins, perform an impressive variety of metabolic jobs for the body. They build, activate, regulate, transmit, and control. For example, sodium and potassium control water balance. Calcium and phosphorus build the body framework. Iron helps build the vital oxygen carrier hemoglobin. Cobalt is the central core of vitamin B_{12}. Iodine builds thyroid hormone, which in turn regulates the overall rate of all body metabolism. Thus, far from being static and inert, minerals are active essential participants, helping to control many of the body's overall metabolic processes.

Variety in amount needed

As described in the previous chapter, all vitamins are required in very small amounts to do their jobs. On the contrary, minerals occur in varying amounts in the body. For example, calcium forms a relatively large amount of the body weight—about 2%. Most of this amount is in bone tissue. An adult who weighs 150 pounds has about 3 pounds of calcium in the body. On the other hand, iron occurs in very small amounts. The same adult has only about 3 g (about 1/10 ounce) of iron in the body. In both cases, the amount of each mineral is essential for its specific task.

Classes of body minerals

The varying amount of individual minerals in the body provides the basis for classifying them into two main groups.

Major minerals. Some elements are referred to as major minerals not because they are more important, but simply because they occur in larger amounts in the body. These seven major minerals are calcium, phosphorus, sodium, potassium, magnesium, chlorine, and sulfur.

Trace elements. The remaining 18 elements make up the group of trace elements. These minerals are not less important, but they occur in very small traces or amounts in the body. They are equally essential for their specific tasks. You will find Table 7-1 a helpful study guide as you proceed through the chapter.

Control of amount and distribution

The correct amount of minerals for body needs is usually controlled either at the point of absorption or at points of tissue uptake.

❖ **TABLE 7-1**   *Major minerals and trace elements in human nutrition*

	Trace elements	
Major minerals (required intake over 100 mg/day)	Essential (required intake under 100 mg/day)	Essentiality unclear
Calcium (Ca)	Iron (Fe)	Silicon (Si)
Phosphorus (P)	Iodine (I)	Vanadium (V)
Sodium (Na)	Zinc (Zn)	Nickel (Ni)
Potassium (K)	Copper (Cu)	Tin (Sn)
Magnesium (Mg)	Manganese (Mn)	Cadmium (Cd)
Chlorine (Cl)	Chromium (Cr)	Arsenic (As)
Sulfur (S)	Cobalt (Co)	Aluminum (Al)
	Selenium (Se)	Boron (B)
	Molybdenum (Mo)	
	Fluoride (Fl)	

Absorption. Minerals are absorbed and used in the body in their activated *ionic* (carrying an electrical charge, + or −) form. Three general factors influence how much of a mineral is actually absorbed into the body system from the gastrointestinal tract: (1) *food form*—minerals in animal foods are usually more readily absorbed than those in plant foods; (2) *body need*—if the body is deficient, more is absorbed than if the body has enough; and (3) *tissue health*—if the absorbing tissue surface is affected by disease, its absorptive capacity is greatly diminished.

Tissue uptake. Some minerals are controlled at the point of their "target" tissue uptake by regulating hormones, with the excess being excreted in the urine. For example, the thyroid-stimulating hormone (TSH) controls the uptake of iodine from the blood according to the amount needed to make the thyroid hormone *thyroxine*. When more thyroxine is needed, more iodine is taken up by the thyroid gland under TSH stimulation and less is excreted. At other times, when blood levels of thyroxine are normal, less iodine is taken up by the thyroid gland and more is excreted.

Occurrence in the body. Body minerals are found in several forms in places related to their functions. There are two basic forms in which minerals occur in the body: (1) *free*—particles may exist free as *ions* (meaning that they carry an electrical charge) in body fluids, such as sodium in tissue fluids, which helps to control water balance; and (2) *combined*—minerals may exist combined with other minerals, such as calcium with phosphorus to form bone, or combined with organic substances, such as iron with heme and globin to form the organic compound hemoglobin.

ISSUE OF MINERAL SUPPLEMENTATION

The same principles discussed in the previous chapter in relation to vitamin supplements also guide the use of mineral supplements. Special needs during growth periods and in clinical situations may require individual supplements of specific major minerals or trace elements.

Life cycle needs. Added minerals may be needed during rapid growth periods in the life cycle.

1. *Pregnancy and lactation.* Women require added calcium, phosphorus, and iron to meet the demands of rapid fetal growth and milk production, and the breast-feeding infant may need added fluoride.

2. *Adolescence.* The rapid growth during adolescence requires increased calcium for long bone growth. If the teenager's diet provides insufficient calcium, added amounts may be indicated to increase bone density and decrease risk in later adult years of bone density problems such as osteoporosis.[1,2]

3. *Adulthood.* Healthy adults do not need mineral supplementation. However, questions have been raised in media and advertising about calcium needs in relation to prevention and treatment of osteoporosis. As currently marketed to prevent osteoporosis, calcium supplements alone have little effect. A young adult idiopathic (cause unknown) form of osteoporosis does not respond to calcium supplements. At any adult age, calcium supplements alone neither prevent nor successfully treat osteoporosis, the cause of which is not clear. Calcium may be used as part of a treatment program together with vitamin D hormone, estrogen, and increased physical activity.

Clinical needs. Several clinical problems, or persons at high risk of developing these problems, require mineral supplementation.

1. *Iron-deficiency anemia.* One of the most prevalent health problems encountered in population surveys is iron-deficiency anemia. The need for iron supplements has long been established for pregnant and breast-feeding women.[1] Other high-risk groups may also need to supplement their diets: adolescent girls, low-income adolescent boys, athletes, and elderly persons eating poor diets.

2. *Zinc deficiency.* Increased use of processed foods and vegetarian diets have increased concern about possible zinc deficiency, especially among pregnant and lactating women, children, and elderly persons. Signs of deficiency are slow growth, impaired taste and smell, poor wound healing, and skin problems, but it takes 3 to 24 weeks for symptoms to appear. Others at risk include alcoholics, persons on long-term low-caloric diets, and elderly persons in long-term institutional care.

3. *Potassium-losing drugs.* Persons requiring long-term use of potassium-losing diuretic drugs for treatment of hypertension may need potassium replacement supplements. Increased intake of foods high in potassium is also needed.

MAJOR MINERALS
Calcium

Functions. Most of the U.S. food and nutrition surveys, such as those conducted regularly by the U.S. Department of Agriculture and the National Center for Health Statistics, indicate that calcium is one of the minerals most likely to be deficient, as measured by the RDA standards. Men and boys are more likely to take in adequate amounts of calcium than are women and girls, simply because men and boys usually eat larger amounts of food. The absorption of the dietary calcium depends on (1) the food form—plant forms are usually bound with other substances and not readily available; and (2) the interaction of three hormones that directly control absorption—vitamin D hormone calcitriol, parathyroid hormone (PTH), and calcitonin (from the thyroid gland), with indirect metabolic stimuli from the estrogen hormones (sex hormones produced in the ovaries and testes). Once absorbed, calcium functions in four basic ways in the body.

1. *Bone and tooth formation.* Most of the body calcium, 99%, is found in bone tissues. When calcium phosphate is removed from bone, the remaining tissue is flexible cartilage. If dietary calcium is insufficient during childhood growth, especially during initial fetal skeletal formation and rapid growth of long bones during adolescence, the production of healthy bone tissue is hindered. The calcification of teeth occurs before their eruption from the gums, so later dietary calcium does not affect tooth structure as it does the continuing balance of calcium in bone tissue.[3]

2. *Blood clotting.* Calcium is essential for the formation of fibrin that makes up the blood clot.

3. *Muscle and nerve action.* Calcium ions stimulate muscle contraction and transmit impulses along nerve fibers.

4. *Metabolic reactions.* Calcium is required for many general metabolic functions in the body. These include absorption of vitamin B_{12}, activation of the fat-splitting enzyme pancreatic lipase, and secretion of insulin from special cells in the pancreas where it is synthesized. Calcium also occurs in cell membranes, where it governs the permeability of the membrane to nutrients.

Requirements. The RDA standard for calcium is 1200 mg/day for both sexes from ages 11 to 24.[1] For older age groups, the previous allowance of 800 mg is retained. The recommended intake for all women throughout pregnancy and lactation is 1200 mg, irrespective of age. For children ages 1 to 10 years the allowance is 800 mg.

Food sources. Milk and milk products are the most important sources of readily available calcium (Fig. 7-1). The calcium in these dairy products is well absorbed, whereas the calcium in most plant sources is not readily available. Not all of the milk in the diet needs to be consumed as a beverage. It may be used in cooking, as in soups, sauces, puddings, or in milk products such as yogurt, cheese, and ice cream. Secondary sources of calcium include egg yolks, grains, legumes, and nuts. In Swiss chard and beet greens, the calcium is bound with oxalic acid and not available. However, other green vegetables such as broccoli, kale, and mustard and turnip greens are better sources because they do not contain oxalic acid. Excessive fiber can decrease calcium absorption.

Deficiency states. If available calcium is insufficient during growth years, various bone deformities occur. The gross deficiency disease *rickets* is related to a deficiency of vitamin D to support adequate calcium absorption. A decrease of calcium in the blood, in relation to its serum partner phosphorus, results in *tetany*, a condition characterized by abnormal muscle spasms. The condition of *osteoporosis*, an abnormal thinning of the bones in adult years resulting from bone calcium loss, is not a primary calcium deficiency disease as such. Rather it results from a combination of hormonal factors controlling calcium absorption and metabolism. The precise cause of this imbalance in bone calcium deposit and resorption, which most adults maintain normally, is not as yet known. Thus increased calcium *alone*, in diet or supplements, will not prevent osteoporosis in susceptible adults nor successfully treat diagnosed cases. Therapies reported to reduce bone loss in osteoporosis include combi-

❖ **FIG. 7-1**

Milk is the major food source of calcium.

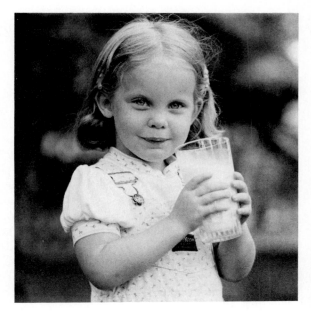

nations of the various factors involved: calcium, the active hormonal form of vitamin D, and estrogens.[3]

Phosphorus

Functions. Phosphorus serves as a partner with calcium in the major task of bone formation but also functions in other metabolic processes.

1. Bone and tooth formation. The calcification of bones and teeth depends on the fixing of phosphorus in the bone-forming tissue as calcium phosphate.

2. Energy metabolism. Phosphate is necessary for the controlled oxidation of carbohydrate, fat, and protein in producing and storing available energy for the body. It also contributes to energy and protein metabolism, as well as cell function and genetic inheritance, as an essential component of cell enzymes, thiamin, and the critical cell compounds deoxyribonucleic acid (DNA) and ribonucleic acid (RNA), which control cell reproduction.

3. Acid-base balance. Phosphate is an important buffer material to prevent changes in the acidity of body fluids.

Requirements. The RDA standard of phosphorus is 800 mg for children 1 to 10 years, 1200 mg for ages 11 to 24 years, and 800 mg for ages beyond 24.[1] The precise requirement is unknown, but a 1:1 ratio of calcium/phosphorus provides sufficient phosphorus for most age groups, although if the calcium intake is adequate, the precise ratio is unimportant.

Food sources. High-protein foods are rich in phosphorus. Hence milk and milk products, meat, eggs, and cereal grains are the primary sources of phosphorus in the average diet. Additional sources include legumes and nuts.

Deficiency states. Because of the widespread distribution of phosphorus in foods, dietary phosphorus deficiency does not usually occur. The only evidence of deficiency has been among persons consuming large amounts of aluminum hydroxide as an antacid for prolonged periods of time. Aluminum hydroxide binds phosphorus, making it unavailable for absorption. Phosphorus deficiency results in bone loss and is characterized by weakness, loss of appetite, fatigue, and pain.[1]

Sodium

Functions. The main function of sodium is body water balance, as discussed in Chapter 8. Sodium also has important tasks in acid-base balance and in muscle action.

1. *Water balance.* Sodium is the major electrolyte controlling the amount of body water *outside* of cells. As such, it helps prevent dehydration. It is also an integral part of all the digestive secretions into the gastrointestinal tract, most of which are then reabsorbed.

2. *Acid-base balance.* Sodium accounts for about 90% of the alkalinity of fluids outside of cells and helps to balance acid-forming elements. Alkalosis may result from a continued use of antacid drugs containing sodium.

3. *Muscle action.* Sodium ions are necessary for normal transmission of nerve impulses to stimulate muscle action. The resulting muscle contraction also involves sodium.

4. *Glucose absorption.* Sodium is essential as a transport substance for the absorption of glucose across absorbing membranes in the small intestine.

Requirements. There is no stated RDA standard for dietary sodium, since needs vary with growth, sweat losses, and loss of other secretions, as in diarrhea. However, the Diet and Health Committee of the Food and Nutrition Board has recently recommended that daily intakes of salt (sodium chloride), our main dietary source of sodium, be limited to 6 g (2.4 g sodium) or less.[2] The average American diet far exceeds basic body needs, about two to five times the recommended amount, depending on the individual use of added salt.

Food sources. Sodium occurs naturally in foods, being most prevalent generally in foods of animal origin. There is an ample amount in such natural food sources to meet body needs. However, by far the greatest amount of dietary sodium, too much in fact, comes from added salt and other sodium compounds in processed foods. For example, cured ham has about 20 times as much sodium as raw pork. (See Appendix for sodium and potassium content of foods.)

Deficiency states. Because the body sodium need is low, a deficiency state rarely occurs. Exceptions occur, however, in heavy body sweating. This may be the case with those engaged in heavy labor or with athletes doing strenuous physical exercise in a hot environment. Such persons may need additional salt to replace these heavy sodium losses.

Potassium

Functions. Potassium is a partner with sodium in body water balance but also has many metabolic functions.

1. *Water balance.* Potassium is the major electrolyte controlling the water *inside* cells. It balances with sodium concentration in the water outside of cells.

2. *Metabolic reactions.* Potassium is involved in the synthesis of glycogen and protein in the cell and in energy production.

3. Muscle action. Potassium ions also play a role in nerve impulse transmission to stimulate muscle action. Then, along with magnesium and sodium, potassium acts as a muscle relaxant in balance with calcium, which causes muscle contraction.

4. Insulin release. Potassium is involved in insulin release from the pancreas when it is triggered by a rise in blood glucose level.

5. Blood pressure. Sodium is a main dietary factor related to elevated blood pressure. However, there is evidence that this relation may be more involved with the sodium/potassium ratio rather than with the actual amount of dietary sodium alone. A potassium intake equal to that of sodium may be the protecting factor.

Requirements. Although potassium has been established as a dietary essential, there is little information on basic needs and no stated requirement is given. However, the minimum need appears to be approximately 2000 mg/day, and the recommendations of the National Research Council for increased intake of fruits and vegetables would raise potassium intake of adults to about 3500 mg, which is ample for average needs.[1,2]

Food sources. The richest dietary sources of potassium are unprocessed foods, especially fruits, many vegetables, and fresh meats.[1] Since the plant form is very soluble, much of the potassium content may be lost in excessive-water cooking unless the water is retained. The comparative potassium content of some selected foods is given in Table 7-2.

Deficiency states. Potassium deficiency symptoms are well defined but seldom related to inadequate dietary intake. Deficiency is more likely to occur in losses that result from situations such as prolonged vomiting or diarrhea,

❖ **TABLE 7-2**   *Potassium content per average serving of some selected foods*

Group A (600 mg)	Group B (400 mg)	Group C (300 mg)	Group D (200 mg)
Dried apricots	Bananas	Avocados	Fruit cocktail
Dried peaches	Grapefruit	Cantaloupe	Grapes
Lima beans	Orange juice	Cherries	Peaches
Parsnips	Artichokes	Green beans	Pineapple
Spinach, fresh	Broccoli	Fresh tomatoes	Plums
Tomato juice	Brussels sprouts	Milk	Prunes, dried
Sweet potatoes	Carrots		Strawberries
	Cauliflower		Asparagus
	Corn		Cabbage
	Winter squash		Green peas
	Turnip greens		
	White potatoes		
	Liver		
	Pork		
	Beef		
	Chicken		
	Fish		
	Peanut butter		
	Cashew nuts		

use of diuretic drugs, severe malnutrition, and surgery. It is of concern in the use of potassium-losing diuretic drugs in the treatment of hypertension. Characteristic symptoms of deficiency include overall muscle weakness, poor intestinal muscle tone with resulting bloating, heart muscle problems with possible cardiac arrest, and weakness of respiratory muscles with breathing difficulties. Excessive use of potassium replacement drugs by persons taking diuretics may also be a problem in potassium balance. This is especially true with an elderly person having impaired kidney function and thus difficulty in excreting potassium.

Magnesium

Functions. The functions of magnesium are widespread throughout body metabolism, in tissue synthesis, and in muscle action.

1. *General metabolism.* Magnesium serves as a significant catalyst in hundreds of reactions in cells through which energy is produced, body compounds are synthesized, or nutrients are absorbed and transported.

2. *Protein synthesis.* Magnesium activates amino acids for protein synthesis and facilitates the synthesis and maintenance of the cell genetic material DNA.

3. *Muscle action.* Magnesium ions help conduct nerve impulses to muscles for normal contraction. In the action of muscles, magnesium then acts as a relaxant, in balance with calcium, which works as a stimulant to contraction.

4. *Basal metabolic rate.* Magnesium influences the secretion of the thyroid hormone thyroxine and thus helps in the maintenance of a normal metabolic rate and adaptation of the body to cold temperatures.

Requirements. The RDA standard for adults is 350 mg/day for men and 280 mg for women, with an increase to 320 mg during pregnancy and 355 mg for lactation.

Food sources. The highest concentrations of magnesium are found in whole seeds such as nuts, legumes, and unrefined grains. More than 80% of the magnesium is lost by removal of the germ and outer layers of cereal grains.[1] Green vegetables are another good source of magnesium, much of it is contained in the plant's chlorophyll.

Deficiency states. Purely dietary magnesium deficiency has not been reported in people consuming natural diets.[1] Magnesium deficiency symptoms have been observed in clinical situations such as starvation, persistent vomiting or diarrhea with loss of magnesium-rich gastrointestinal fluids, surgical trauma and prolonged postoperative use of magnesium-free fluids, and in excessive use of alcohol, which increases magnesium excretion. In such cases, deficiency symptoms include muscle weakness and a tetany-like state progressing from early tremors to convulsive seizures. Injections of magnesium sulfate relieve these symptoms.

Chloride

Functions. Chloride is widely distributed throughout body tissues. Its two significant functions involve digestion and respiration.

1. *Digestion.* Chloride is a necessary element in the hydrochloric acid secreted in the gastric juices. This constant secretion maintains the acidity of

stomach fluids necessary for the action of gastric enzymes. This acid secretion also helps maintain the acid-base balance in body fluids.

2. Respiration. Chloride ions help red blood cells transport large amounts of carbon dioxide to the lungs for release in breathing. The chloride ions move easily in and out of red blood cells in balance with the carbon dioxide, to counteract any potential changes in the acid-base balance. This ready movement of chloride in and out of red blood cells is called the *chloride shift.*

Requirements. Both the intake of chloride from food and its losses from the body under normal circumstances parallel those of sodium. Thus the RDA for all ages except infants parallel those of sodium.[1]

Food sources. Dietary chloride is provided almost entirely by sodium chloride, or table salt. The kidney is very efficient in reabsorbing chloride when the dietary intake is low.

Deficiency states. Dietary deficiency of chloride does not occur under normal circumstances. Chloride loss parallels losses of sodium in situations such as diarrhea, vomiting, or heavy sweating.

Sulfur

Functions. Sulfur is present in all body cells, contributing to widespread metabolic and structural functions.

1. Hair, skin, and nails. Sulfur is involved in the structure of hair, skin, and nails through its presence in two amino acids, methionine and cystine, which are concentrated in the tissue protein keratin.

2. General metabolic functions. Combined with hydrogen, sulfur is an important high-energy bond in building many tissue compounds. It helps transfer energy as needed in various tissues.

3. Vitamin structure. Sulfur is a part of several vitamins—thiamin, pantothenic acid, and biotin—which in turn act as coenzymes in cell metabolism.

4. Collagen structure. Sulfur is necessary for collagen synthesis, and thus is important in building connective tissue.

Requirements. There are no stated requirements for dietary sulfur as such, since it is supplied by protein foods containing the amino acids methionine and cystine.

Food sources. Sulfur is available to the body primarily as the organic sulfur compounds in its two amino acid carriers, methionine and cystine. Thus animal protein foods would be the main dietary sources.

Deficiency states. No deficiency states have been reported. Such conditions would relate only to general protein malnutrition and absence of the sulfur-carrying amino acids methionine and cystine.

A summary of the major minerals is given in Table 7-3.

TRACE ELEMENTS
Iron

Functions. Iron functions both in the synthesis of hemoglobin and in general body metabolism.

1. Hemoglobin synthesis. Iron is an essential component of heme, the nonprotein part of the hemoglobin structure. Hemoglobin in the red blood cell carries oxygen to the cells for cell oxidation and metabolism. Iron is also a

❖ **TABLE 7-3**   *A summary of major minerals*

Mineral	Metabolism	Physiologic functions	Clinical application	Requirements	Food sources
Calcium (Ca)	Absorption according to body need, aided by vitamin D; hindered by binding agents (oxalates), or excessive fiber Parathyroid hormone controls absorption and mobilization	Bone formation Teeth Blood clotting Muscle contraction and relaxation Heart action Nerve transmission	Tetany—decrease in ionized serum calcium Rickets Osteoporosis	Adults: 1200 mg Pregnancy and lactation: 1200 mg Infants: 400-600 mg Children: 800-1200 mg	Milk Cheese Whole grains Egg yolk Legumes, nuts Green leafy vegetables
Phosphorus (P)	Absorption with calcium aided by vitamin D; hindered by excess binding agents (aluminum)	Bone and tooth formation Overall metabolism Energy metabolism (enzymes) Acid-base balance	Bone loss Poor growth	Adults: 1200-800 mg Pregnancy and lactation: 1200 mg Infants: 300-500 mg Children: 800-1200 mg	Milk Cheese Meat Egg yolk Whole grains Legumes, nuts
Sodium (Na)	Readily absorbed	Major extracellular fluid control Water balance Acid-base balance Muscle action; transmission of nerve impulse and resulting contraction	Fluid shifts and control Buffer system Losses in gastrointestinal disorders Dehydration	Limit to 2.4 g or less	Table salt (NaCl) Milk Meat Egg Baking soda Baking powder Carrots, beets, spinach, celery

Mineral	Metabolism	Physiological Functions	Clinical Applications	Requirement	Food Sources
Potassium (K)	Secreted and reabsorbed in digestive juices	Major intracellular fluid control; Acid-base balance; Regulates nerve impulse and muscle contraction; Glycogen formation; Protein synthesis; Energy metabolism	Fluid shifts; Heart action—low serum potassium (cardiac arrest); Insulin release; Blood pressure factor	About 1000-3500 mg; Diet adequate in protein, calcium, and iron contains adequate potassium	Fruits; Vegetables; Meats; Whole grains; Legumes
Magnesium (Mg)	Absorption increased by parathyroid hormone	Aids thyroid hormone secretion, normal BMR; Activator and coenzyme in carbohydrate and protein metabolism; Muscle, nerve action	Tremor, spasm; low serum level following gastrointestinal losses or renal losses from alcoholism; convulsions	Adults: 280-350 mg; Pregnancy and lactation: 320-355 mg; Deficiency in humans unlikely	Whole grains; Nuts; Legumes; Green vegetables (chlorophyll)
Chlorine (Cl)	Absorbed readily	Acid-base balance—chloride shift; Gastric hydrochloric acid—digestion	Hypochloremic alkalosis in prolonged vomiting, diarrhea, tube drainage	Parallel requirement of sodium	Table salt
Sulfur (S)	Absorbed as such and as constituent of sulfur-containing amino acids methionine and cystine	Essential constituent of cell protein; Hair, skin, nails; Vitamin structure; Collagen structure; High-energy sulfur bonds in energy metabolism	General protein malnutrition	Diet adequate in protein contains adequate sulfur	Meat; Egg; Cheese; Milk; Nuts, legumes

necessary part of myoglobin, a similar compound in muscle tissue. Approximately 75% of the total body iron is found in hemoglobin.

2. *General metabolism.* General metabolic functions that require iron include glucose metabolism in the cell, antibody production, detoxification of drugs in the liver, conversion of carotene to vitamin A, collagen synthesis, and purine synthesis. The amount of iron in the body is regulated according to the body's need, specifically to accomplish these vital functions.

Requirements. Adult requirements for iron differ between men and women. The RDA standard suggests a general iron intake of 10 mg/day for men and 15 mg/day for women, given usual diets in the United States.[1] The greater amount for women is needed to cover menstrual losses and the iron demands of pregnancy. During pregnancy the woman's RDA for iron doubles to 30 mg/day, an increase usually requiring an iron supplement because neither the usual American diets nor iron stores of many women can meet the increased iron demands.

Food sources. Iron is widely distributed in the U.S. food supply, mainly in meat, especially liver, eggs, vegetables, and cereals, especially fortified cereal products.[1] Although fruits, vegetables, and juices contain varying amounts of iron, as a group they contribute another major source of dietary iron. Iron availability in foods may be enhanced by use of foods containing vitamin C. The iron in food sources occurs in two forms, *heme* and *nonheme*, a factor that affects its absorption and hence its availability to the body. Heme iron is the most easily absorbed form of dietary iron, but it contributes the smallest amount of the total dietary iron, coming from none of the plant food sources and only 40% of the animal food sources (Table 7-4). Nonheme iron is less easily absorbed because it occurs in foods in a more tightly bound form, yet the majority of our food sources—60% of the animal food sources and all of the plant food sources— contain this form. Including food sources of vitamin C, moderate amounts of lean meats, and enriched cereal products in the diet would help enhance the absorption and availability of this larger amount of dietary nonheme iron.

Deficiency states. The major condition indicating a deficiency of iron is **anemia**, characterized by a decrease in the number of red blood cells or in the amount of cell hemoglobin or both. Iron deficiency anemia is the most prevalent nutritional problem in the world today. This lack of iron or ability to use it may result from several causes: (1) inadequate supply of dietary iron; (2)

❖ **TABLE 7-4**   *Characteristics of heme and nonheme portions of dietary iron*

Heme (smallest portion)	Nonheme (largest portion)
Food sources	
None in plant sources; 40% of iron in animal sources	All iron in plant sources; 60% of iron in animal sources
Absorption rate	
Rapid; transported and absorbed intact	Slow; tightly bound in organic molecules

excessive blood loss; (3) inability to form hemoglobin in the absence of other necessary factors such as vitamin B_{12} (pernicious anemia); (4) lack of gastric hydrochloric acid necessary to help liberate iron for absorption; (5) presence of various inhibitors of iron absorption, such as phosphate or phytate; or (6) mucosal lesions affecting the absorbing surface area.

Iodine

Functions. The only known function of iodine in human nutrition is in the synthesis of the thyroid hormone thyroxine. The uptake of iodine by the thyroid gland is controlled by the thyroid-stimulating hormone (TSH) from the pituitary gland, in direct response to the level of thyroxine circulating in the blood. When the blood level of thyroxine decreases below normal, more TSH is secreted by the pituitary gland, stimulating the thyroid gland to take up more iodine so that it can make more thyroxine. The transport form of iodine in the blood is called serum *protein-bound iodine* (PBI). After thyroxine (in its two forms having hormonal activity— T_3 and T_4) is used to stimulate metabolic processes in cells, it is broken down in the liver and the iodine portion is excreted in bile as inorganic iodine. Thus the basic overall function of iodine relates to control of the body's basal metabolic rate (BMR), through its role in the synthesis of the controlling hormone thyroxine.

Requirements. The RDA standard for iodine is 150 μg/day for adults of both sexes and for rapidly growing adolescents. For pregnant women the need increases to 175 μg and to 200 μg during lactation.

Food sources. The amount of iodine in natural food sources varies considerably depending on the iodine content of the soil. Foods from the sea provide a good amount of iodine. The major reliable source, however, is iodized table salt—76 μg iodine per gram of salt[1].

Deficiency states. A lack of iodine contributes to several deficiency diseases.

1. Goiter. The classic condition of goiter, as shown in Fig. 7-2, is caused by lack of iodine in the diet. It is characterized by enlargement of the thyroid gland, sometimes to tremendous size. It occurs in areas where the water and soil contain little iodine. The person's thyroid gland is starved for iodine and cannot produce a normal amount of thyroxine. With this low level of thyroxine in the blood, the pituitary gland continues to secrete more and more TSH. These large amounts of TSH continually stimulate the nonproductive thyroid gland, causing it to increase greatly in size. Such an iodine-starved thyroid gland may weigh as much as 0.45 to 0.67 kg (1 to 1.5 lbs) or more.

2. Cretinism. The condition of cretinism occurs among children born to mothers who have had limited iodine intake during adolescence and pregnancy. During her pregnancy, the mother's iodine need takes precedence over that of the developing child. Thus the fetus suffers from iodine deficiency, and the lack continues after birth. These children are retarded in both physical and mental development. However, if the condition is discovered at birth and treatment is started immediately, many of the symptoms are reversible. If the condition continues beyond early childhood, the physical and mental retardation becomes permanent.

3. Hypothyroidism. A poorly functioning thyroid gland cannot make enough thyroxine and the BMR is greatly reduced, resulting in an adult form

❖ **Fig. 7-2**

Goiter. The extreme enlargment shown here is a result of
extended duration of iodine deficiency.

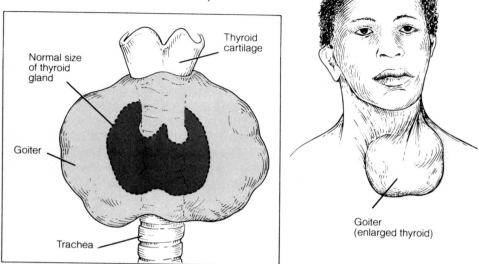

of hypothyroidism called *myxedema*. The symptoms of this condition are thin
coarse hair, dry skin, poor tolerance for cold, weight gain, and a low husky
voice.

4. *Hyperthyroidism.* An opposite condition, hyperthyroidism, in which the
accelerated thyroid produces excessive thyroxine and the BMR is greatly increased, may also occur in adults. It is known as Graves' disease, or *exoph-
thalmic goiter.* Symptoms include weight loss, hand tremors and general ner-
vousness, increased appetite, intolerance of heat, and protruding eyeballs.

Iodine overload. Increased incidental intake of iodine may cause an overload for some persons. Iodates are used as dough oxidizers in the continuous
bread making process, adding about 500 μg/100 g of bread. Most of this
excess comes through dairy products.[4] These dairy sources include iodized salt
licks for the animals and the use of iodine-containing disinfectants on cows'
udders, milking machines, and milk storage tanks. Other iodine-containing
compounds are used as additives to the animals' feeds. Excess iodine may result
in acnelike skin lesions or may worsen preexisting acne of adolescents or young
adults. Excessive amounts may also cause "iodine goiter," which could be
misdiagnosed as goiter caused by insufficient iodine. However, continued use
of iodized salt is still a wise practice for several reasons: (1) moderately excessive iodine is relatively harmless, (2) persons living in certain regions may
be at greater risk of goiter, and (3) individual iodine intake is highly variable
and may at times be insufficient depending on geographic location and food
supply.

Zinc

Functions. The widespread nature of zinc's functions in the human body
is reflected in its distribution in many of the body tissues, including the pan-

creas, liver, kidneys, lungs, muscles, bones, eyes, endocrine glands, prostate secretions, and spermatozoa. In these tissues zinc participates in three different types of metabolic functions.

1. *Enzyme constituent.* Zinc functions throughout the body as an essential part of cell enzyme systems. Over 70 such zinc enzymes have been identified. In its role in protein metabolism zinc is associated with wound healing and healthy skin. It has great influence on any rapidly growing tissues. Therefore its effect on reproduction is highly significant.

2. *Insulin storage.* Zinc combines readily with insulin in the pancreas and serves as a storage form of the hormone. The pancreas of a person with diabetes contains about half of the normal amount of zinc.

3. *Immune system.* A considerable amount of zinc bound to protein is present in the leukocytes (white blood cells), a major component of the body's immune system. Zinc affects the immune system through its essential role in

---

BOX 7-1

❖ ——————— **CLINICAL APPLICATION** ——————— ❖

Zinc Barriers

Are people eating more zinc but absorbing it less? Current trends toward a "heart-healthy" diet may be one of the reasons. Some Americans may be at risk for developing a zinc deficiency, not because they avoid zinc-rich foods, but because they are choosing foods and supplements that reduce its availability for absorption. For example:

- Animal foods, rich in readily available zinc, are consumed less by an increasingly cholesterol-conscious public.
- Fiber, being promoted by some persons as a cardiovascular panacea, may create a negative zinc balance when used in excessive amounts.
- Vitamin-mineral supplements may contain iron/zinc ratios greater than 3:1 and provide enough iron to inhibit zinc absorption.

The risk for zinc deficiency is greatest among pregnant and breast-feeding women. Low levels can reduce the amount of protein available to carry iron and vitamin A to the target tissues and reduce the mother's appetite and taste for foods. As a result, the fetus is at even greater risk for inadequate growth and development.

All of these conditions, plus milling processes that remove excessive amounts of zinc from grains, have resulted in an average adult intake between 10 and 15 mg/day, with elderly adults consuming only 7 to 10 mg zinc daily. The average adult intake is less than the 15 to 19 mg/day recommended for pregnant and lactating women and the 12 to 15 mg/day for older adults.

To increase zinc in their diets, persons may:

- Include some form of animal food—meat, milk, eggs—in the diet each day to ensure a minimal intake of zinc.
- Avoid "crash" diets and extensive use of alcohol.

Signs of zinc deficiency are fairly rare in the United States but are becoming more apparent among at-risk persons, such as older adults with long-term chronic illness and hospitalization. There is no need, however, for the general public to overprotect themselves with massive supplements. These can lead to nausea, abdominal pain, anemia, and impairment of the immune system. As with all other nutrients, too much of a good thing can sometimes be as bad as too little—or even worse.

the synthesis of nucleic acids (DNA and RNA) and protein. It is also needed for lymphocyte transformation. Also, lymphoid tissue, which gives rise to lymphocytes, the major white cell populations involved in the body's immune system, contains a large amount of zinc. The leukocytes of patients with leukemia, for example, contain about 10% less zinc than normal.

Requirements. The RDA standard for adult men is 15 mg/day and for women, because of their smaller size, the zinc allowance is 12 mg/day. Pregnant women require 15 mg/day to meet fetal growth needs and 19 mg/day for lactation. The zinc content of typical mixed diets of adults in the United States has been reported to furnish between 10 and 15 mg/day.[1]

Food sources. Approximately 70% of the zinc consumed by most people in the United States is provided by animal products, especially meat. Seafoods, particularly oysters, are excellent sources of zinc. Additional sources, although less available to the body, are legumes and whole grains. Consistent use of a well-balanced diet usually meets adult needs for zinc, but there is considerable evidence that diets high in processed foods may be low in zinc.

Deficiency states. Zinc is a nutritional imperative during periods of rapid tissue growth. In some populations where dietary intake of zinc is low, retarded physical growth (dwarfism) and retarded sexual maturation, especially in males, has been observed. Also, impaired taste and smell (hypogeusia and hyposmia) are improved with increased zinc intake. Poor wound healing in patients with zinc deficiency seems to be common in the average hospital. Supplements may be needed for surgical patients and for older patients.[5] Those having poor appetites, subsisting on marginal diets in the face of chronic wounds and illnesses and tissue breakdown, may be particularly vulnerable to zinc deficiency. (See Box 7-1.)

Selenium

Functions. Selenium functions as an essential part of an antioxidant enzyme that protects cells and their lipid membranes against oxidative damage. In this role, selenium balances with vitamin E, each sparing the other (p. 70). It also has a structural function as it is part of the protein center of teeth. In addition, recent work in China seeking the cause of Keshan disease, a heart muscle disease affecting young children and women of child-bearing age, has indicated that selenium plays a role in preventing this disease.[1,2] Selenium deficiency clearly predisposes people to Keshan disease, named for the area in China in which it was discovered, possibly by making them more vulnerable to a cardiotoxic virus.[6]

Requirements. Based on information about selenium needs gained from the studies of Keshan disease in China, adjusted for selenium's adult requirement relationship to body weight and individual variation, the U.S. RDA standard for adults has been established as 70 µg/day for men and 55 µg/day for women. A daily increment of 10 µg is needed during pregnancy and an additional 20 µg during lactation.[1]

Food sources. Seafoods, kidney, and liver, and to a lesser extent other meats, are consistently good sources of selenium. Grains and other seeds are more variable, depending on the selenium content of the soils in which they are grown.[1] Fruits and vegetables generally contain little selenium.

Deficiency states. Two conditions have been associated with selenium deficiency: (1) heart failure as a result of cardiomyopathy (degeneration of the heart muscle), as described in relation to Keshan disease, and (2) muscular discomfort or weakness and low blood levels of the selenium-containing antioxidant exzyme (glutathione peroxide), as well as low levels of selenium in plasma and red cells, observed in patients receiving total parenteral nutrition (TPN). Some cases of heart muscle damage have also occurred in patients receiving TPN. In both of these situations patients have responded to selenium supplementation.[6,7]

Other essential trace elements

Because of difficulties in quantifying their human requirements, five other essential trace elements do not as yet have established RDA standards. Instead the RDA committee has recommended "safe and adequate" ranges of intake. These five trace elements are copper, manganese, fluoride, chromium, and molybdenum. (See summary table inside book cover.) The one remaining essential trace element cobalt has no recommended intake of its own because it is supplied in vitamin B_{12}. These six essential trace elements are briefly reviewed.

Copper. This element has frequently been called the "iron twin." The two are metabolized in much the same way and share functions as cell enzyme components. Both are related to energy production and hemoglobin synthesis. A recent dietary survey, the Food and Drug Administration's Total Diet Study, showed relatively lower levels of copper in Americans' diets than had previously been estimated, increasing a nutritional concern for its adequacy.[8] However, severe copper deficiency is rare because of individual adaptation to somewhat lower intakes, but copper depletion sufficient to cause low blood levels has been observed during TPN and in cases of anemia.[1] The RDA committee's safe and adequate copper recommendation for adults is 1.5 to 3.0 mg/day. The richest food sources of copper are organ meats, especially liver, followed by seafoods, nuts, and seeds, including legumes and grains.

Manganese. The small amount of manganese in the body, about 20 mg, occurs mainly in the liver, pancreas, pituitary gland, and bone. It functions like other trace elements as an essential part of cell enzymes that catalyze many important metabolic reactions. Manganese deficiency is rare but has been reported in diabetes and pancreatic insufficiency as well as in protein-energy malnutrition states such as *kwashiorkor*.Toxicity occurs as an industrial disease, *inhalation toxicity*, in miners and other workers with prolonged exposure to manganese dust. The excess manganese accumulates in the liver and central nervous system, producing severe neuromuscular symptoms similar to those of Parkinson's disease. The RDA committee's safe and adequate range for manganese in adult diets is 2.5 to 5.0 mg/day, with 1.0 to 2.0 mg/day for children. The best food sources of manganese are of plant origin. Whole grains and cereal products are the richest food sources, and fruits and vegetables are somewhat less so. Dairy products, meat, fish, and poultry are poor sources. Tea is also a rich source.

Fluoride. Fluoride accumulates in calcified body tissues, mostly in bones and teeth. In human nutrition fluoride functions mainly to prevent dental caries. Fluoride treatment strengthens the ability of the tooth structure to withstand

❖ **TABLE 7-5** A summary of selected trace elements

Element	Metabolism	Physiologic functions	Clinical application	Requirements	Food sources
Iron (Fe)	Absorption according to body need; aided by vitamin C. Heme and nonheme forms. Excretion from tissue in minute quantities; body conserves then reuses	Hemoglobin formation. Cellular oxidation of glucose. Myoglobin in muscle. Antibody production. Drug detoxification. Carotene conversion to vitamin A. Collagen synthesis	Growth. Pregnancy demands. Deficiency—anemia	Men: 10 mg. Women: 15 mg. Pregnancy: 30 mg. Lactation: 15 mg. Children: 10-15 mg	Liver. Meats. Egg yolk. Whole grains. Enriched bread and cereal. Dark green vegetables. Legumes, nuts
Iodine (I)	Absorbed as iodides, taken up by thyroid gland under control of thyroid-stimulating hormone (TSH). Excretion by kidney	Synthesis of thyroxine, the thyroid hormone, which regulates cell oxidation. BMR regulation	Deficiency—endemic colloid goiter; cretinism. Hypothyroidism. Hyperthyroidism	Men: 150 µg. Women: 150 µg. Infants: 35-45 µg. Children: 70-150 µg	Iodized salt. Seafood
Zinc (Zn)	Transported with plasma proteins. Excretion largely intestinal. Stored in liver, muscle, bone, and organs	Essential enzyme constituent: Combined with insulin for storage of the hormone. Immune system leukocytes	Wound healing. Taste and smell acuity. Retarded sexual and physical development	Men: 15 mg. Women: 12 mg. Children: 10-15 mg. Infants: 5 mg	Meat. Seafood, especially oysters. Eggs. Milk. Whole grains. Legumes
Copper (Cu)	Stored in muscle, bone, liver, heart, kidney, and central nervous system. Iron twin	Associated with iron in energy production. Hemoglobin synthesis. Absorption and transport of iron	TPN deficiency. Anemia	Adults: 1.5-3.0 mg. Children: 1.0-2.5 mg (estimated)	Liver. Seafood. Whole grains. Legumes, nuts

Mineral	Metabolism	Function	Deficiency/Toxicity	Requirement	Sources
Manganese (Mn)	Absorption limited Excretion mainly by intestine	Activates reactions in Urea formation Protein metabolism Glucose oxidation Lipoprotein clearance and synthesis of fatty acids	Clinical deficiency in protein-energy malnutrition Inhalation toxicity in miners	Adults: 2-5 mg (estimated) Children: 1-5 mg	Cereals, whole grain Soybeans Legumes, nuts Tea Vegetables Fruits
Chromium (Cr)	Improves faulty uptake of glucose by body tissues as part of glucose tolerance factor	Associated with glucose metabolism; raises abnormally low fasting blood sugar levels	Possible link with cardiovascular disorders and diabetes	Adults: 50-200 µg Children: 20-200 µg (estimated)	Whole grains Cereal products
Cobalt (Co)	Absorbed chiefly as constituent of vitamin B_{12}	Constituent of vitamin B_{12}; essential factor in red blood cell formation	Deficiency associated with deficiency of vitamin B_{12}—pernicious anemia	Unknown	Supplied by pre-formed vitamin B_{12}
Selenium (Se)	Active as cofactor in cell oxidation enzyme systems	Associated with vitamin E as antioxidant; protects lipid in cell membrane	Keshan disease, heart muscle failure TPN deficiency	Men: 70 µg Women: 55 µg Children: 20 µg	Seafoods Kidney Liver Meats Whole grains
Molybdenum (Mo)	Minute traces in the body	Constituent of specific enzymes involved in Purine conversion to uric acid Aldehyde oxidation		Adults: 75-250 µg (estimated)	Organ meats Milk Whole grains Leafy vegetables Legumes
Fluorine (Fl)	Deposited in bones and teeth	Associated with dental health	Small amount prevents dental caries Excess causes endemic dental fluorosis	Adults: 1.5-4 mg (estimated) Children: 0.5-2.5 mg	Fluoridated water (1 ppm Fl)

the erosive effect of bacterial acids on the tooth. Three factors have contributed to the decreased incidence of caries in young children: (1) fluoridation of public water supply (1 ppm), (2) use of fluoridated toothpaste (0.1%), and (3) improved dental hygiene habits. Definitive evidence for a similar fluoride role in protecting adult bone or preventing osteoporosis is lacking. The RDA committee's recommended safe and adequate range of fluoride intake for adults is 1.5 to 4.0 mg/day. Fish, fish products, and tea contain the highest concentration of fluoride. Cooking with fluoridated water raises the levels in many foods.

Chromium. Chromium functions as an essential component of the organic complex *glucose tolerance factor* (GTF), which stimulates the action of insulin. Insulin resistance shown by impaired glucose tolerance has responded positively to chromium supplements, restoring normal blood glucose levels. Also, significant reduction of elevated serum cholesterol has been observed in persons treated with chromium supplements, lowering low-density lipoprotein (LDL) cholesterol and increasing high-density lipoprotein (HDL) cholesterol. The RDA committee's recommended safe and adequate range of chromium intake for adults is 50 to 200 μg/day. Brewer's yeast is a rich source of chromium, and most grains and cereal products contain significant amounts.

Molybdenum. Molybdenum functions as a catalyst component in several cell enzyme systems. As such it is essential for a number of metabolic reactions. The RDA committee's recommended safe and adequate range of molybdenum intake for adults is 75 to 250 μg/day. Food sources include legumes, whole grains, milk, leafy vegetables, and organ meats.

Cobalt. As an essential part of vitamin B_{12} (cobalamin), cobalt's only known function is associated with red blood cell formation. It is provided in the human diet only by vitamin B_{12}. The human requirement is unknown, but is exceeding small. For example, as little as 0.045 to 0.09 μg/day maintains bone marrow function in persons with pernicious anemia. Cobalt is widely distributed in nature. However, for our needs—as an essential part of vitamin B_{12}—cobalt is obtained in the preformed vitamin, which is synthesized in animals by intestinal bacteria.

Probably essential trace elements

The eight remaining trace elements found in human tissue are silicon, vanadium, nickel, tin, cadmium, arsenic, aluminum, and boron. These elements are being studied to determine their precise functions in the body. Most have already been found to be essential in specific animal nutrition, and are probably essential in human nutrition as well, although their metabolism in humans is not yet fully defined. Because they occur in such small amounts they are more difficult to study and primary dietary deficiency is highly unlikely. However, with increased use of long-term TPN therapy, they may be of increasing clinical concern.

A summary of selected trace elements is given in Table 7-5.

SUMMARY

Minerals are single inorganic elements widely distributed in nature. In their ionized form they build body tissue; activate, regulate, and control metabolic processes; and transmit neurologic messages.

Minerals are classified according to their relative amounts in the body. *Major minerals* are required in larger quantities and make up 60% to 80% of all the inorganic material in the body. *Trace elements* are required in much smaller amounts, as small as a microgram, and make up less than 1% of the body's inorganic material. There are seven major minerals and 10 trace elements known to be essential in human nutrition. Another eight trace elements present in the body are also probably essential and are being studied to define their function more precisely.

❖ REVIEW QUESTIONS

1. List the seven major minerals, describing their functions and problems created by dietary deficiency or excess.
2. List the 10 trace elements with proven essentiality in human nutrition. Which ones have established RDA standards? Which ones have "safe and adequate intakes" suggested? Why is it difficult to establish RDA for everyone?

❖ SELF-TEST QUESTIONS

True-false

For each item you answer "false," write the correct statement.

1. The majority of the calcium in the diet is absorbed and used by the body for bone formation.
2. The adult use of sodium is about 10 times the amount the body actually requires for metabolic balance.
3. Most of the dietary iron is absorbed, and then the body's iron balance is controlled by urinary excretion.
4. Liver is the body's main storage site for iron.
5. Iron is widespread in food sources, so a deficiency problem is rare.
6. The best food source of iron is milk.
7. Iodine has many metabolic functions, the most important of which is its role in thyroxine synthesis.
8. Dental caries can be largely prevented by the use of small amounts of fluoride.

Multiple choice

1. Overall calcium balance is maintained mainly by two interbalanced regulatory agents:
   a. Vitamin A and thyroid hormone
   b. Ascorbic acid and growth hormone
   c. Vitamin D and parathyroid hormone
   d. Phosphorus and TSH
2. Optimum levels of body iron are controlled at the point of absorption, interrelated with a system of transport and storage. Which of the following statements correctly describes this iron-regulating process:
   a. The iron form in foods requires an acid medium to reduce it to the form required for absorption.
   b. Most of the iron ingested in food—about 70% to 90%—is absorbed.
   c. Vitamin C acts as a binding and carrying agent to transport and store iron.
   d. When red blood cells are destroyed, the iron used in making the hemoglobin is excreted.

3. The only known function of fluorine in human nutrition is with dental health. Which of the following statements correctly describes this relation?
   a. Small amounts of fluoride produce mottled discolored teeth.
   b. Fluoridation of public water supply in small amounts (1 ppm) helps prevent dental caries.
   c. Topical application of fluoride to young teeth is not effective.
   d. Fluoride works with calcium to build strong teeth.

❖ SUGGESTIONS FOR ADDITIONAL STUDY

1. Survey food products in a community supermarket to identify items that are fortified with minerals. Read the labels carefully to determine the mineral form added and the quantity used. Do you think this mineral addition is good for the consumer? If so, why?
2. Visit a health food store, using the same procedure you followed in your vitamin study, this time to survey various mineral supplements. Discuss your findings and your evaluations with your class.
3. Using the Appendix food value table, compute the iron in each of the following foods and compare your results: (1) 3 ounces of beef liver, (2) 3 ounces of beef round steak, (3) 1 tablespoon molasses, (4) 1 tablespoon raisins, (5) 1 cup cooked kale, and (6) six dried prunes (plain or cooked).
4. Prepare a chart showing the comparative calcium values of several of the main food sources of calcium and some of the less rich sources. List some ways you can incorporate more dairy products into your diet besides drinking milk.

References

1. National Research Council, Food and Nutrition Board: Recommended dietary allowances, ed 10, Washington, DC, 1989, National Academy Press.
2. National Research Council, Committee on Diet and Health: Diet and health, implications for reducing chronic diseases, Washington, DC, 1989, National Academy Press.
3. Anderson JJB: Dietary calcium and bone mass through the lifecycle, Nutr Today 25(2):9, 1990.
4. Holt HC and others: The iodine concentration of market milk in Tennessee, J Food Protection 52:115, Jan 1989.
5. Bogden JD and others: Effects of one year of supplementation with zinc and other micronutrients on cellular immunity in the elderly, J Am Coll Nutr 9:214, June 1990.
6. Yang G and others: Selenium-related endemic diseases and the daily selenium requirement of humans, World Rev Nutr Diet 55:98, 1988.
7. Brown MR and others: Proximal muscle weakness and selenium deficiency associated with long term parenteral nutrition, Am J Clin Nutr 43:549, 1986.
8. Pennington JAT and others: Nutritional elements in U.S. diets: results from the Total Diet Study, 1982 to 1986, J Am Diet Assoc 89(5):659, 1989.

Further Reading

Anderson JJB: Dietary calcium and bone mass through the lifecycle, Nutr Today 25(2):9, 1990.

Freeland-Graves JH: Manganese: an essential nutrient for humans, Nutr Today 23(6):13, 1988.

Johnson MA and Kays SE: Copper: its role in human nutrition, Nutr Today 25(1):6, 1990.

These three articles from *Nutrition Today*, a popular journal of up-to-date happenings in the world of nutrition, describe in graphic fashion the roles of calcium, manganese, and copper in human nutrition.

8

❖

Water Balance

KEY CONCEPTS

*Water exists throughout the body as one unified whole with constant
ebb and flow among its interfacing parts.*

*Collective body water compartments, inside and outside of cells,
maintain a balanced distribution of total body water.*

*The concentration of various solute particles in the body water
solution determines internal shifts and balances of water.*

*A state of dynamic equilibrium, homeostasis, among all parts
of the body's water balance system sustains life.*

$\mathcal{W}$ ater is the one nutrient most vital to human existence.
In fact, the majority of the earth's surface is covered by water. Our lives, and
those of all other life forms sharing this planet, depend on a constant supply
of water from the earth's ever-moving cycle. We can survive far longer without
food than we can without water. Only our constant need for air is more
demanding.

One of our most basic nutritional tasks is meeting this need for a continuous
supply of water. Ensuring a balancing distribution of this precious water to
all our body cells is a primary physiologic function.

In this chapter we look at the finely developed water balance system in the body. We see how this system works and the various parts and processes that sustain it and thereby sustain life itself.

BODY WATER FUNCTIONS AND REQUIREMENTS
Water: the fundamental nutrient

Basic principles. Three basic principles are essential to an understanding of the balance and uses of water in the human body.

1. A unified whole. The human body forms one continuous body of water. The "sea within" is contained by a protective envelope of skin. Within this enclosing skin, body water moves freely to all parts, its movement controlled only by the water's own chemical nature. Thus in this warm, watery chemical environment, all the processes necessary to life can be sustained.

2. Body water compartments. The key word *compartment* is generally used in body physiology to indicate a collective whole in body systems, the parts of which are separated and distributed throughout the whole. Water compartments throughout the body are separated by *membranes*. Certain quantities of water contained by these membranes in various places in the body are balanced by forces that maintain an equilibrium among all the parts.

3. Particles in the water solution. The concentration and distribution of *particles* in the water solution in various places throughout the body determines all internal shifts and balances in the total body water.

Homeostasis. Thus you can picture body water as a unified whole, sustained in critical balance to protect life. This state of dynamic balance in the body has been called **homeostasis.** Many years ago a thoughtful physiologist, W.B. Cannon, viewed these balance principles as "body wisdom."[1] He applied the term *homeostasis* to the wise capacity built into the body to maintain its life systems, despite what enters the system from the outside. The first part of the word, *homeo-*, is from a Greek word meaning "similar." The second half of the word, *-stasis*, is also from a Greek root, meaning "balance." The body has a marvelous capacity to employ numerous, finely balanced *homeostatic mechanisms* to protect its vital water supply within.

Body water functions

To serve life-sustaining functions, our important body water supply acts as a solvent, serves as a means of transport, and provides form and structure, temperature control, and lubrication for the body.

Solvent. Water provides the basic liquid solvent for all the body's chemical processes. The word *hydrolysis* is used to describe this water-based chemical activity in the body. The first part of the word, *hydro-*, means "water," and the second part, *-lysis*, means "to break apart." Thus with water as the basic solvent, multiple water solutions may be formed as needed throughout the body to allow all of its life-sustaining metabolic activities, such as energy production and tissue building, to proceed.

Transport. Water circulates throughout the body in the form of blood and in the form of various body secretions and tissue fluids. In this circulating fluid, the many nutrients, secretions, metabolites—products formed in body metabolism—and other materials can be carried freely about to meet the needs of all the body cells. The body cell is the functional unit of life. Its fundamental needs for oxygen and nourishment, as well as needs for all its chemical activities, must be met at all times.

Body form and structure. Water also helps to give structure and form to the body by filling in spaces within body tissues. For example, striated muscle contains more water than any other body tissue except blood.

Body temperature. Water is necessary to help maintain a stable body temperature. As the temperature rises, sweat increases and evaporates, thus cooling the body.

Body lubricant. Water also has a lubricating effect on moving parts of the body. For example, fluid within the body joints helps to provide smooth movement of the many joint parts. This fluid in the body joints is called *synovial* fluid.

Body water requirements. The body's requirement for water varies according to several factors: temperature, activity level, functional losses, metabolic needs, and age.

Temperature. As the temperature rises in the surrounding environment, body water is lost to help maintain the body temperature, and thus more water intake is required to offset it. This increasing temperature may be caused by the natural climate, or by the heat of a work environment.

Activity level. Heavy work or extensive physical activity, such as in sports, increases the water requirement for two reasons: (1) more water is lost as sweat, and (2) more water is required for the increased metabolic work involved in the physical activity.

Functional losses. When any disease process interferes with the normal functioning of the body, water requirements are affected. For example, in gastrointestinal problems such as prolonged diarrhea, large amounts of water may be lost. In such cases, replacement of this lost water is vital to prevent dehydration.

Metabolic needs. The work of body metabolism requires water. A general rule is that about 1000 ml of water is required for every 1000 kcalories in the diet. On the average, beverages supply about two thirds of the water intake. Solid foods eaten supply the remaining one third.

Age. Age plays an important role in determining body needs, especially in the case of an infant. An infant needs about 1500 ml of water per day. Water intake is critical for an infant because (1) the infant's body content of water is large—about 70% to 75% of the total body weight and (2) a relatively large amount of this total body water is outside of the cells and thus is more easily lost.

THE HUMAN WATER BALANCE SYSTEM
Body water: the solvent

Amount and distribution. In a man's body 55% to 65% of the total body weight is water, and a woman's body is from 50% to 55% water.[2] The higher water content in men generally results from their greater muscle mass, a tissue that contains a relatively large amount of water. This total body water is divided into two major categories or *compartments*, depending on its placement in the body.

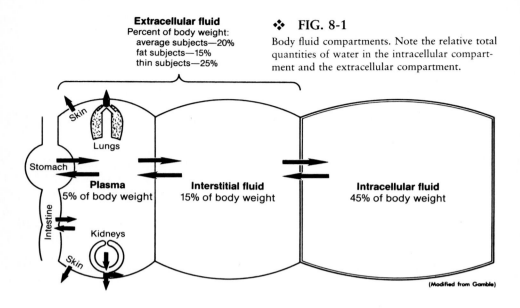

Extracellular fluid
Percent of body weight:
average subjects—20%
fat subjects—15%
thin subjects—25%

❖ **FIG. 8-1**

Body fluid compartments. Note the relative total quantities of water in the intracellular compartment and the extracellular compartment.

(Modified from Gamble)

1. *Total water outside cells.* The total body water outside of the cells is called the *extracellular fluid* (ECF). This collective water throughout the body outside the cells makes up about 20% of the total body weight. About one fourth of this water, 5% of the body weight, is contained in the blood plasma. The remaining three fourths, 15% of the body weight, is composed of (1) water surrounding the cells and bathing the tissues, (2) water in dense tissue such as bone, and (3) water moving through the body in various tissue secretions. The water in the blood plasma includes the total fluid within the heart and all the blood vessels. The fluid surrounding the cells in the tissues is called *interstitial* fluid. This tissue circulation helps to move materials in and out of the body cells to sustain life. Fluid in transit includes all the water in various body fluids and secretions, such as those of the salivary glands, thyroid gland, liver, pancreas, gallbladder, gastrointestinal tract, gonads, various mucous membranes, skin, kidneys, and eye spaces.

2. *Total water inside cells.* Total body water inside the cells is called the *intracellular fluid* (ICF). This total collective water inside the cells amounts to about twice that outside the cells, making up about 45% of the total body weight. This is not surprising, since the cell is the basic unit of life and all life-sustaining work—metabolism—is done within the cells.

The relative amounts of water in the different body water compartments are compared in Fig. 8-1.

Overall water balance. Normally water enters and leaves the body by various routes, controlled by basic mechanisms such as thirst and hormonal controls. Special attention must be given to the water needs of the elderly whose thirst sensation may be decreased.[3] The average adult metabolizes 2.5 to 3 L/day of water in a balance between intake and output.

1. *Water intake.* Water enters the body in three main forms: (1) as preformed water in liquids that are drunk, (2) as preformed water in foods that

❖ **TABLE 8-1**   *Approximate daily adult intake and output of water*

	Intake (replacement) ml/day		Output (loss)	
			Obligatory (insensible) ml/day	Optional (according to need) ml/day
Preformed		Lungs	350	
Liquids	1200-1500	Skin		
In foods	700-1000	Diffusion	350	
Metabolism	200-300	Sweat	100	± 250
(oxidation		Kidneys	900	± 500
of food)		Feces	150	
TOTAL	2100-2800	TOTAL	1850	750
(approx. 2600 ml/day)			(approx. 2600 ml/day)	

are eaten, and (3) as a product of cell oxidation when nutrients are burned in the body for energy—"water of oxidation." Approximate water intake is 2600 ml/day.

2. *Water output.* Water leaves the body through the kidneys, skin, lungs, and feces. Of these output routes, the largest amount of water exits through the kidneys. A certain amount of water is necessary for urinary excretion to carry out the various products of metabolism that are not needed by the body. This is called *obligatory* water loss and must occur daily for health. An additional amount of water may also be secreted by the kidneys each day depending on body activities and needs. This additional or *optional* water loss depends on the climate and physical activity. On the average the daily water output from the body totals about 2600 ml.

The comparative intake and output of body water balance is summarized in Table 8-1.

Solute particles in solution

Solutes in body water are a variety of particles in solution in varying concentrations. Two main types of particles control water balance in the body: electrolytes and plasma protein.

Electrolytes. Electrolytes are small inorganic substances, either single mineral elements or small compounds, that can dissociate or break apart in a solution and carry an electrical charge. These charged particles are called *ions*, from the Greek word meaning "wanderer." Thus these charged particles are free to wander throughout a solution to maintain its chemical balance. In any chemical solution the separate particles are constantly in balance between cations and anions.

1. *Cations.* These are ions carrying a positive charge, for example, sodium (Na^+), potassium (K^+), calcium (Ca^{++}), and magnesium (Mg^{++}).

2. *Anions.* These are ions carrying a negative charge, for example, chloride (Cl^-), carbonate (HCO_3^-), phosphate (HPO_4^-), and sulfate (SO_4^-).

The constant balance between the two major electrolytes, sodium (Na^+) outside the cell and potassium (K^+) inside the cell, maintains water balance between these two water compartments. Because of their small size, these

❖ TABLE 8-2   *Balance of cation and anion concentrations in extracellular fluid (ECF) and intracellular fluid (ICF), which maintains electroneutrality within each compartment*

	ECF (mEq/L)	ICF (mEq/L)
Cation		
Sodium (Na^+)	142	35
Potassium (K^+)	5	123
Calcium (Ca^{++})	5	15
Magnesium (Mg^{++})	3	2
TOTAL	155	175
Anion		
Chloride (Cl^-)	104	5
Phosphate (HPO_4^-)	2	80
Sulfate (SO_4^-)	1	10
Protein	16	70
Carbonate (HCO_3^-)	27	10
Organic acids	5	
TOTAL	155	175

electrolytes can diffuse freely across most membranes of the body. In this way they constantly maintain a balance between the water outside the cell and the water inside the cell.

The balance between cation and anion concentrations in the body fluids maintains a state of chemical neutrality in these fluids that is necessary to life. Electrolyte concentration in body fluids is measured in terms of *milliequivalents* (mEq). The number of these particles in solution per unit of fluid is expressed as mEq/L. Table 8-2 outlines the balance between cations and anions in the two body fluid compartments. The number of particles in each compartment exactly balances with that of the other.

Plasma proteins. Plasma proteins, mainly in the form of albumin and globulin, are organic compounds of large molecular size. They do not move as freely across membranes as do electrolytes, which are much smaller. Thus plasma protein molecules are retained in the blood vessel and make up a major substance in circulating blood that controls water movement in the body and guards the blood volume by influencing the shift of water in and out of capillaries in balance with their surrounding water. In this function, these plasma proteins are called *colloids*, from the Greek word *kolla*, meaning glue, and form *colloidal solutions*. Because of their large size, these particles or molecules normally remain in the blood vessels, where they exert **colloidal osmotic pressure** (COP) to maintain the integrity of the blood volume. In a similar manner cell protein helps to guard cell water.

Small organic compounds. In addition to electrolytes and plasma protein, other organic compounds of small size are in solution in body water. However, they do not ordinarily influence shifts of water because their concentration is too small. In some instances, however, they are found in abnormally large concentrations and do influence water movement. For example, glucose is one of these small particles in body fluids, and only when it is in abnormal concentrations, as in uncontrolled diabetes, does it influence water loss from the body.

Separating membranes

Two quite different types of membranes separate and contain body water in various places throughout the body. These types of membranes are the capillary membrane and the cell membrane.

Capillary membrane. The walls of the capillaries are fairly free membranes because they are thin and porous. Thus water molecules and small particles in solution can move freely across these membranes. Such small particles having free capillary passage include electrolytes and various nutrient materials. However, as indicated, larger particles such as plasma protein molecules cannot pass through the small pores in the capillary membrane. These molecules remain in the capillary vessel and exert an important pressure control, colloidal osmotic pressure, to keep the water circulating between capillaries and the surrounding tissue cells.

Cell membrane. The walls of the cell are thicker membranes, especially constructed to protect and nourish the cell contents. To accomplish these tasks, the cell membranes are structured almost in sandwich fashion, with outer layers and penetrating channels of protein and an inner structure of fat material. Special transport mechanisms are necessary to carry substances across cell membranes.

Forces moving water and solutes across membranes

As a result of the presence of these separating membranes, the capillary membrane and the cell membrane, certain physical and chemical forces are created that control the movement of body water and particles in solution across these membranes.

Osmosis. The term *osmosis* comes from the Greek word *osmos*, which means "a driving or pushing force, an impulse." It describes a fundamental impulse of nature to balance or equalize opposing forces. In human physiology the term **osmosis** is used to describe the process or force—"osmotic pressure"—that impels water molecules to move about throughout the body. When solutions of differing concentrations exist on either side of these semipermeable body membranes, the pressure of crowded water molecules moves them across the membrane to help equalize the solutions on both sides. Thus we can define osmosis as the force that moves water molecules from a space of greater concentration of water molecules (hence fewer particles in solution) to a space of lesser concentration of water molecules (hence more particles in solution). The effect of this movement is to distribute water molecules more evenly throughout the body—water balance—and thus provide a solvent base for materials the water must carry.

Diffusion. The force of diffusion operates in a similar way to osmosis but applies instead to the particles in solution in the water. It is the force by which these particles move outward in all directions from a space of greater concentration of particles to a space of lesser concentration of particles. The relative movements of water molecules and solute particles in the water by osmosis and diffusion effectively balance solution concentrations, and hence pressures,

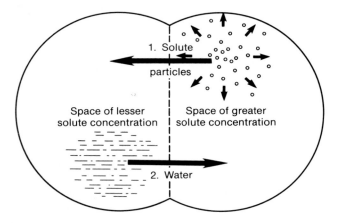

❖ **Fig. 8-2**

Movement of molecules, water, and solutes by osmosis and diffusion.

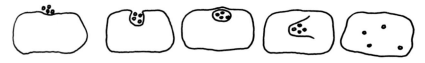

❖ **Fig. 8-3**

Pinocytosis—engulfing of large molecules by the cell.

on both sides of the separating membrane. These two balancing forces of osmosis and diffusion are shown in Fig. 8-2.

Filtration. Water is forced or filtered through the pores of membranes when there is a difference in pressures on the two sides of the membrane. This difference in pressure results from the differences in concentration of particles in the two solutions. It would cause water and small particles to move in the direction of the greater pressure.

Active transport. Particles in solution that are vital to body processes must move across membranes throughout the body at all times, even when the pressures are against their flow. Thus some means of energy-driven *active transport* are necessary to carry these particles "upstream" across the separating membranes. Usually these active transport mechanisms require some sort of carrier partner to help "ferry" them across the membrane. For example, glucose enters absorbing cells through an active transport mechanism involving sodium (Na^+) as a "ferrying" partner.

Pinocytosis. Sometimes larger particles, such as proteins and fats, enter absorbing cells by the process of *pinocytosis* (Fig. 8-3). This term means "cell drinking." In this process larger molecules attach themselves to the thicker cell membrane and are then engulfed by the cell. In this way they are carried into the center of the cell membrane and across it into the cell. For example, this is one of the mechanisms by which fat is absorbed from the small intestine.

Tissue water circulation: capillary fluid shift mechanism

One of the most important controls in the body that maintains overall water balance throughout is the *capillary fluid shift mechanism*. Its purpose is to nourish the life of the cell. It operates a balancing act between opposing fluid pressures.

Purpose. Water and other nutrients are constantly circulated through the body tissues by the blood vessels. However, to nourish cells, the water and nutrients must get out of the blood vessels—capillaries—and into the cells. Then water and the products of cell metabolism—metabolites—leaving the cell must get back into capillaries to circulate all over the body. In other words, essential water, nutrients and oxygen must be pushed out of blood circulation into tissue circulation; then water, cell metabolites, and carbon dioxide must be pulled back into the blood circulation to distribute their goods throughout the body and dispose of metabolic wastes through the kidneys. The body maintains this constant flow of water through the tissues, carrying materials to and from the cells, by means of a balance of opposing fluid pressures: *hydrostatic pressure*, an intracapillary blood pressure from the contracting muscle of the heart pushing blood into circulation, and *colloidal osmotic pressure* from the plasma proteins drawing tissue fluids back into ongoing circulation. A filtration process operates according to the differences in osmotic pressure on either side of the capillary membrane.

Process. When blood first enters the capillary system from the larger vessels coming from the heart, the arterioles, the greater blood pressure from the pumping heart muscle forces water and small particles (for example, glucose) out into the tissues to bathe and nourish the cells. This force of blood pressure is an example of *hydrostatic* pressure—*hydro-* meaning "water" and *-static* meaning "balance." Plasma protein particles, however, are too large to go through the pores of capillary membranes. When the circulating tissue fluids are ready to reenter the blood capillaries, the initial blood pressure is diminished. The *colloidal osmotic pressure* of concentrated protein particles remaining in the capillary vessel is now the greater pressure. It draws the water and its returning metabolites back into the ending capillary circulation after they have served the cells and on to the receiving larger vessels, the venules, for blood circulation back to the heart. A small amount of normal resisting tissue turgor pressure of the capillary membrane remains the same and operates throughout the system. This fundamental fluid shift mechanism constantly controls water balance through its capillary-tissue circulation to nourish cells all over the body. This vital tissue fluid flow is maintained by the balance between blood pressure and osmotic pressure of the plasma protein particles. This key balance is illustrated in Fig. 8-4.

Organ systems involved

In addition to the blood circulation, the human water balance system uses two other major organ system circulations to control overall body water balance. These are the gastrointestinal circulation, which supports digestion and absorption of nutrients, and the renal circulation, which maintains normal blood levels of various nutrients and metabolites.

Gastrointestinal circulation. Water from the blood plasma, containing vital electrolytes, is secreted constantly into the gastrointestinal tract to aid the processes of digesting our food and absorbing its nutrients. This circulation of water and electrolytes moves constantly between the blood plasma, the secreting cells, and the gastrointestinal tract. In the latter portion of the in-

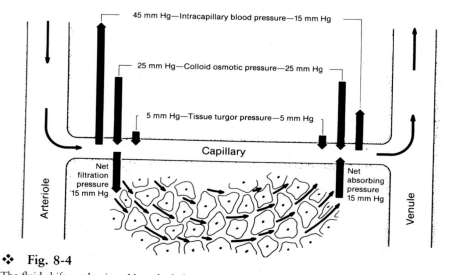

❖ **Fig. 8-4**

The fluid shift mechanism. Note the balance of pressures that controls the flow of fluid.

testine, most of the water and electrolytes are then reabsorbed into the blood to circulate over and over again. This constant movement of a large volume of water and its electrolytes among the blood, the secreting cells, and the gastrointestinal tract is called the *gastrointestinal circulation*. The sheer magnitude of this gastrointestinal circulation, as shown in Table 8-3, indicates the seriousness of fluid loss from the upper or lower portion of the gastrointestinal tract. This circulation is maintained in *isotonicity* with the surrounding water outside of cells, including the blood, and carries risk of clinical imbalances.

1. *Law of isotonicity.* The gastrointestinal fluids are part of the water compartment outside of cells, which includes the blood circulation. All of these fluids are held in *isotonicity*, meaning a state of equal osmotic pressure resulting from equal concentrations of electrolytes and other solute particles. For example, when a person drinks water, plain water without any solutes or accompanying food, electrolytes and salts enter the intestine from the surrounding blood plasma fluid to equalize pressures. If a concentrated solution of food mix is ingested, additional water will then be drawn into the intestine from the surrounding blood plasma to dilute the intestinal contents. In each instance water and electrolytes move among the parts of the extracellular fluid compartment to maintain solutions in the gastrointestinal tract that are *isotonic*,

❖ **TABLE 8-3**   *Approximate total volume of digestive secretions produced in 24 hours by an adult of average size*

Secretion	Volume (ml)
Saliva	1500
Gastric	2500
Bile	500
Pancreatic	700
Intestinal	3000
TOTAL	8200

meaning equal concentration of particles, with the surrounding fluid. If an imbalance of pressures involved continued unchecked, it would eventually draw on the intracellular fluid compartment in an effort to restore balances, creating the risk of critical cell dehydration.

2. *Clinical applications.* The law of isotonicity has many clinical implications. For example, what would happen if a patient undergoing gastric suctioning drank water? Or what would happen if a patient being fed by tube were given the formula too rapidly at too concentrated a dilution? In the first case, the water would cause the stomach to produce more secretions containing electrolytes. Then the electrolytes would be lost in the suctioning. In turn the plasma, from which the electrolytes were supplied, would be gradually depleted of these electrolytes and unable to supply them to tissue cells. In the second case, the concentrated—*hypertonic*—solution being given by tube would cause a shift of water into the intestine to dilute it, which would in turn rapidly shrink the surrounding blood volume. This condition would then produce symptoms of shock, which reflect the body's effort to restore blood volume.

Because of the large amounts of water and electrolytes involved, upper and lower gastrointestinal losses constitute the most common cause of clinical fluid and electrolyte problems. Such problems would exist, for example, in persistent vomiting or prolonged diarrhea, in which large amounts of precious water and electrolytes are lost (Box 8-1). The large numbers of electrolytes involved in gastrointestinal circulation are shown in Table 8-4.

Renal circulation. The kidneys maintain appropriate levels of all the various constituents of blood by filtering the blood and then selectively reabsorbing water and needed materials to be carried throughout the body. Through this continual "laundering" of the blood by the millions of nephrons in the kidneys, the blood is maintained in its proper solution and water balance is continued. When disease occurs in the kidneys and this filtration process does not operate normally, water imbalances occur.

Hormonal controls. Two basic hormonal controls operate in the kidneys to help maintain constant body water balance.

1. *ADH mechanism.* Antidiuretic hormone (ADH), also called *vasopressin*, is produced by the pituitary gland. It operates on the kidneys' nephrons to cause reabsorption of water. Hence it is a water-conserving mechanism. In any stress situation with threatened or real loss of body water, ADH is triggered to conserve vital body water.

2. *Aldosterone mechanism.* The hormone *aldosterone* is produced by the adrenal glands in response to a reduced renal filtration rate or decreased sodium level. It operates on the kidneys' nephrons to cause reabsorption of sodium.

❖ **TABLE 8-4** *Approximate concentration of certain electrolytes in digestive fluids (mEq/L)*

Secretion	Na$^+$	K$^+$	Cl$^-$	HCO
Saliva	10	25	10	15
Gastric	40	10	145	0
Pancreatic	140	5	40	110
Jejunal	135	5	110	30
Bile	140	10	110	40

BOX 8-1

❖ ──────── **CLINICAL APPLICATION** ──────── ❖

Principles of Oral Rehydration Therapy

The principles of electrolyte absorption are used as the basis for developing a method of rehydrating children with diarrhea. A problem usually considered trivial in Western developed countries, diarrhea is responsible worldwide for the deaths of one fourth to one half of all children under 4 years of age. Although 90% of the mortality is associated with fluid loss, the mere provision of water alone can be dangerous.

Intravenous (IV) therapy, developed by Darrow in the 1940s, provided sodium chloride, a base, and potassium in water and proved very successful. Unfortunately, IV therapy is not readily available to those who need it most. A large number of isolated poor rural families, in both developed countries such as America and developing countries around the world, lack access to health care facilities because of lack of transportation or money. Fortunately, however, the World Health Organization (WHO) has developed an *oral rehydration therapy* (ORT) that is much less expensive that is being used in the United States as well as undeveloped countries. If safe drinking water is made available, the solution can easily be mixed at home with guidance by a public health worker and administered by a family member. Its ingredients are 1 L of safe water, 3.5 g table salt (sodium chloride), 2.5 g baking soda (sodium bicarbonate), 1.5 g potassium chloride, and 20 g anhydrous glucose (2%). This oral rehydration therapy is based on principles of sodium absorption in the small intestine.

Transport of metabolic compounds. A number of metabolic compounds depend on sodium to cross the intestinal wall, principally glucose but also certain amino acids, dipeptides, and disaccharides.

Additive effects. The more substrates present, the better the absorption of sodium. The rate at which sodium is absorbed depends on the presence of substrates such as glucose or other protein metabolic products.

Water absorption. The rate of water absorption is enhanced as sodium absorption improves. Thus giving an oral solution of sodium and potassium salts plus glucose equals an IV solution, but the mixture can be given orally.

In addition to the oral rehydration therapy, infants and older children with acute diarrhea should also be fed, not undoing the added malnutrition from fasting that was based on the former belief that recovery was more effective if the bowel was allowed to rest and heal. Children should be fed their regular age diets—breastfeeding, formula, solid foods—being allowed to determine the amount of food they need and extra food as the diarrhea lessens to recover nutritional deficits, food choices should be guided by individual tolerances. Use of the old BRAT diet (bananas, rice, applesauce, and tea or toast) is not recommended because it does not include typical foods consumed by infants and small children and only compounds the energy-nutrient decline.

References

Commentary: Diarrhoeal dehydration—easy to treat but best prevented, World Health Forum 10(1):110, 1989.

Review: Feeding during diarrhea, Nutr Rev 44:102, 1986.

Roberson, LM, and others: Promoting oral rehydration therapy for acute diarrhea, J Am Diet Assoc 87(4):496, Apr 1987.

Self, TW: Pitfalls of the "BRAT" diet, Nutr and the M.D., 12:1, 1986.

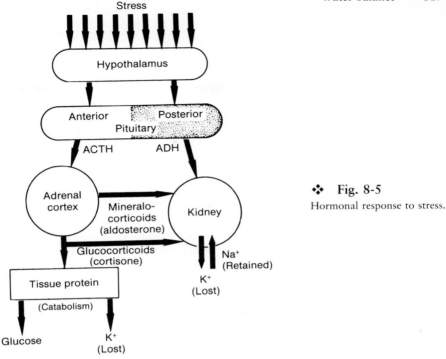

❖ **Fig. 8-5**

Hormonal response to stress.

Hence it is primarily a sodium-conserving mechanism, but in so doing it also exerts a secondary control over water reabsorption.

Both ADH and aldosterone may be activated by stress situations such as body injury or surgery (Fig. 8-5).

HUMAN ACID-BASE BALANCE SYSTEM

The optimal degree of acidity or alkalinity must be maintained in various body water solutions and secretions to support human life. This balance is achieved by solutions of both acids and bases with the correct proportions of each partner controlled by a buffer system.

Acids and bases

The concept of acids and bases relates to *hydrogen* ions, both in its measurement symbol—pH—and in its defining of the terms *acid* and *base*.

Measurement. A substance is *more or less* acid, according to the degree of its concentration of hydrogen ions. Its degree of acidity is therefore expressed in terms of **pH**. The symbol pH is derived from a mathematical term, which refers to the power of the Hydrogen ion concentration. A pH of 7 is the neutral point between an acid and a base. Since the pH is in effect a negative mathematical factor, the higher the hydrogen ion concentration (more acid), the lower the pH. In the same manner, the lower the hydrogen ion concentration (less acid), the higher the pH. Since pH 7 is the neutral point, substances with a pH *lower* than 7 are *acid*. Substances with a pH *higher* than 7 are *alkaline*. More precise definitions of acids and bases are based on the hydrogen ion concentration.

1. Acids. An acid is defined as a compound that has more hydrogen ions, enough to give some away. When in solution, it releases extra hydrogen ions.

2. *Bases.* A base is a compound that has fewer hydrogen ions. Thus in solution it takes up extra hydrogen ions, effectively reducing the solution's acidity.

Acid-base buffer system

The body deals with degrees of acidity by maintaining buffer systems to handle excess acid. A buffer system is a mixture of acidic and alkaline components, an acid partner and a base partner, which together protect a solution against wide variations in its pH, even when strong bases or acids are added to it. For example, if a strong acid is added to a buffered solution, the base partner reacts with the acid to form a weaker acid. If a strong base is added to the solution, the acid partner combines with the intruder to form a weaker base. In both cases, the pH is restored to its starting balance point.

Main buffer system. The human body contains many buffer systems because only a relatively narrow range of pH is compatible with life. However, its main one is the **carbonic acid (H_2CO_3)/base bicarbonate ($NaHCO_3$) buffer system**. The body selects this partnership as its principal buffer system for three reasons:

1. *Available materials.* The raw materials for producing the acid partner carbonic acid (H_2CO_3) are readily available. Water (H_2O) and carbon dioxide (CO_2) are always at hand.

2. *Ease of adjustment.* The lungs and the kidneys can easily adjust to changes in the acid and base partners, quickly returning the body fluids to normal pH level. The normal pH of the ECF is 7.4, with a range of 7.35 to 7.45. Maintenance of the pH within this narrow range is necessary to sustain the life of the cells.

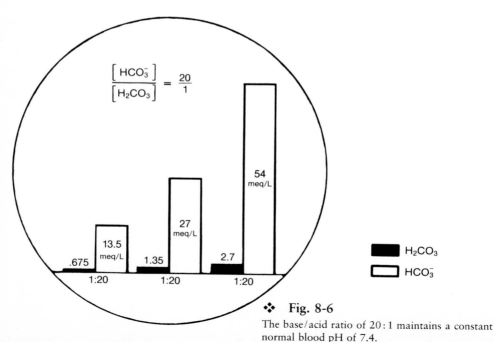

❖ **Fig. 8-6**

The base/acid ratio of 20:1 maintains a constant normal blood pH of 7.4.

3. Base-to-acid ratio. The carbonic acid/base bicarbonate buffer system is able to maintain this essential degree of acidity in the body fluids because the base bicarbonate partner in this buffer system is about 20 times as abundant as the carbonic acid partner. This **20:1 ratio** is maintained even though the absolute amounts of the two partners may fluctuate during adjustment periods. Whether or not added base or acid enters the system, as long as the 20:1 ratio is maintained, the ECF acid-base balance is held constant (Fig. 8-6). In this way the life of the cells is protected.

SUMMARY

The human body is approximately 50% to 60% water. The primary functions of body water are to give form and structure to the body tissue, provide the water environment necessary for cell work, and control body temperature. Body water is distributed in two collective body water compartments: intra-cellular and extracellular. Water inside cells is the larger portion, accounting for about 40% of the total body weight. Water outside cells consists of fluid in spaces between cells (interstitial fluid and lymph), the blood plasma, the secretions in transit such as the gastrointestinal circulation, and the smaller amount in cartilage and bone.

Overall body water balance is maintained by fluid intake and output. The distribution of body water is controlled by two types of solute particles: (1) electrolytes, mainly charged mineral elements, and (2) plasma protein, mainly albumin. These solute particles influence the movement of water across cell or capillary membranes, allowing tissue circulation to nourish cells.

The acid-base buffer system, controlled mainly by the lungs and the kidneys, uses electrolytes and hydrogen ions to maintain a normal ECF pH of about 7.4. This level is necessary to sustain cell life.

❖ REVIEW QUESTIONS

1. Why is the total body water considered a unified whole? What does the term "body compartment" mean? How does this term apply to body water balance?
2. Define the term *homeostasis*. Give examples of how this state is maintained in the body.
3. List and describe five functions of body water. Describe five factors that influence water requirements to supply these body water functions.
4. Apply your present knowledge of the capillary fluid shift mechanism to account for the gross body edema seen in starving children.

❖ SELF-TEST QUESTIONS

Matching
Match the terms provided below with the corresponding items listed here:

_____ 1. Chief electrolyte guarding the water outside of cells.
_____ 2. An ion carrying a negative electrical charge.
_____ 3. Sodium-conserving mechanism or control agent.
_____ 4. Simple passage of water molecules through a membrane separating so-lutions of different concentrations, from the side of lower concentration of solute particles to that of higher concentration of particles, thus tending to equalize the solutions.
_____ 5. A substance (element or compound) that, in solution, conducts an electrical current and is dissociated into cations and anions.

_____ 6. Particles in solution, such as electrolytes and protein.
_____ 7. State of dynamic equilibrium maintained by an organism among all its parts and controlled by many finely balanced mechanisms.
_____ 8. Chief electrolyte guarding the water inside of cells.
_____ 9. Major plasma protein that guards and maintains the blood volume.
_____ 10. Abnormal increase in water held in body tissues.
_____ 11. An ion carrying a positive electrical charge.
_____ 12. The body's means of maintaining tissue water circulation by means of opposing fluid pressures.
_____ 13. Force exerted by a contained fluid, for example, blood pressure.
_____ 14. Movement of particles throughout a solution and across membranes from from the area of denser concentration of particles outward to all surrounding spaces.
_____ 15. A type of fluid outside of cells.
_____ 16. Movement of particles in solution across cell membranes against normal osmotic pressures, involving a carrier and energy for the work.

a. Osmosis
b. Solutes
c. Diffusion
d. Cation
e. Interstitial fluid
f. Homeostasis
g. Anion
h. K^+

i. Albumin
j. Hydrostatic pressure
k. Na^+
l. Electrolyte
m. Active transport
n. Aldosterone
o. Capillary fluid shift mechanism
p. Edema

❖ SUGGESTIONS FOR ADDITIONAL STUDY

1. Keep a 3-day record of your total fluid intake from any sources, including water. Note the circumstances in which you took in these fluids. How did thirst influence your intake? Evaluate your intake in terms of total amount of fluid consumed and the nutrients contributed by each source.
2. Observe some type of athletic competition. What provision do you see to cover water loss by the participants? Does it appear to be adequate? Why would athletes require increased water intake? Record your observations and discuss them in class.

References

1. Cannon WB: The wisdom of the body, New York, 1932, W W Norton and Co, Inc.
2. Randall HT: Water, electrolytes, and acid-base balance. In Shils ME and Young VR, editors: Modern nutrition in health and disease, ed 7, Philadelphia, 1988, Lea & Febiger.
3. National Research Council, Food and Nutrition Board: Recommended dietary allowances, ed 10, Washington, DC, 1989, National Academy Press.

Further reading

McCleary K: The fitness report: when water works and when it doesn't, Am Health 5(5):26, 1986.

This is a helpful article describing the need for more water for activities in the summer's heat, especially the dangers of dehydration and water intoxication.

Robinson JR: Water, the indispensable nutrient, Nutr Today 5(1):16, 1970.

This now classic but still current article by a world authority New Zealand physician describes clearly the processes involved in body water balance. It is filled with excellent charts and diagrams to illustrate key principles.

9

❖

Digestion and absorption

K E Y   C O N C E P T S

*Through a balanced system of mechanical and chemical change, our
food is broken down into simpler substances and its nutrients
released and reformed for the body's use.*

*Special organ structures and functions conduct these changes
through the successive parts of the overall system.*

$\mathcal{A}$ s described earlier, the nutrients our bodies require do
not come to us ready to use. Instead they come packaged as foods in a wide
variety of forms. Our body cells cannot use nutrients in these forms, and our
foods need to be changed to simpler substances. In the process we must free
the food nutrients, reform and reroute them for our special life needs.

In this chapter we see how this marvelous process of change takes place.
We view the overall process of food digestion and nutrient absorption as one
continuous *whole* made up of a series of successive events. Throughout we
review the unique body structures and functions that make all of this process—
and our lives—possible.

DIGESTION
Basic principles

Principle of change. Foods as we eat them cannot be used by our body
cells. They must be changed into simpler substances and then into other, still
simpler, substances that our cells can use to sustain our lives. Preparing food

for our body's use involves many changes that make up the overall digestion-absorption-metabolism process.

1. *Digestion* is the process that breaks up food in the gastrointestinal tract, releasing many nutrients in forms the body can use.

2. *Absorption* is the process that carries these many nutrients into the body's circulation system and delivers them to the cells.

3. *Cell metabolism* is the sum of the vast number of chemical changes in the cell—the functional unit of life—that finally produces the essential materials we need for energy, tissue building, and metabolic controls.

Principle of wholeness. The parts of this overall process of change do not exist separately. They make up one continuous *whole*. The different parts of the gastrointestinal tract and their relative positions in the overall system are shown in Fig. 9-1. Food components travel *together* through this system for delivery to the cells.

Mechanical and chemical changes

In order for nutrients to be delivered to cells, the food we eat must go through a series of mechanical and chemical changes. These two types of actions, working together, make up the overall process of digestion.

Mechanical digestion: gastrointestinal motility. Muscles and nerves in the walls of the gastrointestinal tract coordinate their actions to provide the necessary motility for digestion to proceed. The word *motility* means the ability to move spontaneously. This automatic response to the presence of food enables the system to break up the food mass and move it along the digestive pathway at the best rate. Muscles and nerves work together to produce this smoothly running motility.

1. *Muscles.* The layers of smooth muscle making up the gastrointestinal wall interact to provide two general types of movement: (1) *muscle tone* or tonic contraction, which ensures continuous passage of the food mass and valve control along the way; and (2) *periodic muscle contraction and relaxation*, in rhythmic waves, which mix the food mass and move it forward. These alternating muscular contractions and relaxations that force the contents forward are known as *peristalsis*, a term from two Greek words—*peri-* meaning "around" and *-stalsis* meaning "contraction."

2. *Nerves.* Specific nerves regulate these muscle actions. A complex network of nerves within the gastrointestinal wall extends from the esophagus to the anus. These nerves do three things: (1) control muscle tone in the wall, (2) regulate the rate and intensity of the alternating muscle contractions, and (3) coordinate all of the various movements. When all is well, these finely tuned movements flow together like those of a great symphony and you are unaware of them. But when all is not well, you feel the discord as pain.

Chemical digestion: gastrointestinal secretions. A number of secretions work together to make chemical digestion possible. Generally, there are five types of substances involved, the basic enzymes that break down the food materials, and four other substances that help them do their specific jobs.

1. *Enzymes.* Digestive enzymes are proteins, specific in kind and quantity for the breaking down of specific nutrients.

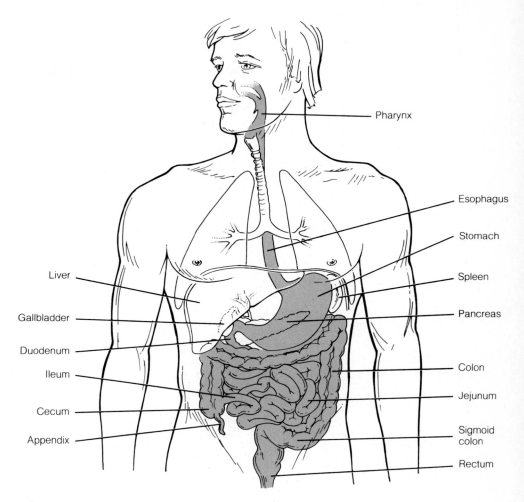

Pharynx

Esophagus

Stomach

Liver

Spleen

Gallbladder

Pancreas

Duodenum

Ileum

Colon

Cecum

Jejunum

Appendix

Sigmoid
colon

Rectum

❖ **FIG. 9-1**

The gastrointestinal system. Through the successive parts of the system, multiple activities of
digestion liberate and reform food nutrients to our use.

2. Hydrochloric acid and buffer ions. Hydrochloric acid and buffer ions
are needed to produce the pH, degree of acidity or alkalinity, required for
enzyme activity.

3. Mucus. Secretions of mucus lubricate and protect the mucosal tissues
lining the gastrointestinal tract and also aid in mixing the food mass.

4. Water and electrolytes. The products of digestion are carried and circulated through the tract and into the tissues by water and electrolytes.

5. Bile. Made in the liver and stored in the gallbladder, bile divides fat into
smaller pieces to expose more surface area for the fat enzyme actions.

Special secretory cells in the intestinal tract itself and in nearby accessory
organs—pancreas and liver—produce these secretions for their specific jobs

in chemical digestion. The secretory action of these special cells or glands is stimulated by (1) the presence of food, (2) nerve impulse, or (3) hormones specific for certain nutrients.

Digestion in the mouth and esophagus

Mechanical digestion. In the mouth the process of *mastication*, biting and chewing, begins to break up the food into smaller particles. The teeth and oral structures are particularly suited for this work. After the food is chewed, the mixed mass of food particles is swallowed and passes down the esophagus largely by peristaltic waves controlled by nerve reflexes. Muscles at the base of the tongue help the swallowing process. Then, in the usual upright position, gravity aids the movement of food down the esophagus. At the entry into the stomach, the gastroesophageal sphincter muscle controlling food passage relaxes to allow the food to enter, then constricts again to retain the food. If this muscle does not work properly, or if a part of the stomach protrudes upward into the chest (thorax) causing the fairly common *hiatal hernia*, the person feels "heartburn" after eating, from the bit of now acid-mixed food pushed back up into the lower esophagus. This condition, of course, has nothing to do with the heart, but has been called this because sensations are perceived as originating in the region of the heart.

Chemical digestion. The salivary glands secrete material containing a **salivary amylase** called *ptyalin*. *Amylase* is the general name for any starch-splitting enzyme. However, in this case the food remains in the mouth too briefly for much chemical action to occur. The salivary glands also secrete a mucous material that lubricates and binds food particles to help in swallowing each food *bolus*, or lump of food material. Mucous glands also line the esophagus, and their secretions help move the food mass toward the stomach.

Digestion in the stomach

Mechanical digestion. The major parts of the stomach are shown in Fig. 9-2. Under sphincter muscle control from the esophagus, joining the stomach at the cardiac notch, the food enters the *fundus*, the upper portion of the stomach, in individual bolus lumps swallowed. In the body of the stomach, muscles in the stomach wall gradually knead, store, mix, and propel the food mass forward in slow, controlled movements. By the time the food mass reaches the *antrum*, the lower portion of the stomach, it is now a semiliquid acid food mix called **chyme**. A constricting sphincter muscle at the end of the stomach, the *pyloric valve*, controls the flow at this point. It releases the acid chyme slowly so that it can be buffered quickly by the alkaline intestinal secretions and not irritate the mucosal lining of the *duodenum*, the first section of the small intestine. The caloric density of a meal, due mainly to its fat component, not just its volume or particular composition, influences the rate of stomach emptying at the pyloric valve.[1]

Chemical digestion. The gastric secretions contain three types of materials that aid chemical digestion in the stomach.

1. Acid. Special cells produce hydrochloric acid to create the necessary degree of acidity for gastric enzymes to work.

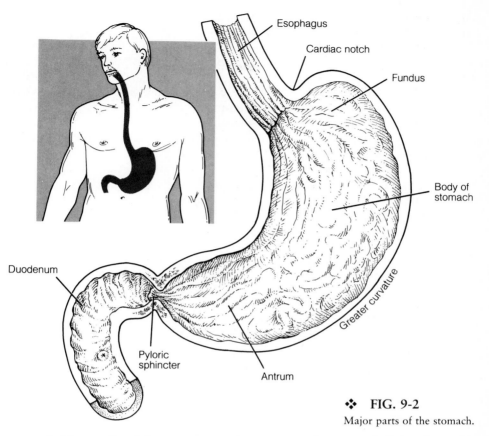

❖ **FIG. 9-2**

Major parts of the stomach.

2. Mucus. Special mucous secretions protect the stomach lining from the eroding effect of the acid. Secretions also bind and mix the food mass and help move it along.

3. Enzymes. The inactive enzyme form *pepsinogen* is secreted by special cells and activated by the acid to the major protein-splitting enzyme **pepsin**. Still other cells produce small amounts of a specific **gastric lipase** called *tributyrinase* because it works on tributyrin (butterfat). *Lipase* is the general name of all fat-splitting enzymes. However, this is a relatively minor activity here in the stomach.

Various sensations, emotions, and food intake stimulate nerve impulses that trigger these secretions. It is not without reason that the stomach is said to "mirror the person within." For example, anger and hostility increase secretions. Fear and depression decrease secretions and inhibit blood flow and motility as well. Additional hormonal stimulus comes with entrance of food into the stomach.

Digestion in the small intestine

Up to this point, digestion of food consumed has been largely mechanical, delivering to the small intestine a semifluid mixture of fine food particles and watery secretions. Chemical digestion has been minimal. Thus the major task of digestion, and of absorption that follows, occurs in the small intestine. Its structural parts, its synchronized movements, and its array of specific enzymes are highly developed for this all-important final task of mechanical and chemical digestion.

Mechanical digestion. Under the control of nerve impulses, wall stretch from the food mass, or hormonal stimuli, the intestinal muscles produce several types of movement that aid digestion.

1. Peristaltic waves push the food mass slowly forward, sometimes with long sweeping waves over the entire length of the intestine.

2. Pendular movements from small local muscles sweep back and forth, stirring the chyme at the mucosal surface.

3. Segmentation rings from alternate contraction and relaxation of circular muscles progressively chop the food mass into successive soft lumps and mix them with secretions.

4. Longitudinal rotation by long muscles running the length of the intestine rolls the slowly moving food mass in a spiral motion, mixing it and exposing new surfaces for absorption.

5. Motion of surface villi stirs and mixes chyme at the intestinal wall, exposing additional nutrient material for absorption.

Chemical digestion. To meet the major burden of chemical digestion, this portion of the gastrointestinal system, together with its accessory organs—the pancreas, liver, and gallbladder—supplies many secretory materials.

1. Enzymes from intestinal glands

CARBOHYDRATE. **Disaccharidases** (maltase, lactase, sucrase) convert their respective disaccharides (maltose, lactose, sucrose) to the monosaccharides (glucose, fructose, galactose). A majority of the world's population actually produces insufficient lactase to digest lactose (milk sugar) and cannot tolerate milk and milk products very well, unless they are in some "predigested" form, such as yogurt, buttermilk, or cheese, or lactase-treated milk.

PROTEIN. The intestinal enzyme enterokinase activates trypsinogen (from the pancreas) to the protein-splitting enzyme trypsin. **Amino peptidase** removes the end amino acid from polypeptides. **Dipeptidase** splits dipeptides into their two remaining amino acids.

FAT. **Intestinal lipase** splits fat into glycerides and fatty acids.

2. Enzymes from the pancreas

CARBOHYDRATE. **Pancreatic amylase** converts starch to the dissacharides maltose and sucrose.

PROTEIN. **Trypsin** and **chymotrypsin** split large protein molecules into smaller and smaller peptide fragments and finally into single amino acids. **Carboxypeptidase** removes an end amino acid from peptide chains.

FAT. **Pancreatic lipase** converts fat to glycerides and fatty acids.

3. Mucus. Large quantities of mucus, secreted by intestinal glands, protect the mucosal lining from irritation and erosion by the highly acidic gastric contents entering the duodenum.

4. Bile. An important aid to fat digestion and absorption is the emulsifying agent bile. It is produced by the liver and stored in the adjacent gallbladder, ready for use when fat enters the intestine.

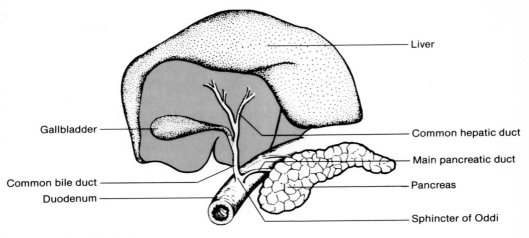

❖ **FIG. 9-3**

Organs of the biliary system and the pancreatic ducts.

5. *Hormones.* The hormone *secretin*, produced by mucosal glands in the first part of the intestine, controls secretion of enzymes from the pancreas and their acidity. The resulting alkaline environment in the small intestine— pH 8—is necessary for activity of the pancreatic enzymes. The hormone *cholecystokinin*, secreted by intestinal mucosal glands when fat enters, triggers release of bile from the gallbladder to emulsify the fat.

The arrangement of the accessory organs to the duodenum, the first section of the small intestine, is shown in Fig. 9-3. These organs comprise the biliary system and have vital roles in digestion and metabolism. The liver especially is sometimes called the "metabolic capital" of the body with numerous functions in the metabolism of all the converging nutrients. The portal blood circulation drains the small intestine directly to the liver for immediate cell enzyme work in energy production, protein metabolism, and rapid conversion of fat into lipoproteins for transport to body cells. A metabolic "pool" of nutrients and metabolites is maintained for constant cell supply and special provision for metabolic waste removal, such as the unique **urea cycle** for the ultimate removal of nitrogen and maintenance of nitrogen balance. The liver's many metabolic functions are reviewed in greater detail in Chapter 18.

The various nerve and hormone controls of digestion are illustrated in Fig. 9-4. Although small individual summaries of digestion are given in each of the chapters on major nutrients, a general summary of the entire digestive processes is given in Table 9-1 to help view the overall process as it is—one continuous integrated *whole.*

ABSORPTION

When digestion is complete, our original food is changed into simple end products that are the nutrients ready for the cells to use. Carbohydrate foods are reduced to the *simple sugars* glucose, fructose, and galactose. Fats are transformed into *fatty acids* and *glycerides.* Protein foods are changed to single *amino acids.* Vitamins and minerals are also liberated. With a water base for

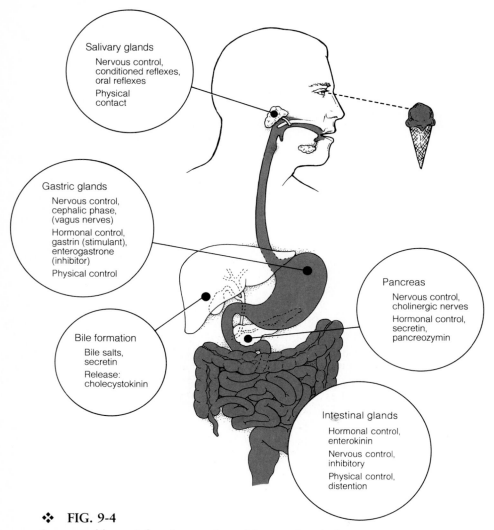

❖ FIG. 9-4

Summary of factors influencing secretions of the gastrointestinal tract.

solution and transport plus the necessary electrolytes, the total fluid food-derived mass is now prepared for absorption as part of the large "gastrointestinal circulation." The large 10-liter volume of this daily circulating absorption is shown in Table 9-2. For many nutrients, especially certain vitamins and minerals, the point of absorption becomes the vital "gatekeeper" that determines how much of a given nutrient will be kept for body use.[2] This degree of *bioavailability* is a factor in setting dietary intake standards.[3,4]

Absorption in the small intestine

Special absorbing structures. Three important structures of the surface of the intestinal wall are particularly adapted to ensure maximum absorption of essential nutrients freed from food in the digestive process (Fig. 9-5).

❖ **TABLE 9-1** *Summary of digestive processes*

	Carbohydrate	Protein	Fat
Mouth	Starch $\xrightarrow{\text{Ptyalin}}$ Dextrins		
Stomach		Protein $\xrightarrow[\text{Hydrochloric acid}]{\text{Pepsin}}$ Polypeptides	Tributyrin (butterfat) $\xrightarrow{\text{Tributyrinase}}$ Glycerol, Fatty acids
Small intestine	*Pancreas* (Disaccharides)	*Pancreas*	*Pancreas*
	Starch $\xrightarrow{\text{Amylase}}$ Maltose and sucrose	Protein, Polypeptides $\xrightarrow{\text{Trypsin}}$ Dipeptides	Fat $\xrightarrow{\text{Lipase}}$ Glycerol, Glycerides (di-, mono-), Fatty acids
	Intestine (Monosaccharides)	Protein, Polypeptides $\xrightarrow{\text{Chymotrypsin}}$ Dipeptides	*Intestine*
	Lactose $\xrightarrow{\text{Lactase}}$ Glucose and galactose	Polypeptides, Dipeptides $\xrightarrow{\text{Carboxypeptidase}}$ Amino acids	Fat $\xrightarrow{\text{Lipase}}$ Glycerol, Glycerides (di-, mono-), Fatty acids
	Sucrose $\xrightarrow{\text{Sucrase}}$ Glucose and fructose	*Intestine*	*Liver and gallbladder*
	Maltose $\xrightarrow{\text{Maltase}}$ Glucose and glucose	Polypeptides, Dipeptides $\xrightarrow{\text{Aminopeptidase}}$ Amino acids	Fat $\xrightarrow{\text{Bile}}$ Emulsified fat
		Dipeptides $\xrightarrow{\text{Dipeptidase}}$ Amino acids	

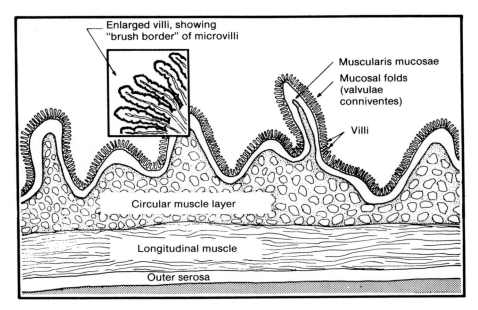

Enlarged villi, showing "brush border" of microvilli

Muscularis mucosae

Mucosal folds (valvulae conniventes)

Villi

Circular muscle layer

Longitudinal muscle

Outer serosa

❖ **FIG. 9-5**

Intestinal wall. Note the arrangement of muscle layers and the structures of the mucosa that increase the surface area for absorption—mucosal folds, villi, and microvilli.

❖ **TABLE 9-2**   *Daily absorption volume in human gastrointestinal system*

	Intake (L)	Intestinal absorption (L)	Elimination (L)
Food ingested	1.5		
Gastrointestinal secretions	8.5		
TOTAL	10.0		
Fluid absorbed in small intestine		9.5	
Fluid absorbed in large intestine		0.4	
TOTAL		9.9	
Feces			.01

1. *Mucosal folds.* Like so many hills and valleys in a mountain range, the surface of the small intestine piles into many folds. These folds can easily be seen when such tissue is examined.

2. *Villi.* Closer examination by a regular light microscope reveals small fingerlike projections, the **villi**, covering these piled-up folds of mucosal lining. These little villi further increase the area of exposed surface. Each villus has an ample supply of blood vessels to receive protein and carbohydrate materials, and a special lymph vessel to receive fat materials. This lymph vessel is called a *lacteal* because the fatty chyme at this point is creamy and looks like milk.

3. *Microvilli.* Still closer examination with an electron microscope reveals

a multiple covering of still smaller projections on the surface of each tiny villus. This covering of **microvilli** on each minute villus is called a *brush border* because it looks like bristles on a brush.

These three unique structures of the inner intestinal wall—folds, villi, and microvilli—combine to make the inner surface some 600 times the area of the outer surface of the intestine. Also, the length of the small intestine is about 660 cm (22 feet). It is evident that this remarkable organ is well adapted to deliver its precious nutrients to the body cells. In fact, as a feat in providing such a tremendous absorbing surface area in so compact a space, it can scarcely be equaled. It has been estimated that if this entire surface were spread out on a flat plane, the total surface area would be as large or larger than half a basketball court. Far from being the lowly "gut," this is actually one of the most highly developed, exquisitely fashioned, specialized tissues in the human body.

Absorption processes. A number of absorbing processes complete the task of moving vital nutrients across the inner intestinal wall and into body circulation. These processes include diffusion, both passive or simple for small materials and carrier-assisted for larger items, energy-driven active transport with the help of a "ferrying" substance, and penetration of larger materials through engulfing pinocytosis. (See Chapter 8.)

Routes of absorption. Most of the products of digestion are water-soluble nutrients and so can be absorbed directly into the bloodstream. Since fatty materials are not water-soluble, another route must be provided. These fat molecules pass into the lymph vessels in the villi, the lacteals, flow into the larger lymph vessels of the body, and eventually enter the blood.

Absorption in the large intestine

Water. The main absorption task remaining for the large intestine is that of taking up needed body water. The major portion of the water in the chyme entering the large intestine is absorbed in the first half of the colon. Only a small amount remains, about 100 ml, to form and eliminate the feces.

Dietary fiber. Food fiber is not digested because humans lack the specific enzymes required. However, dietary fiber contributes important bulk to the food mass throughout the digestion-absorption process and helps to form the feces. The formation and passage of intestinal gas is a normal process but embarrassing to some persons (Box 9-1).

Table 9-3 summarizes major features of intestinal nutrient absorption.

SUMMARY

Necessary nutrients as they occur in food are not available to us. They must be changed, released, regrouped, and rerouted in forms our body cells can use. Two closely related activities—digestion and absorption—ensure delivery of key food nutrients to the cells for their multiple metabolic tasks that sustain our lives.

Mechanical digestion consists of spontaneous muscular activity that is responsible for (1) initial mechanical breakdown by such means as mastication, and (2) movement of the food mass along the gastrointestinal tract by such

---

BOX 9-1

❖ ——————— **CLINICAL APPLICATION** ——————— ❖

Digestion-Absorption's Sometimes Embarrassing Effects

A common complaint of many persons after eating a meal or certain foods is the discomfort, and sometimes embarrassment, of "gas." This gas is a normal by-product of digestion, but when it becomes painful or apparent to others it may become a physical and social problem.

The gastrointestinal tract normally holds about 3 ounces of gas, moving along with the food mass and silently absorbed into the bloodstream. Sometimes extra gas collects in the stomach or intestine, creating an embarrassing, though usually harmless, situation.

Stomach gas

Gas in the stomach results from uncomfortable air bubbles trapped there. It occurs when a person eats too fast, drinks through a straw, or otherwise takes in extra air while eating. Burping relieves it. But these tips may help to avoid this social slip:

- Avoid carbonated beverages
- Don't gulp
- Chew with your mouth closed
- Don't drink from a can or through a straw
- Don't eat when you're nervous

Intestinal gas

The passing of gas from the intestine is usually a social embarrassment. This gas is formed in the colon, where bacteria attack nondigested items, causing them to decompose and produce gas. Carbohydrates release hydrogen, carbon dioxide, and in some people with certain types of bacteria in the gut, *methane*. All three of these products are odorless (though noisy) gases. Protein produces *hydrogen sulfide* and such volatile compounds as *indole* and *skatole*, which add a distinctive aroma to the expelled air. However, these suggestions may help control the problem:

- Cut down on simple carbohydrates—sugars. Especially observe milk's effect because *lactose intolerance* may be the real culprit. Substitute cultured forms such as yogurt or milk treated with a lactase product such as LactAid.
- Eliminate known food offenders. These vary among individuals but some of the most common ones are beans, onions, cabbage, and high-fiber wheat products.

Once relief is achieved, add more complex carbohydrates and high-fiber foods back to the diet—*slowly*. Once small amounts are tolerated, try moderate increases. If there is still no relief, medical help may be needed to rule out or treat an overactive gastrointestinal tract.

---

motions as peristalsis. Chemical digestion involves enzymatic action that breaks food down into smaller and smaller components and releases its nutrients for absorption.

Absorption involves the passage of food nutrients from the intestines to the bloodstream across the intestinal wall. It occurs mainly in the small intestine by means of highly efficient intestinal wall structures that greatly increase the absorbing surface area, together with a number of effective absorbing mechanisms.

❖ **TABLE 9-3**   *Intestinal absorption of some major nutrients*

Nutrient	Form	Means of absorption	Control agent or required cofactor	Route
Carbohydrate	Monosaccharides (glucose and galactose)	Competitive	—	Blood
		Selective	—	
		Active transport via sodium pump	Sodium	
Protein	Amino acids	Selective	—	Blood
	Some dipeptides	Carrier transport systems	Pyridoxine (pyridoxal phosphate)	Blood
	Whole protein (rare)	Pinocytosis	—	Blood
Fat	Fatty acids	Fatty acid-bile complex (micelles)	Bile	Lymph
	Glycerides (mono-, di-)		—	Lymph
	Few triglycerides (neutral fat)	Pinocytosis	—	Lymph
Vitamins	B_{12}	Carrier transport	Intrinsic factor (IF)	Blood
	A	Bile complex	Bile	Blood
	K	Bile complex	Bile	From large intestine to blood
Minerals	Sodium	Active transport via sodium pump	—	Blood
	Calcium	Active transport	Vitamin D	Blood
	Iron	Active transport	Ferritin mechanism	Blood (as transferritin)
Water	Water	Osmosis	—	Blood, lymph, interstitial fluid

❖ REVIEW QUESTIONS

1. Describe the types of muscle movement involved in mechanical digestion. What does the word "motility" mean? How are the nerves involved?
2. Identify digestive enzymes and any related substances secreted by the following glands: salivary, mucosal, pancreas, and liver. What activity do they perform on carbohydrates, proteins, and fats? What stimulates their release? What inhibits their activity?

3. Describe four mechanisms of nutrient absorption from the small intestine. Describe the routes taken by the breakdown products of carbohydrates, proteins, and fats after absorption. Why must an alternate route to the bloodstream be provided?
4. What functions does the large intestine perform?

❖ SELF-TEST QUESTIONS

True-false

For each item you answer "false," write the correct statement.

1. The digestive products of a large meal are difficult to absorb because the overall area of the intestinal absorbing surface is relatively small.
2. Some enzymes must be activated by hydrochloric acid or other enzymes before they can work.
3. Bile is a specific enzyme for fat breakdown.
4. The "gastrointestinal circulation" provides a constant supply of water and electrolytes to carry digestive secretions and substances being produced.
5. Secretions from the gastrointestinal accessory organs, the gallbladder and the pancreas, mix with gastric secretions to aid digestion.
6. One enzyme may work on more than one nutrient.
7. Bile is released from the gallbladder in response to hormonal stimulus.

Multiple choice

1. During digestion the major muscle action that moves the food mass forward by regular rhythmic waves is called:
   a. Valve contraction
   b. Segmentation ring motion
   c. Muscle tone
   d. Peristalsis
2. Gastrointestinal secretory action is triggered by:
   (1) Hormones
   (2) Enzymes
   (3) Nerve network
   (4) Senses of sight, smell, taste
       a. 1 and 2
       b. 2 and 4
       c. 1, 3, and 4
       d. 2 and 3
3. Mucus is an important gastrointestinal secretion because it:
   a. Causes chemical changes in substances to prepare for enzyme action.
   b. Helps create proper degree of acidity for enzymes to act.
   c. Lubricates and protects the gastrointestinal lining.
   d. Helps to emulsify fats for enzyme action.
4. Pepsin is:
   a. Produced in the small intestine to act on protein.
   b. A gastric enzyme that acts on protein.
   c. Produced in the pancreas to act on fat.
   d. Produced in the small intestine to act on fat.
5. Bile is an important secretion that is:
   a. Produced by the gallbladder.
   b. Stored in the liver.
   c. An aid to protein digestion.
   d. A fat emulsifying agent.

6. The route of fat absorption is:
   a. The lymphatic system via the villi lacteals.
   b. Directly into the portal blood circulation.
   c. With the aid of bile directly into the villi blood capillaries.
   d. With the aid of protein directly into the portal blood circulation.

❖ SUGGESTIONS FOR ADDITIONAL STUDY

1. On 3 successive days eat the following breakfasts:
   Day 1: All fruit breakfast. Eat several fruits and fruit juices only.
   Day 2: Eat only fruit juice, one or two slices of white toast with jelly, and hot tea or coffee with sugar.
   Day 3: Eat only one or two slices of toast with a generous amount of butter or margarine, two to four slices of bacon, two eggs scrambled in the bacon fat, and tea or coffee with cream.
2. On each day, record the time that you first felt hungry. Compare each breakfast's food combination. Which food combination satisfied you for the longest period of time? How do you account for this difference?

References

1. Wilson PC and Greene HL: The gastrointestinal tract: portal to nutrient utilization. In Shils ME and Young VR, editors: Modern nutrition and disease, ed 7, Philadelphia, 1988, Lea & Febiger.
2. Sauberlich HE: Vitamins—how much is for keeps? Nutr Today 22(1):20, 1987.
3. National Research Council, Food and Nutrition Board: Recommended dietary allowances, ed 10, Washington, DC, 1989, National Academy Press.
4. National Research Council, Food and Nutrition Board, Committee on diet and health: Diet and health, implications for reducing chronic disease risks, Washington, DC, 1989, National Academy Press.

Further Reading

Fosmire GJ: Possible hazards associated with zinc supplementation, Nutr Today 24(3):15, 1989.

Johnson MA and Kays SE: Copper: Its role in human nutrition, Nutr Today 25(1):6, 1990.

Sauberlich HE: Vitamins—how much is for keeps? Nutr Today 22(1):20, 1987.

Thomson ABR: Intestinal aspects of lipid absorption, Nutr Today 24(4):16, 1989.

These articles from the well-known journal *Nutrition Today* provide good reviews of the many factors that influence the absorption of key nutrients. Fosmire describes the induced deficiency of copper by large supplemental doses of zinc as they compete for absorbing sites. Johnson and Kays review the interrelated homeostatic controls of copper absorption. Sauberlich explains how vital balance of nutrients such as vitamins is controlled at the absorption point. Thomson explains the complexities of lipid absorption and the relation of these processes to health.

CHAPTER 10

Nutrition during pregnancy and lactation

KEY CONCEPTS

The mother's food habits and nutritional status before conception, as well as during her pregnancy, influence the pregnancy's outcome.

Pregnancy is a prime example of physiologic synergism in which mother, fetus, and placenta collaborate to sustain and nurture new life.

Through the food a pregnant woman eats, she gives to her unborn child the nourishment required to begin and sustain fetal growth and development.

Through her diet, a breast-feeding woman continues to provide all the nutritional needs of her nursing baby.

*H*ealthy body tissues depend directly on certain essential nutrients in food. This is especially true during pregnancy because a whole new body is being formed. The tremendous growth of a baby from the moment of conception to the time of birth depends entirely on nourishment from the mother's food. The complex processes of rapid, specialized human growth demand increased amounts of nutrients from the mother.

In this chapter we look at the beginnings of life. We see that the infant's fetal development and the maternal supporting tissues relate directly to the mother's diet. We explore these nutritional needs of pregnancy and the lactation period that follows and recognize the vital role they play in producing a healthy infant.

MATERNAL NUTRITION AND THE OUTCOME OF PREGNANCY

Not many years ago, traditional practices and diet during pregnancy were highly restrictive in nature, built on assumptions and folklore of the past, having little or no basis in scientific fact. Early obstetricians had even developed the incredible notion that semistarvation of the mother during pregnancy was a blessing in disguise because it produced a small, lightweight baby who was easy to deliver. To this end they used a diet restricted in kcalories, protein, water, and salt.

Developments in both nutritional and medical science have refuted these prior false ideas and laid a sound base for positive nutrition in current maternal care. However, old dogma dies hard. Shreds of the old beliefs are sometimes still in evidence, but do not be misled by these false concepts. We now know that it is very important to the health of both mother and child that a prospective mother eat a well-balanced diet with increased amounts of all the essential nutrients. In fact, the woman who has always eaten a well-balanced diet is in a good state of nutrition at conception before she even knows she is pregnant. This woman has a better chance of having a healthy baby and of remaining in good health herself than the woman who has been undernourished.

POSITIVE NUTRITIONAL DEMANDS OF PREGNANCY

The 9 months between the time of conception and the birth of a fully formed baby is a marvelous period of rapid growth and intricate functional development. All of these tremendous activities require increased energy and nutrient support to produce a positive healthy outcome. General guidelines for these increases are provided in the RDA standard (see tables inside book covers).[1,2]

The RDA guidelines are based on general needs for healthy populations. Individual women, such as those poorly nourished when they become pregnant or those carrying additional risks (p. 143), demand more nutritional support. First, we will review the basic nutritional needs for positive support of a normal pregnancy, with emphasis on critical energy and protein requirements and key mineral and vitamin needs. In each case, there are reasons for the increased demand, the general amount of that increase, and food sources to supply it. In the following section we will underscore the importance of sufficient weight gain and the problems facing high-risk mothers and infants.

Energy needs

Reasons for increased need. The energy intake during pregnancy is measured in terms of the kcalorie value of the food the mother eats. She needs more kcalories for two important reasons: (1) to supply the increased fuel demanded by the enlarged metabolic workload, and (2) to spare protein for the added tissue-building requirements. At least 36 kcal/kg is required for efficient use of protein during pregnancy. For these reasons, the mother must have more food, especially more nutrient-dense food.

Amount of energy increase. The RDA standard recommends an increase of about 300 kcalories during pregnancy. This amounts to about a 15% to 20% increase over the previous prepregnant energy need, from 2200 to about 2500 kcalories. Even more is needed by an active, large, or nutritionally deficient woman, who may require as many as 2700 to 3000 kcalories. The emphasis should always be a positive one on ample kcalories to secure the necessary nutrient and energy needs. Sufficient weight gain is vital to a successful pregnancy, and will indicate whether or not sufficient kcalories are provided.

Protein needs

Reasons for increased needs. Protein is a primary need during pregnancy because it is the growth element for body tissues. Reasons for this increased need reflect the tremendous growth involved in pregnancy.

1. *Rapid growth of the baby.* The mere increase in size of the infant from one cell to millions of cells in a 3.2 kg (7 pounds) child in only 9 months indicates the large amount of protein required for such rapid growth.

2. *Development of the placenta.* The placenta is literally the fetus's lifeline to the mother. The mature placenta requires sufficient protein for its complete development as a vital unique organ to sustain, support, and nourish the fetus during growth.

3. *Growth of maternal tissues.* To support the pregnancy, increased development of breast and uterine tissue is required.

4. *Increased maternal blood volume.* The mother's blood volume increases 20% to 50% during pregnancy. This greater amount of circulating blood is necessary to nourish the child and support the vast amount of increased metabolic workload.With extra blood volume comes a need for greater synthesis of blood components, especially hemoglobin and plasma protein, which are proteins vital to the support of the pregnancy. **Hemoglobin** increase supplies oxygen to the growing number of cells, and **plasma protein** (**albumin**) increase helps the greater blood volume circulate sufficient tissue fluids between the capillaries and the cells. Albumin in the blood provides the osmotic force constantly needed to pull the tissue fluids back into circulation after they have bathed and nourished the cells, thus preventing an abnormal accumulation of water in the tissues beyond the normal physiologic edema of pregnancy.

5. *Amniotic fluid.* Amniotic fluid surrounds the fetus during growth and guards it against shock or injury. It contains proteins, hence its formation requires still more protein.

6. *Storage reserves.* Increased tissue storage reserves, especially fuel stores as adipose fat tissues, are needed in the mother's body to prepare for a large energy requirement during labor, delivery, the immediate postpartum period, and lactation.

Amount of increase. The RDA standard recommends an increase of 10 g of protein during pregnancy, making a total protein need of 60 g/day. This indicates about a 20% increase over the average adult requirement. However, a large number of high-risk or active pregnant women need even more protein.

Food sources. The only *complete* protein foods of high biologic value are milk, egg, cheese, and meat (p. 39). Certain other *incomplete* proteins from plant sources such as legumes and grains contribute additional secondary amounts. Protein-rich foods also contribute other nutrients such as calcium, iron, and B vitamins. The amounts of these foods that will supply the needed protein are indicated in the daily core food plan given in Table 10-1.

Key mineral and vitamin needs

Increases in all the minerals and vitamins are needed during pregnancy to meet the greater structural and metabolic requirements. These increases are indicated in the RDA tables inside the book covers. However, several of these essential substances have key roles in pregnancy and require special attention.

Calcium. A good supply of calcium, along with phosphorus and vitamin D, is essential for fetal development of bones and teeth, as well as the mother's own body needs. Calcium is also necessary for proper clotting of blood. A diet that includes 1 quart fortified milk daily plus generous amounts of green vegetables, whole grains, and eggs will usually supply sufficient calcium. In cases of poor maternal stores or pregnancies involving more than one fetus, supplements are needed. Since food sources of the major minerals calcium and phosphorus are almost the same, a diet sufficient in calcium would also provide enough phosphorus.

Iron and iodine. Particular attention is given to iron and iodine intake during pregnancy. Iron is essential for increased hemoglobin synthesis required for the greater maternal blood volume, as well as for the necessary prenatal storage of iron in the baby. Since iron occurs in small amounts in food sources, and much of this intake is not in a form readily absorbed, the maternal diet alone can rarely meet needs. Thus the RDA standard recommends a daily iron intake of 30 g, twice the woman's prepregnant need. However, since the increased pregnancy requirement cannot be met by the iron content of usual U.S. diets or by the iron stores of at least some women, daily iron supplements are usually recommended.[1] Adequate iodine intake is essential for producing more thyroxine, the thyroid hormone needed in greater amounts to control the increased basal metabolic rate during pregnancy. This increased iodine need is easily ensured by the use of iodized salt.

Vitamins. Vitamins A and C are needed in increased amounts during pregnancy because they are both important elements in tissue growth. The B vitamins are needed in increased amounts because of their vital roles as coenzyme factors in energy production and protein metabolism. Folate is especially needed to build mature red blood cells. The RDA standard recommends a daily folate intake of 400 μg, more than double the nonpregnant woman's need of 180 μg/day. For women who are not well fed or have less than optimal food habits, a folate supplement may be needed during the pregnancy. The increased vitamin D need to ensure absorption and utilization of calcium and phosphorus for fetal bone growth is met by the mother's intake of 1 quart fortified milk per day in her daily food plan. Fortified milk contains 10 μg (400 IU) of cholecalciferol (vitamin D) per quart, just the RDA amount. The mother's general exposure to sunlight will produce more.

Daily food plan

General basic plan. Some form of a food plan needs to be developed for each pregnant woman on an individual basis if it is to meet her increased nutritional needs. A core plan, such as the one given in Table 10-1, can serve

❖ **TABLE 10-1** *Core food plan for daily intake during pregnancy and lactation**

Food	Nonpregnant woman	Pregnancy	Lactation
Milk, cheese, ice cream, skimmed or buttermilk (food made with milk can supply part of requirement)	2 cups	3-4 cups	4-5 cups
Meat (lean meat, fish, poultry, cheese, occasional dried beans or peas)	1 serving (3-4 oz)	2 servings (6-8 oz); include liver frequently	2½ servings (8 oz)
Eggs	1	1-2	1-2
Vegetable† (dark green or deep yellow)	1 serving	1 serving	1-2 servings
Vitamin C-rich food†	1 good source or 2 fair sources	1 good source and 1 fair source or 2 good sources	1 good source and 1 fair source or 2 good sources
Good source: citrus fruit, berries, cantaloupe			
Fair source: tomatoes, cabbage, greens, potatoes in skin			
Other vegetables, fruits, juices	2 servings	4-6 servings	4-6 servings
Bread‡ and cereals (enriched or whole grain)	6 servings	10 servings	10 servings
Butter or fortified margarine	Moderate amount	Moderate amount	Moderate amount

* Meets nutrient needs; add additional foods as needed for energy (kcalorie) demands.
† Use some raw daily.
‡ One slice of bread or ½ cup starch (grains or vegetables) equals 1 serving.

as a guideline, with additional amounts of foods as needed for sufficient kcalories. This general core food plan is built on regular basic foods in American markets, designed to supply necessary nutrient increases. The RDA standards for individual nutrients apply throughout the pregnancy, so a core food guide such as this with additional foods as needed should provide for the required nutrients. Energy needs increase as the pregnancy progresses, and the RDA increment of 300 kcal/day applies to the second and third trimesters. However, adolescent mothers, underweight, or malnourished women would need special attention to increased energy needs from the outset of the pregnancy.

Alternate food patterns. For women with alternate food patterns the core food plan may be only a starting point. Other food patterns exist among women from different ethnic backgrounds, belief systems, and life-styles, making individual diet counseling essential. *Specific nutrients*, not necessarily specific foods, are required for successful pregnancies, and these nutrients may be found in a wide variety of foods. Wise health workers encourage pregnant women to use foods that serve both their personal needs and their nutritional needs, whatever those foods may be. Many resources have been developed to serve as guides for a variety of alternative food patterns, such as ethnic and vegetarian.(See Chapter 4, further reading list and Box 4-1.) If the vegetarian pattern includes dairy products and eggs (lacto-ovo), there is no problem in achieving a sound diet for pregnancy needs by increasing the use of these animal proteins. Strict vegan vegetarians who are pregnant are at greater risk.[1] Vitamin B_{12} supplements are mandatory at RDA levels of 2.2 µg/day during pregnancy and 2.6 µg/day during lactation.[2,3] Specific counseling concerning avoidance of alcohol, caffeine, tobacco, and drugs during pregnancy is essential. Information about the direct fetal effects of poor nutrition, especially related to brain development and later learning problems and developmental delays, will help motivate many pregnant women to choose a well-selected diet of optimal nutritional value. Certainly, given the American obsession with thinness, especially among teenage girls, pregnancy is no time to diet.

Basic principles. Whatever the food pattern, two important principles govern the prenatal diet: (1) the pregnant woman must eat a sufficient *quantity* of food, and (2) she needs to eat *regular meals and snacks*, avoiding any habit of fasting or skipping meals—especially breakfast.

GENERAL CONCERNS
Functional gastrointestinal problems

Nausea and vomiting. The so-called morning sickness of early pregnancy is usually mild, only occurring briefly during the first trimester. It is caused by hormonal adaptations in the first weeks and may be increased by stress or anxieties about the pregnancy itself. Simple treatment usually helps relieve symptoms: small frequent meals and snacks that are fairly dry, consisting mostly of easily digested energy foods such as carbohydrates, with liquids between, not with, meals. If the condition becomes severe and prolonged, it requires medical treatment.

Constipation. Usually a minor complaint, constipation may occur in the latter part of pregnancy as a result of increasing pressure of the enlarging uterus and the muscle-relaxing effect of placental hormones on the gastroin-

❖ **TABLE 10-2**   *Approximate weight of products of a normal pregnancy*

Products	Weight
Fetus	3400 g (7.5 lb)
Placenta	450 g (1 lb)
Amniotic fluid	900 g (2 lb)
Uterus (weight increase)	1100 g (2.5 lb)
Breast tissue (weight increase)	1400 g (3 lb)
Blood volume (weight increase)	1800 g (4 lb) (1500 ml)
Maternal stores	1800-3600 g (4-8 lb)
TOTAL	11000-13000 g
	(11-13 kg; 24 to 28 lb)

testinal tract, which reduce normal peristalsis. Helpful remedies include adequate exercise, increased fluid intake, and naturally laxative foods such as whole grains, dried fruits (especially prunes and figs), and other fruits and juices. The pregnant woman is advised to avoid artificial laxatives.

Weight gain during pregnancy

Amount and quality. The mother's optimal weight gain during pregnancy, sufficient to support and nurture her and the fetus, is essential. Weight gain should not be viewed negatively. Rather it is an important reflection of good nutritional status and contributes to a successful course and outcome of pregnancy. Generally the average weight gained is about 11 to 13 kg (25 to 30 pounds) as indicated in Table 10-2. A current report of the National Academy of Sciences, *Nutrition During Pregnancy*, recommends setting weight gain goals together with the pregnant woman according to her prepregnant nutritional status and weight for height: normal weight, 25 to 35 pounds; underweight, 28 to 40 pounds; overweight, 15 to 25 pounds. Adolescent mothers should strive for the upper end of the recommended range, and a total target weight gain for a woman carrying twins of 35 to 45 pounds.[4] But the important consideration in each case is not only the quantity of weight gain but also the *quality* of the gain and the foods consumed to bring it about. There is a definite connection between high-risk, low-birth-weight babies, and inadequate maternal weight gain during the pregnancy.[4,5] Clearly, severe caloric restriction during pregnancy is physiologically unsound and potentially harmful to both the developing fetus and the mother. Such a restricted diet cannot supply all the energy and nutrient demands essential to the growth process during pregnancy. Thus weight reduction should *never* be undertaken during pregnancy. To the contrary, adequate weight gain, more for the underweight woman, should be supported with the use of a nourishing, well-balanced diet.[6]

Rate of weight gain. About 2 to 4 pounds (0.9 to 1.8 kg) is an average weight gain during the first trimester of pregnancy. Thereafter about 1 pound (0.45 kg) a week during the remainder of the pregnancy is usual, although some women will need to gain more. It is only unusual patterns of gain, such as a sudden sharp increase in weight after the 20th week of pregnancy, which may indicate excessive and abnormal water retention, that should be monitored.

Role of sodium. Just as with restriction of kcalories, routine restriction of sodium during pregnancy is physiologically unsound and unfounded. A regular moderate amount of dietary sodium is needed, about 2 to 3 g/day. This can be achieved through general use of salt in cooking and seasoning, but limiting extra use—a "heavy hand with the shaker"—at the table, as well as controlling extra use of obviously salty processed foods. Maintenance of the increased circulating maternal blood volume, which is normal during pregnancy to support the increased metabolic work, requires adequate amounts of both sodium and protein. The National Research Council and both the professional nutrition and obstetrics guidelines have labeled routine use of salt-free diets and diuretics as potentially dangerous.

High risk mothers and infants

Identify risk factors involved. To avoid the results of poor nutrition during pregnancy, mothers at risk should be identified as early as possible. Risk factors that identify women with special nutritional needs during pregnancy are shown in Box 10-1. These nutrition-related factors are based on clinical evidence of inadequate nutrition. Do not wait for clinical symptoms of poor nutrition to appear. The best approach is to identify poor food patterns and prevent nutritional problems from developing. Three types of dietary patterns that will not support optimal maternal and fetal nutrition are: (1) insufficient food intake, (2) poor food selection, and (3) poor food distribution throughout the day.

Plan personal care. Every pregnant woman needs personalized care and support during her pregnancy. However, women with risk factors such as those listed in Box 10-1 have special counseling needs. In each case we need to work with the mother in a sensitive, supportive manner to help her develop a healthy food plan that is both practical and nourishing for her. Dangerous practices need to be identified, such as diet fads, extreme macrobiotic diets, or *pica*.[7] Pica is the name given a perverted appetite or craving for unnatural foods, for example, chalk, laundry starch, or clay, a practice sometimes seen in pregnancy or in malnourished children.

Recognize special counseling needs. In addition to avoiding dangerous practices such as those listed above, several special needs require sensitive counseling, including those related to age and parity, detrimental life-style habits, and socioeconomic problems.

1. Age and parity. Pregnancies at either age extreme of the reproductive cycle carry special problems. The adolescent pregnancy adds many social and nutrition-related risks as its social upheaval and physical demands are imposed on a still immature teenaged girl. Sensitive counseling must involve both information and emotional support with good prenatal care throughout. On the other hand, the older pregnant woman, over 35 years of age and having her first child, also requires special attention. She may be more at risk for high blood pressure, either pre-existing or pregnancy-induced, and need guidance about rate of weight gain and excessive use of sodium. In addition, the woman with a high *parity* rate, who has had several pregnancies within a limited number of years, enters each successive pregnancy at a higher risk, drained of nutritional resources and usually facing increasing physical and economic pres-

Nutritional Risk Factors in Pregnancy

Risk factors presented at the onset of pregnancy
Age
  15 years or younger
  35 years or older
Frequent pregnancies: three or more during a 2-year period
Poor obstetric history or poor fetal performance
Poverty
Bizarre or faddist food habits
Abuse of nicotine, alcohol, or drugs
Therapeutic diet required for a chronic disorder
Weight
  Less than 85% of standard weight
  More than 120% of standard weight
Risk factors occurring during pregnancy
Low hemoglobin and/or hematocrit
  Hemoglobin less than 12.0 g
  Hematocrit less than 35.0 mg/dl
Inadequate weight gain
  Any weight loss
  Weight gain of less than 2 lb per month after the first trimester
Excessive weight gain: greater than 1 kg (2 lb) per week after the first trimester

sures of child care. Counseling may well include discussions of acceptable means of contraception and nutrition information and support.

2. Social habits: alcohol, cigarettes, and drugs. These three personal lifestyle habits cause fetal damage and are contraindicated during pregnancy. Extensive habitual alcohol use leads to the well-described and documented *fetal alcohol syndrome (FAS)*, which has become a leading cause of mental retardation and other birth defects.[8,9] Cigarette smoking during pregnancy causes placental abnormalities and fetal damage, including prematurity and low birthweight (Box 10-2), largely as a result of impaired oxygen transport.[10]

Drug use, both medicinal and recreational, poses many problems. Self-medication with over-the-counter drugs carries potential adverse effects. The use of "street drugs" is especially dangerous to the developing fetus, causing the baby to be born addicted or with acquired immunodeficiency syndrome (AIDS) from the mother's use of contaminated needles in her drug injections. Dangers come not only from use of the drug itself or contaminated needles but also from the impurities such street drugs contain.[11] In addition, drug abuse from megadoses of basic nutrients such as vitamin A during pregnancy may also cause fetal damage. Especially dangerous are drugs made from vitamin A compounds, retinoids such as *etretinoin* (Accutane), prescribed for severe acne, which have caused spontaneous abortion of malformed fetuses by women who conceived during such acne treatment.[12] Thus the use of these drugs without contraception is definitely contraindicated.

3. Caffeine. Depending on extent of its use, caffeine's effect during pregnancy is much milder than effects of the agents just discussed. However, caf-

BOX 10-2

❖ ——————— **CLINICAL APPLICATION** ——————— ❖

Who Will Have The Low-Birth-Weight Baby?

The number of babies weighing less than 2500 g (5 pounds) at birth is still a problem. Perinatal nutritionists are well aware of the dietary factors that influence this increase, especially poor weight gain during pregnancy. The prevalence of the turn-of-the-century adage to "grow the baby to fit the pelvis" continues to influence some physicians, nurses, and expectant mothers to limit prenatal weight gain to 9 kg (20 pounds) or less to avoid obstetric problems at delivery. This practice is harmful and is refuted by current evidence that a weight gain of 25 to 35 pounds for normal weight women and more, 28 to 40 pounds, for underweight women is correlated with birth weight of greater than 2500 g (5 pounds).

The obsession with weight control during pregnancy can lead to harmful restrictions of vital energy and nutrients. Weight reduction should *never* be attempted during pregnancy. Such diets are extremely dangerous to the fetus. Even the common habit of skipping breakfast, especially late in pregnancy, may impair intellectual development by producing a pseudostarvation state very quickly. Increased ketoacidosis from fat breakdown can cause neurologic damage to the fetus.

Nondietary factors influencing this growing trend toward more low-birth-weight (LBW) babies include:

- Rise in number of older primigravid women (over 35 years of age)
- Rise in number of teenage pregnancies
- Previous induced abortions
- Technologic advances in neonatal care, which keeps premature infants alive longer
- Race: nonwhites have higher rates of LBW infants than whites

To reduce the risk of LBW infants in mothers you may be counseling, you may want to:

- Explain the reasons for gaining sufficient weight as recommended
- Help mothers who smoke or drink to stop using cigarettes or alcohol
- Monitor excessive weight gain and sodium intake in older primigravid women, who are at risk for prenatal essential hypertension and obesity
- Explore eating habits of adolescents, working with the girl and her "significant others" to include nutrient-dense foods in her meal and snack selections
- Keep informed of federal, state, and local supplemental food programs available to low-income women to ensure an adequate intake of nutrients
- Encourage regular eating patterns throughout pregnancy

Brown, JE: Improving pregnancy outcomes in the United States, The importance of preventive nutrition services, J Am Diet Assoc 89(5):631, May 1989.
Brown, JE: "Let them eat cake" or a prescription for improving the outcome of pregnancy? Nutr Today 25(6):18, Nov/Dec 1990.
National Academy of Sciences, Committee on Nutritional Status During Pregnancy and Lactation, Food and Nutrition Board: Nutrition during pregnancy, Washington, DC, 1990.

feine is still a widely used drug that can cross the placenta and enter fetal circulation. Its use at pharmacologic levels has been associated with low-birth-weight babies.[13] A pharmacologic dose of caffeine—250 mg—is contained in 2 cups of coffee, 3.5 cups of tea, or 5 12-ounce colas, so such use is not recommended.[14] Responsible health agencies have recommended that pregnant women avoid caffeine-containing beverages, and that products containing caffeine be plainly labeled to inform consumers.

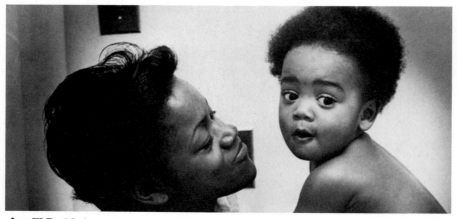

❖   **FIG. 10-1**
This mother is a participant in the WIC program.

4. Socioeconomic problems. Special counseling is required for women and young girls living in low-income situations. Poverty, especially, puts pregnant women in grave difficulty. They need resources for financial assistance and food procurement. Nutritionists and social workers on the health care team can provide special counseling and referrals. Community resources include programs such as the special Supplemental Food Program for Women, Infants, and Children (WIC), which has helped many low income mothers have healthy babies.

Complications of pregnancy

Anemia. Anemia is common during pregnancy. About 10% of the women in large U.S. prenatal clinics have low hemoglobin and hematocrit levels. Anemia is far more prevalent among poor women, many of whom live on marginal diets barely adequate for subsistence. However, anemia is by no means restricted to the lower economic groups. A deficiency of iron or folate in the mother's diet can cause nutritional anemia, so dietary intake needs to be determined and supplements used as indicated.[4] During the second and third trimesters of pregnancy, a low-dose iron supplement of 30 mg of ferrous iron daily can provide the amount of extra iron needed. Although routine folate supplementation is not recommended, 300 μg/day may be given when individual dietary adequacy is doubtful. Women who do not eat fruit, juices, whole-grain or fortified cereals, and green vegetables frequently are likely to have low folate intake and need supplements.

Pregnancy-induced hypertension (PIH). Formerly called *toxemia*, pregnancy-induced hypertension (PIH) is primarily a disease of malnutrition, especially related to diets low in protein, kcalories, calcium, and salt. Such malnutrition affects the liver and its metabolic activities. In a classic sense, it is associated with poverty and found most often in women subsisting on inadequate diets with little or no prenatal care. Symptoms of PIH, which occur in late pregnancy near term, are elevated blood pressure, abnormal and excessive water retention, albumin in the urine, and in severe cases, convulsions. Specific treatment varies according to individual symptoms and needs, but in any case optimal nutrition is basic. Emphasis is given to adequate dietary protein, kcalories, salt, minerals, and vitamins.

Pre-existing disease. Pre-existing clinical conditions, such as hypertension, diabetes, phenylketonuria (PKU), or other disease, complicate pregnancy. In each case, the woman's pregnancy is managed, usually by a team of specialists, according to the principles of care related to pregnancy and to the particular disease involved.

LACTATION
Trends

In America and other developed countries, the number of mothers choosing to breast-feed their babies had been increasing but recently has leveled off somewhat, with about 62% of white women and about 25% of black women nursing their babies and finding it a pleasurable experience (Fig. 10-2). Several factors have contributed to this choice: (1) more mothers are informed about the benefits of breast-feeding, (2) practitioners recognize the ability of human milk to meet unique infant needs (as shown in Table 10-3), (3) maternity wards and alternative birth centers are being modified to support successful lactation, and (4) community support is more available, even in workplaces. Almost all women who choose to breast-feed their infants can do so. Exclusive breast-feeding by well-nourished mothers provides adequate nutrition for periods varying from 2 to 15 months, with solid foods usually added to the baby's diet at about 6 months of age.

Nutritional needs

The basic diet followed during pregnancy, as well as the prenatal nutrient supplement used, can be continued through the lactation period. In general, attention to three lactation supports is needed.

Diet. Milk production requires energy, about 800 kcal/day, for both the process and the product. Thus more food for more kcalories is needed. Since some of this energy need may be partially met by extra fat stored during pregnancy, the RDA standard is an additional 500 kcal/day throughout lactation above the mother's nonpregnant need of about 2200 kcalories, or a total of 2700 kcal/day. The RDA for protein during lactation is an additional 15 g/day above the mother's usual need of 50 g, or a total of 65 g/day. These lactation energy and nutrient increases are shown in the RDA standards (see tables inside book covers). The core food plan for meeting these lactation needs, as shown in Table 10-1, includes 4 to 5 cups milk, 6 to 8 ounces lean meat, 1 to 2 eggs, 1 to 2 servings dark green or yellow vegetables, 2 servings vitamin C-rich fruits and vegetables, 4 to 6 servings other vegetables, fruits, and juices, 10 servings whole-grain or enriched breads and cereals, and moderate amounts of butter or fortified margarine. Compare these increases in each food group with the amounts needed for nonpregnant women and for pregnancy.

Fluids. Since milk is a fluid tissue, the breast-feeding mother needs more fluids for adequate milk production. Water and other beverages such as juices and milk add to the fluid necessary to produce milk. Alcohol and caffeine-containing beverages should be limited or avoided since they are secreted to some extent in the mother's milk.

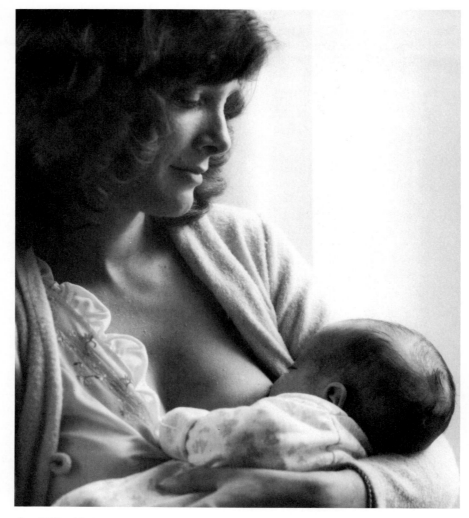

❖   **FIG. 10-2**
Breast-feeding mother and infant.

Rest and relaxation.   In addition to the increased diet and fluids, the breast-feeding mother requires rest, moderate exercise, and relaxation. Often the nurse and the nutritionist help by counseling her about her new family situation. Together they may develop plans to meet these personal needs.

Advantages of breast-feeding.   There are many physiologic and practical advantages to breast-feeding, including: (1) *fewer infections*, since the mother transfers certain antibodies or immune properties in human milk to her nursing infant, (2) *fewer allergies and intolerances*, especially in allergy-prone infants, since cow's milk contains a number of potentially allergy-causing proteins that are human milk does not have, (3) *ease of digestion*, since human milk forms a softer curd in the gastrointestinal tract that is easier for the infant to digest, (4) *convenience and economy*, as the mother is free from the time and expense

❖ **TABLE 10-3**   *Nutritional components of human milk (per 100 ml)*

Milk component	Colostrum*	Transitional†	Mature‡	Cow's milk
Kilocalories	57.0	63.0	65.0	65.0
Vitamins, fat-soluble:				
A (μg)	151.0	88.0	75.0	41.0
D (IU)	—	—	5.0	2.5
E (mg)	1.5	0.9	0.25	0.07
K (μg)	—	—	1.5	6.0
Vitamins, water-soluble:				
Thiamin (μg)	1.9	5.9	14.0	43.0
Riboflavin (μg)	30.0	37.0	40.0	145.0
Niacin (μg)	75.0	175.0	160.0	82.0
Panthothenic acid (μg)	183.0	288.0	246.0	340.0
Biotin (μg)	0.06	0.35	0.6	2.8
Vitamin B₁₂ (μg)	0.05	0.04	0.1	0.6
Vitamin C (mg)	5.9	7.1	5.0	1.1

*On delivery.
†Delivery to approximately 4 weeks.
‡Human milk after approximately 4 weeks.

involved in buying and preparing formula, and her breast milk is always ready and sterile.

SUMMARY

Pregnancy involves fundamental interactions among three distinct yet unified biologic entities—the fetus, the placenta, and the mother. Maternal needs also reflect the increasing nutritional needs of the fetus and the placenta. An optimal weight gain varies with the prepregnant nutritional status and weight of the mother, with a goal of about 25 to 35 pounds for a normal-weight woman and more for an underweight woman and less for an overweight woman. Sufficient weight gain is important during pregnancy to support the rapid growth taking place. As significant as the actual weight gain is the nutritional quality of the diet.

Common problems during pregnancy include first-trimester nausea and vomiting associated with hormonal adaptations, and later constipation resulting from pressure of the enlarging uterus. In most cases they are relieved without medication by simple, often temporary changes in the diet. Unusual or irregular eating habits, age, parity, prepartum weight status, and low income are among the many related conditions that identify pregnant women at risk for complications.

The ultimate goal of prenatal care is a healthy infant and a healthy mother who is physically capable of breast-feeding her child, should she choose to do so. Human milk provides essential nutrients in quantities uniquely suited for optimal infant growth and development.

❖ REVIEW QUESTIONS

1. List six nutrients that are required in larger amounts during pregnancy. Describe their special role and identify four food sources of each.

2. Identify two common gastrointestinal problems associated with pregnancy and describe the diet management of each.
3. List and describe five major nutritional factors for the support of lactation. What additional nonnutritional needs does the breast-feeding mother have, and what suggestions can you give to help her meet them?

❖ SELF-TEST QUESTIONS

True-false
For each item answered "false," write the correct statement.
1. The development of the fetus is directly related to the diet of the mother.
2. Strict weight control during pregnancy is needed to avoid complications.
3. Salt should be removed from the pregnant woman's diet to prevent edema.
4. A higher risk of pregnancy complications occurs in teenagers and older-age women.
5. A woman's diet before her pregnancy has little effect on the outcome of her pregnancy.
6. No woman should ever gain more than 15 to 20 pounds during her pregnancy.
7. Rapid growth of the fetal skeleton requires increased calcium in the mother's diet.
8. Inadequate vitamin D during pregnancy contributes to faulty skeletal development in the fetus.
9. Anemia is common during pregnancy because iron requirements are increased.
10. Additional kcalories and fluids are needed during lactation.

Multiple choice
1. Blood volume during pregnancy:
   a. Increases
   b. Decreases
   c. Remains unchanged
   d. Fluctuates widely
2. Which of the following foods are complete proteins of high biologic value and hence should be increased during pregnancy?
   a. Enriched whole grains and breads
   b. Milk, egg, and cheese
   c. Beans, peas, and lentils
   d. Nuts and seeds
3. Which of the following foods has the highest iron content to help meet the increased iron need during pregnancy?
   a. Lean beef
   b. Liver
   c. Orange juice
   d. Milk
4. The increased need for vitamin A during pregnancy may be met by increased use of such foods as:
   a. Nonfat milk
   b. Extra egg whites
   c. Citrus fruits
   d. Carrots

❖ SUGGESTIONS FOR ADDITIONAL STUDY

Nutritional analysis of pregnant woman's diet
1. Using the general guides in your textbook, interview a pregnant woman to learn about her food habits and environment.

2. From your account of her usual day's food intake pattern, calculate her intake of the following key nutrients: kcalories, protein, calcium, iron, vitamin A, and vitamin C.
3. Using the information gained in your interview about her living and family situation and her food habits, plan with her a suitable daily food plan to meet her increased nutritional needs during her pregnancy.

Cultural food pattern in pregnancy

1. Select any one of the various cultural food patterns. Plan a prenatal diet within this pattern to meet the increased nutritional demands of pregnancy.
2. If possible, interview a pregnant woman of this cultural group and analyze her diet.

Diet for lactation

1. Interview a breast-feeding mother of a newborn baby to determine her food habits and questions concerning a diet for lactation.
2. Discuss with her the lactation process and assist her with successful breast-feeding techniques.

References

1. Dwyer J: Vegetarian diets in pregnancy. In National Research Council, Food and Nutrition Board: Alternative dietary practices and nutritional abuses in pregnancy, Washington, DC, 1982, National Academy Press.
2. National Research Council, Food and Nutrition Board: Recommended dietary allowances, ed 10, Washington, DC, 1989, National Academy Press.
3. National Research Council, Food and Nutrition Board, Committee on Diet and Health: Diet and health, Implications for reducing chronic disease risk, Washington, DC, 1989, National Academy Press.
4. National Academy of Sciences, Committee on Nutritional Status During Pregnancy and Lactation, Food and Nutrition Board: Nutrition during pregnancy, Washington, DC, 1990, National Academy Press.
5. Brown JE: Improving pregnancy outcomes in the United States, The importance of preventive nutrition services, J Am Diet Assoc 89(5):631, 1989.
6. Mitchell MC and Lerner E: Weight gain and pregnancy outcome in underweight and normal weight women, J Am Diet Assoc 89(5):634, 1989.
7. Horner RD and others: Pica practices of pregnant women, J Am Diet Assoc 91:34, Mar 1991.
8. Abel EL and Sokol RJ: Fetal alcohol syndrome is now leading cause of mental retardation, Lancet 2:1222, Nov 22, 1986.
9. Raymond CA: Birth defects linked with specific level of maternal alcohol use, but abstinence still the best policy, JAMA 258:177, July 10, 1987.
10. Bureau MA and others: Maternal cigarette smoking and fetal oxygen transport, Pediatrics 72:22, 1983.
11. Enig MG: Pharmacologic basis of drug-nutrient interaction related to drug abuse during pregnancy, Clin Nutr 6:235, 1987.
12. Watson RR: Vitamin A and teratogenesis: recommendations for pregnancy, J Am Diet Assoc 88:364, Mar 1988.
13. Leonard TK and others: The effects of caffeine on various body systems: a review, J Am Diet Assoc 87:1048, Aug 1987.
14. Leonard-Green TK and Watson RR: Caffeine and health risk, J Am Diet Assoc 88:370, Mar 1988.

Further Reading

Brown JE: Nutrition for your pregnancy, Minneapolis, 1983, University of Minnesota Press.

Written in an interesting popular style by an experienced nutritionist and mother, this small book is an excellent resource. It contains many references and tools, and provides a good reference for parents.

Hess MA and Hunt AE: Pickles and ice cream, Winnetka, Ill, 1986, Hess & Hunt, Inc.

Written by a nutritionist and home economist especially for parents, this short paperback combines both substance and style in its helpful material.

11

❖

Nutrition in infancy, childhood, and adolescence

K E Y   C O N C E P T S

Normal growth of individual children varies within a relatively wide range of measures.

Human growth and development require both nutritional and psychosocial support.

A variety of food patterns and habits supply the energy and nutrient requirements of normal growth and development, although basic nutritional needs change with each growth period.

*I*n any culture, for each infant, child, or adolescent, food nurtures both the physical and the personal "growing up" process. Food and feeding and eating during these highly significant years of childhood do not and cannot exist apart from the broader overall process of growth and development. The *whole* process produces the *whole* person.

In this chapter we consider food and feeding in an individual and unique manner, as a basic part of human "growing up" for each person. We then relate the various age-group nutritional needs and food patterns to individual psychosocial development as well as to physical growth.

NUTRITION FOR GROWTH AND DEVELOPMENT
Life cycle growth pattern

The normal human life cycle follows four general stages of overall growth, with individual variances along the way.

Infancy. Growth is rapid during the first year of life, with the rate tapering off somewhat in the latter half of the year. Most infants double their birth weight by the time they are 6 months of age and triple it by the age of 1 year.

Childhood. Between infancy and adolescence, the childhood growth rate slows and becomes irregular. Growth occurs in small spurts and during these times children have increased appetites and eat accordingly. Plateaus occur in between, and during these times children have little or no appetite and eat less. Parents who recognize this as a normal growth pattern in the "latent period of childhood" will relax, enjoy their child, and not make eating a battle issue.

Adolescence. The onset of puberty begins the second rapid growth, which continues until adult maturity. The flooding sex hormones and increased growth hormone bring multiple and often bewildering body changes to young adolescents. During this period long bones grow rapidly, sex characteristics develop, and fat and muscle mass increase.

Adulthood. With physical maturity comes the final phase of a normal life cycle. Physical growth levels off during adulthood and then gradually declines during old age. However, mental and psychosocial development last a lifetime.

Measuring childhood growth

Individual growth rates. Children grow normally at widely varying rates. The best counsel for parents, therefore, is that children are *individuals*. One child should not be compared with another. Growth is not inadequate because the rate does not equal that of another child. General measures of growth in children relate not only to physical development but also to mental, emotional, social, and cultural growth.

Physical growth. Growth charts such as those developed by the National Center for Health Statistics (NCHS) provide a broad base for growth in children today. These charts are based on large numbers of children representing our national population. They are used as guides to see an individual child's pattern of physical growth in relation to the general percentile growth curves on the charts. Individual measures of physical growth in a child include weight and height, body measurements, general signs of health, laboratory tests, and nutritional study of general eating habits.

Psychosocial development. A number of tests are used to measure mental, emotional, social, and cultural growth and development. Food is intimately related to these aspects of psychosocial development as well as to physical growth. The growing child does not learn food attitudes and habits in a vacuum, but in close personal and social relationships.

NUTRITIONAL REQUIREMENTS FOR GROWTH
Energy needs

Kilocalories. The demand for energy, as measured in kcalories from food, is relatively large during childhood. The general recommendations for energy and nutrient needs at different ages are given in the RDA tables inside the book covers. However, individual need varies with age and condition. For example, the total daily caloric intake of a 5-year-old child is spent in the following way:

Basal metabolism	50%
Physical activities	25%
Tissue growth	12%
Fecal loss	8%
Metabolic effect of food	5%

Energy nutrients. Of the total kcalories from the energy-yielding macronutrients carbohydrate, fat, and protein, carbohydrate is the main energy source. It also acts as a protein-sparer so that protein vital for building tissue during childhood growth will not be diverted for energy needs. Fat is a backup energy source, and it also supplies *linoleic acid*, the essential fatty acid necessary for growth.

Protein needs

Protein is the fundamental *tissue-building* substance of the body. It supplies the essential specific building materials—amino acids—for tissue growth and maintenance. As a child grows, the protein requirements per unit of body weight gradually decrease. For example, for the first 6 months of life protein requirements of an infant are 2.2 g/kg of body weight, but the protein needs of a fully grown adult are only 0.8 g/kg. A healthy, active, growing child will usually eat enough in amount and variety of the foods provided to supply the necessary protein and kcalories for overall growth.

Water requirements

Water is an essential nutrient, second only to oxygen for life itself. Metabolic needs during periods of rapid growth especially demand adequate fluid intake. For example, compare the infant and adult water needs. The infant requires more water per unit of body weight than an adult for two important reasons: (1) a greater percentage of the infant's total body weight is made up of water, and (2) a larger proportion of the infant's total body water is outside the cells and hence more easily available for loss, resulting in serious dehydration. Generally an infant consumes daily an amount of water equivalent to 10% to 15% of body weight, whereas an adult consumes a daily amount equivalent to 2% to 4% of body weight. A summary of approximate daily fluid needs during the growth years is given in Table 11-1.

❖ **TABLE 11-1**   *Approximate daily fluid needs during growth years*

Age	ml/kg	Age	ml/kg
0-3 months	120	4-7 years	95
3-6 months	115	7-11 years	90
6-12 months	110	11-19 years	50
1-4 years	100	>19 years	30

Mineral and vitamin needs

As described earlier, though yielding no energy themselves, the micronutrients minerals and vitamins have important roles in tissue growth and maintenance and in overall energy metabolism. Positive childhood growth depends on adequate amounts of all these essential substances, as indicated in the RDA tables (inside book covers), but several of these essential materials are of special concern during rapid growth years.

Calcium. Calcium is needed throughout the growth years, especially during the most rapid growth periods of infancy and adolescence. In infancy, mineralization of the skeleton is completed, bones grow larger, and teeth are formed from initial buds. In adolescence, the skeleton grows most rapidly to its adult size. Bone density, particularly in long bones and in vertebrae, demands adequate calcium, along with phosphorus and vitamin D. In fact, as a preventive measure to reduce risk of osteoporosis in older adult years, both research and clinical experience indicate that emphasis on calcium is needed during adolescence. Calcium intake during rapid adolescent bone growth, both in size and density, is far more effective than the use of more poorly absorbed calcium supplements in older adult years.[1]

Iron. Iron is essential for hemoglobin formation. The infant's fetal store is depleted within 4 to 6 months after birth and the first infant food, milk, provides little iron. However, iron in human milk is more easily absorbed and commercial formulas are usually iron-fortified. Solid food additions at 4 to 6 months of age, such as enriched cereal, egg yolk, and meat, help supply the need for iron.

Hypervitaminosis. Excess amounts of two vitamins, A and D, are of concern in feeding children. Excess intake may occur over prolonged periods as a result of ignorance, carelessness, or misunderstanding. Instruct parents to use only the amount directed and no more.

AGE GROUP NEEDS
Infancy

At birth we begin our development in our particular "world" as unique human beings. As we grow older this process continues throughout our lives. Food is intimately related at each stage, as our physical growth and personal psychosocial development go hand in hand.

Immature infants. Special care is crucial for these tiny, immature babies.[2] The two main types are defined by weight and by gestational age.

1. Weight. Defined by birth weight, low-birth-weight (LBW) babies are those weighing less than 2500 g (5 pounds); very-low-birth-weight (VLBW) babies are those weighing less than 1500 g (3 pounds); extremely-low-birth-weight (ELBW) babies are those weighing less than 990 g (2 pounds).

2. Gestational age. Defined by gestational age, premature babies are those who are born preterm, at fewer than 270 days of gestation, and weigh less than 2500 g (5 pounds). Small-for-gestational-age (SGA) babies are those who are born at full term but have suffered some degree of intrauterine growth failure before birth and have general growth retardation and low birth weight.

All of these infants have problems catching up with growth and nutrition. Because their bodies are not fully formed they differ from full-term, normal-weight infants. They have (1) much more body water and less protein and minerals, (2) little subcutaneous fat and must be kept warm, (3) poorly calcified bones, (4) incomplete nerve and muscle development that makes sucking reflexes weak, (5) limited digestion-absorption ability and renal function, and (6) an immature liver lacking developed metabolic enzyme systems or adequate iron stores. To survive, these "tiniest babies" require special feeding.

1. Type of milk. Immature babies have grown well on both breast milk and special formulas. However, for a number of reasons, most preterm and immature babies are fed special commercial formulas. Table 11-2 shows a comparison of these special formulas with standard full-term infant formulas and human milk.

2. Methods of feeding. Tube feeding and peripheral vein feeding are used in special cases, but both carry hazards and are avoided if possible. For most immature infants, bottle feeding can be successful with much care and support, using one of the newer special formulas.

Full-term infants. Mature newborns have more finely developed body systems and grow rapidly, gaining about 168 g (6 ounces) per week during the first 6 months. The feeding process is an important component of the bonding relationship between parent and child. The mother may choose to breast-feed her baby or to use a formula, with solid foods added later when the baby is able to handle them at about 4 to 6 months of age.

Breast-feeding. The ideal first food for the infant is human milk. It is the primary recommendation of both pediatricians and nutritionists. The nutrients in human milk are uniquely adapted to meet the growth needs of the infant, in forms more easily digested, absorbed, and used. Breast-feeding supports early immunity for the baby, helps the mother's uterus return quickly to normal size, and assists in the important mother-child bonding process (Fig. 11-1).

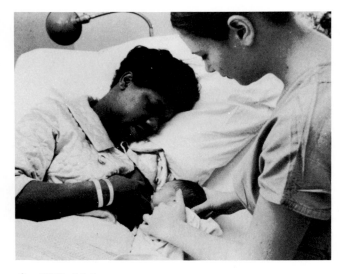

❖ **FIG. 11-1**

Breast-feeding the newborn infant. Note that the nurse, in assisting the mother, avoids touching the infant's outer cheek so as not to counteract his natural rooting reflex at the touch of the breast.

❖ **TABLE 11-2** *Nutritional value of special formulas and human milk for the preterm infant*

| Nutritional component | Advisable intake by birth weight | | Human milk | | Standard formulas | Special premature formulas | | |
	1.0 kg (2.2 lb)	1.5 kg (3.3 lb)	Preterm	Mature	Enfamil* Similac† SMA‡	Enfamil Premature with Whey*	Similac Special Care†	"Preemie" SMA‡
Kilocalories/deciliter			73	73	67	81	81	81
Protein (g/100 kcal)	3.1	2.7	2.3§	1.5	2.2	3.0	2.7	2.5
Vitamins, fat-soluble								
D (IU/120 kcal/kg/day)	600	600	—	4.0	70-75	75	180	76
E (IU/120 kcal/kg/day)	30	30	—	0.3	2-3	2	4	2
Vitamins, water-soluble								
Folic acid (μg/120 kcal/kg/day)	60	60	—	8.0	9-19	36	45	14
Vitamin C (mg/120 kcal/kg/day)	60	60	—	7.0	10	10	45	10
Minerals								
Calcium (mg/100 kcal)	160	140	40	43.0	66-78	117	178	92
Phosphorus (mg/100 kcal)	108	95	18.0	20.0	49-66	58	89	49
Sodium (mEq/100 kcal)	2.7	2.3	1.5‖	0.8	1.0-1.8	1.7	1.9	1.7

*Mead Johnson Nutritional Division, Evansville, Ind.
†Ross Laboratories, Columbus, Ohio.
‡Wyeth Laboratories, Philadelphia.
§Range: 1.9-2.8 g/100 kcal.
‖Range: 0.9-2.3 mEq/100 kcal.

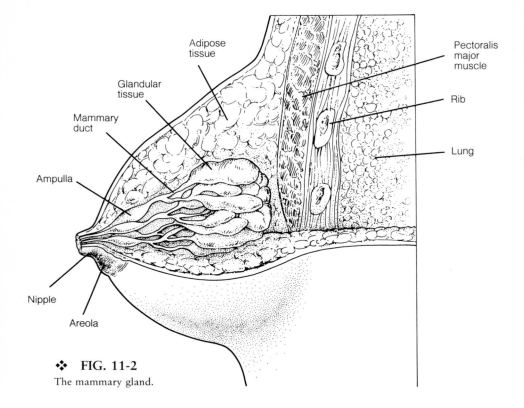

Adipose tissue

Glandular tissue

Mammary duct

Ampulla

Nipple

Areola

Pectoralis major muscle

Rib

Lung

❖ **FIG. 11-2**

The mammary gland.

Breast-feeding can be successfully started and maintained by most women who try, have support, and use an increased diet for lactation (see Chapter 10). The female breasts or mammary glands are highly specialized secretory organs (Fig. 11-2). During pregnancy the breasts are prepared for lactation, and toward term produce a thin fluid pre-milk called *colostrum*. As the infant grows, the breast milk develops and adapts in composition to match the needs of the developing child. The newborn rooting reflex, oral needs for sucking, and the basic hunger drive usually make breast-feeding simple for the healthy, relaxed mother. The working mother who wants to breast-feed her baby can do so by (1) using manual expression and breast pump while at work, and (2) freezing and storing 1- or 2-ounce amounts of milk in sealed plastic baby bottle liners for later use. Child care facilities provided in some business and industry settings support breast-feeding for employed mothers.

Bottle-feeding. If the mother does not choose to breast-feed, or some condition in either mother or baby prevents it, bottle feeding of an appropriate formula is an acceptable alternative. Most mothers use a commercial formula (Table 11-2). Use of home-prepared evaporated milk formula, although least expensive, is usually not recommended because of the increased risk involved from inaccurate measurement and bacterial contamination during preparation. If it must be used, preparation of a single feeding at a time is safer, using the following ingredient proportions: 90 ml (3 ounces) evaporated milk, 135 ml (4.5 ounces) boiled water, and 2 teaspoons corn syrup. A fluoride supplement is recommended if the local water supply is not fluoridated.

Cow's milk. At no time during the first year of life should an infant be fed regular whole cow's milk. Unmodified cow's milk is not suitable for infants. Its concentration may cause gastrointestinal bleeding and is too heavy a solute load for the infant's renal system. Also, infants and young children should not be fed cow's milk of reduced fat content, such as skim or low-fat, for two reasons: (1) *insufficient energy* is provided, and (2) *linoleic acid*, the essential fatty acid for growth in the fat portion, is not available. To meet infant needs during the first year of life, the American Academy of Pediatrics recommends breast milk supplemented by vitamin D and fluoride from birth and iron supplement after 4 months of age, with gradual addition of suitable foods beginning at about 6 months. An alternative appropriate formula may be the mother's choice in place of breast milk.

Solid food additions. There is no nutritional need for adding solid foods to the infant's diet before 4 to 6 months of age. Since the infant's system cannot use foods very well before 4 to 6 months, they are not needed. When solid foods are started, there is no one specific sequence of food additions that must be followed. A general guide is given in Table 11-3, but individual needs and responses vary, and suggestions of individual practitioners are the guide. Single foods are usually introduced first, one at a time in small amounts, so that if there is an adverse reaction, the offending food can be identified. Over time the child will be introduced to a wide variety of foods and come to enjoy many of them (Fig. 11-3). A variety of commercial baby foods are available, now prepared without the formerly added sugar, salt, or monosodium glutamate. Some mothers prefer to prepare their own baby food. Home preparation of

A   B

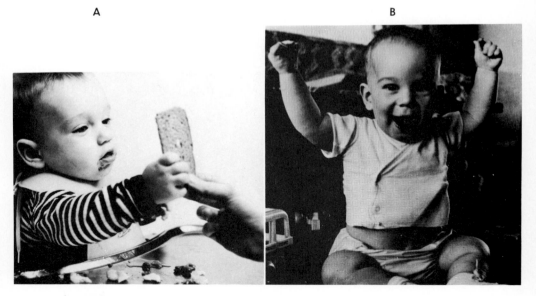

❖ **FIG. 11-3**

A, This 6-month-old boy is taking a variety of solid food additions and is developing wide tastes. Here feeding has become a bond of relationship between mother and child and is serving as a source not only of physical growth but also of psychosocial development. **B,** Optimal physical development and security are evident, the result of sound nutrition and loving care.

❖ **TABLE 11-3**   *Guideline for adding of solid foods to infant's diet during the first year*

Foods added*	Feeding
6 to 7 months	
Cereal and strained cooked fruit	10 AM and 6 PM
Egg yolk (at first, hard boiled and sieved, soft boiled or poached later)	
Strained cooked vegetable and strained meat	2 PM
Zweiback or hard toast	At any feeding
7 to 9 months	
Meat: beef, lamb, or liver (broiled or baked and finely chopped)	10 AM and 6 PM
Potato: baked or boiled and mashed or seived	
9 months to 1 year or older—suggested meal plan	
Milk	7 AM
240 ml (8 oz)	
Cereal	
2-3 tbsp	
Strained fruit	
2-3 tbsp	
Zweiback or dry toast	
Milk	12 NOON
240 ml (8 oz)	
Vegetables	
2-3 tbsp	
Chopped meat or one whole egg	
Puddings or cooked fruit	
2-3 tbsp	
Milk	3 PM
120 ml (4 oz)	
Toast, zweiback, or crackers	
Milk	6 PM
240 ml (8 oz)	
Whole egg or chopped meat	
2 tbsp	
Potato: baked or mashed	
2-3 tbsp	
Pudding or cooked fruit	
Zweiback or toast	

* Semisolid foods should be given immediately before milk feeding. One or two teaspoons should be given at first. If food is accepted and tolerated well, the amount should be increased to 1 to 2 tbsp per feeding.
NOTE: Banana or cottage cheese may be used as substitution for any meal.

baby food can be done easily by cooking and straining vegetables and fruits, freezing a batch at a time in ice cube trays, and storing the cubes in plastic bags in the freezer. Later, a single cube can be reheated conveniently for use at a feeding. Throughout the early feeding period, whatever plan is followed, three basic principles should guide the feeding process: (1) *necessary nutrients* are needed, not any specific food or sequence, (2) food is a basis of *learning*, and (3) *normal physical development* guides the feeding behavior (Box 11-1). Good food habits begin early in life and continue as the child grows older. By 8 or 9 months of age, infants should be able to eat so-called table foods—chopped, cooked, simply seasoned foods—without needing special infant foods.

Summary guidelines. The Nutrition Committee of the American Academy of Pediatrics (AAP) has provided recommendations to guide infant feeding:

1. *Breast-feeding* provides the ideal first food for the infant, continued for the first full year of life supplemented with vitamin D and fluoride from birth and iron supplement after 4 months of age.

2. *Commercial formulas* if desired, provide an alternative choice to breast-feeding during the first year of life; fluoride supplement may be needed for mixing if the local water supply is not fluoridated.

3. *Solid foods* may be introduced at approximately 4 to 6 months of age, after the extrusion reflex of early infancy has disappeared and the ability to swallow nonliquid food has been established.

4. *Whole cow's milk* may be introduced at the end of the first year if breast-feeding has been completely discontinued and infants are consuming one third of their kcalories as a balanced mixture of solid foods including cereals, vegetables, fruits, and other foods to supply adequate sources of vitamin C and iron. Reduced-fat cow's milk is not recommended.

5. *Iron-fortified formula* should be used for older infants more than 6 months of age who are not consuming a significant portion of their kcalories from added solid foods.

6. *Allergens* such as wheat, egg white, citrus juice, nut butters, and chocolate should not be used in early introductions of solid foods, but added later after tolerance has been established in gradual use.

7. *Honey* should not be given to infants less than 1 year of age because botulism spores have been reported in honey and the immune system capacity of young infants cannot resist this infection.

8. *Physically irritating foods* such as hot dogs, nuts, grapes, carrots, and round candy may cause choking and aspiration, so are best delayed for careful use only with older children and should not be given to infants.

Throughout the first year of life the requirements for physical growth and psychosocial development will be met by human milk or formula, a variety of solid food additions, and a loving, trusting relationship between parents and child.

Childhood

Toddlers (1 to 3 years). Once a child learns to walk at about 1 year of age, the toddler is off and away, into everything, and learning new skills. This dawning sense of self, a fundamental foundation for ultimate maturity, carries

BOX 11-1

❖ ————————— CLINICAL APPLICATION ————————— ❖

How Infants Learn to Eat

During their first year of life, guided by reflexes and gradually developing muscle controls, infants learn a great many things about living in their particular environment. A most basic need is food, which they obtain through a normal developmental sequence of feeding behaviors in the process of learning to eat.

Age 1 to 3 Months

Rooting, sucking, and swallowing reflexes are present at birth, along with the tonic neck reflex. Thus infants secure their first food, milk, with a suckling pattern in which the tongue is projected during a swallow. In the beginning head control is poor, but develops by the third month.

Age 4 to 6 Months

The early rooting and biting reflexes fade, and the tonic neck reflex has faded by 16 weeks. Infants now change from a suckling pattern with protruded tongue to a mature stronger suck with liquids and a munching pattern begins. They are able to grasp objects with a fistlike palmar grip, bringing them to the mouth and biting them.

Age 7 to 9 Months

The gag reflex weakens as chewing of solid foods begins and a normal controlled gag develops along with control of the choking reflex. Now munching movements develop as older infants increase their use of solid foods and chew with a rotary motion. They can sit alone, secure items and release them then resecure them, and hold a bottle alone. They begin to develop a pincer grasp to pick up very small items between the thumb and forefinger and put them in the mouth.

Age 10 to 12 Months

Older infants can now reach for a spoon. They bite nipples, spoons, and crunchy foods, can grasp a bottle and foods and bring them to the mouth, and with assistance can drink from a cup that is held. They have tongue control to lick food morsels off the lower lip, and they can finger-feed themselves with a refined pincer grasp.

These normal developmental behaviors form the basis for a progressive pattern of introducing semisolid foods and table foods to the older infant:

4 to 6 months—Add iron-fortified infant cereals, starting with less allergenic rice and progressing to wheat and mixed grains.

6 to 8 months—Add strained fruits, vegetables, and progressing to strained or finely chopped table meats. Add finger foods such as arrowroot biscuits or over-dried toast that can be secured with a palmar grasp.

9 to 12 months—Gradually delete strained foods and introduce a variety of table foods such as well-cooked and chopped vegetables and meats and chopped well-cooked or canned fruits. Increase the use of small-sized finger foods as the pincer grasp develops. Add other well-cooked mashed or chopped table foods, all prepared without added salt or sugar, and assist with moderate amounts of juice by cup.

over into many areas—including food. After parents have become accustomed to the rapid growth and resulting appetite of the first year of life, they may be concerned when they see their toddler eating less food and at times having little appetite, while being easily distracted from food to another activity (see Box 11-2). An increasing variety of foods will help a child develop good food habits. Food preferences of young children grow directly from frequency of use in pleasant surroundings and increased opportunity to become familiar

BOX 11-2

❖ —————————— **CLINICAL APPLICATION** —————————— ❖

Toddler- and Preschooler-Feeding Made Simple

Parents waste a lot of time coaxing, arguing, begging, even threatening their 2- to 5-year-olds to eat more than one and one half green peas at dinner time. You can help them save time, tears, and energy by developing child-feeding strategies based on the normal developmental needs of their little ones.

First, remind them that:

Their children are not growing as fast as they did during the first year of life. Consequently, they need less food.

A child's energy needs are irregular. Just watch their activity level. Then provide food as needed to help their bodies keep up with the many activities they have "planned" each day.

Second, offer a few suggestions that make child-feeding easier:

Offer a variety of foods. After a taste, put a new food aside if not taken. Then try again later to help develop broad tastes.

Serve small portions. Let them ask for seconds if they're still hungry.

Guide them in serving themselves small portions. Like adults, children's eyes tend to be bigger than their stomachs. Constant gentle reminders help them learn when to stop.

Avoid overseasoning. Let tastes develop gradually. If it's too spicy, no amount of screaming or cajoling will make them eat it.

Don't force foods that the child dislikes. Individual food dislikes usually don't last very long. If the child shuns one food, offer a similar one—if it's available at that meal (e.g., a fruit if the child rejects vegetables). At this rate, there's little chance of deficiency signs cropping up anytime soon.

Don't put away the main meal before serving dessert. If there is a dessert, hold on to the main meal food. Amazing but true: some children will ask for more main meal foods *after* finishing dessert, if they're still hungry.

Keep "quick-fix" nutritious foods around for "off-hour" meals. The word "snack" isn't appropriate for the amount of food some youngsters put away between regular meals. To keep from turning into a permanent short-order chef, keep foods such as fruit, cheese, peanut butter, bread, and crackers to serve between meals and provide essential nutrients.

Enroll the child in a nursery school or preschool program. Since food is not always available in the classroom, little students learn to eat at regular times. They also tend to try foods rejected at home, probably because of peer pressure or a desire to impress a new authority figure—the teacher.

Be patient. Remember that while adults may be discussing world events over broccoli, toddlers are just now learning how to pick it up with their forks.

They may take longer. They may not even eat at all. But with flexibility, time, patience, and a sense of humor, most parents find they can get enough nutrients into their children to keep them alive and happy throughout the preschool years.

with a number of foods. Reserve sweets for special occasions, not for habitual use or bribes to get a child to eat.

Preschool children (3 to 5 years). Physical growth—and appetite—continues in spurts. Mental capacities develop and the gradually expanding environment is explored. The child continues to form life patterns in attitudes and basic eating habits as a result of social and emotional experiences. These varying experiences frequently lead to "food jags" that last a few days but are usually short-lived and of no major concern. Again, the key is food variety and relatively small portions. Group eating becomes a significant means of socialization (see Box 11-2). In a preschool experience, for example, food preferences grow according to what the group is eating. In such situations the child learns a widening variety of different food habits and forms new social relationships.

School-age children (5 to 12 years). The generally slow and irregular growth rate continues in the early school years and body changes occur gradually. In the year or two just before adolescence especially, reserves are being laid for the rapid growth period ahead. This is the last lull before the storm. By now body types are established and growth rates vary widely. Girls' development usually outdistances boys' in the latter part of this period. With the stimulus of school and a variety of learning activities, the child experiences increasing mental and social development, ability to work out problems, and competitive activities. The child begins moving from dependence on parental patterns to the standards of peers, in preparation for coming maturity. Food preferences are products of earlier years, but the school-age child is increasingly exposed to new stimuli, including television, that influence food habits. Some favorite foods of American children are listed in Table 11-4. The relation of sound nutrition and learning has long been established, and breakfast is particularly important for a school child. The school lunch program provides a nourishing noon meal for many children who would otherwise lack one. There are also positive learning opportunities in the classroom, particularly when parents provide support at home. An interested and motivated teacher can integrate nutrition into many other learning activities.

Adolescence (12 to 18 years)

Physical growth. The final growth spurt of childhood occurs with the onset of puberty. This rapid growth is evident in increasing body size and development of sex characteristics in response to hormonal influences. The rate of these changes varies widely among individual boys and girls, but it is particularly distinct in growth patterns that emerge. Girls develop an increasing amount of fat deposit, especially in the abdominal area. As the bony pelvis widens in preparation for future childbearing, and subcutaneous fat increases, the size of the hips also increases. This causes much anxiety to many figure-conscious young girls. In boys, physical growth is seen more in increased muscle mass and long-bone growth. At first a boy's growth spurt is slower than that of the girl, but he soon passes her in weight and height.

Eating patterns. Teenagers' eating habits are greatly influenced by their rapid growth, hence need for energy, and their self-conscious peer pressure, hence acceptance of popular food fads. They tend to skip lunch more often than breakfast, derive a great deal of their energy in snacks, eat at fast-food restaurants since these are frequent "hangouts," and are likely to eat any kind of food at any time of day. Unfortunately, some teenagers begin to get a significant portion of their total caloric intake in the form of alcohol. Even a mild form of alcohol abuse, when combined with the elevated nutritional

❖ **TABLE 11-4** *Favorite food choices of American children (listed in order of priority)*

Breakfast	Lunch or dinner	Vegetables	Fruit	Beverage	Desserts	Sandwiches
Cereal	Steak or roast beef	Corn	Apple	Cola or soda	Ice cream	Peanut butter and jelly
Pancakes or waffles	Pizza	Carrots	Orange	Milk	Cake	Meat or cold cuts
Eggs	Spaghetti	Beans	Peach	Fruit punch	Pie	Ham
French toast	Chicken	Tomatoes	Grape	Root beer	Pudding	Tuna fish
Toast	Hamburger	Peas	Banana	Juices (other than orange)	Gelatin dessert	Cheese
Sweet rolls	Fish	Greens, collards, or spinach	Watermelon	Orange juice	Banana split	Bacon, lettuce, and tomato
Doughnuts	Macaroni and cheese	Potatoes	Pear	Lemonade	Brownie	Roast beef

Modified from survey data of Lamme AJ and Lamme LL: Children's food preferences, J Sch Health 50(7):397, 1980.

demands of adolescence, can easily affect their nutritional status. In general overall nutrition, boys usually fare better than girls. Their larger appetite and sheer volume of food consumed usually ensure an adequate intake of nutrients. On the other hand, under a greater social pressure for thinness, girls may tend to restrict their food and have inadequate nutrient intake.

Eating disorders. Social, family, and personal pressures concerning figure control strongly influence many young girls. As a result, they sometimes follow unwise self-imposed "crash" diets for weight loss. In some cases self-starvation occurs. Complex and far-reaching eating disorders such as *anorexia nervosa* and *bulimia* may develop. Traditionally psychologists have identified mothers as the main source of family pressure to remain thin. Current study indicates, however, that fathers have a role also, if they are emotionally distant and do not provide important feedback to build self-worth and self-esteem in their young daughters.[3] The researchers advise fathers to help their daughters see themselves as loved no matter what they weigh, so they will not be as vulnerable to social influences that equate extreme thinness with beauty. Eating disorders can have severe effects, and involve a distorted body image and a morbid, irrational pursuit of thinness. Often they begin in early adolescent years. In one high school survey of over a thousand girls aged 13 to 19, 36% said they were currently "dieting" to lose weight, 69% had been dieting at some time before the survey, 52% had begun dieting before age 14, and 14% were "chronic dieters."[4] Despite the fact that their average weight was below the normal weight for their height, all of these girls saw themselves as "fat." Many had varying degrees of malnutrition.

Teenage pregnancy. Currently, the number of teenage pregnancies is increasing. With a background of inadequate diet, many of these girls are very poorly prepared for the demands of pregnancy. They must complete their own growth and development and at the same time supply the extra needs of the baby. A teenage girl who is poorly prepared nutritionally for pregnancy is at risk for complications such as abortion, premature labor, pregnancy-induced hypertension (PIH), and delivery of an immature, low-birth-weight baby. A girl who has maintained good nutrition has a better chance to deliver a healthy baby. These very young mothers need much counseling, guidance, education, and support to help reduce the infant mortality rate involved (see Chapter 10).

SUMMARY

Positive growth and development of healthy children depend on optimal nutritional support. In turn, this good nutrition depends on many social, psychologic, cultural, and environmental influences that affect individual growth potential throughout the life cycle.

From birth, as children grow older, their nutritional needs change with each unique growth period. *Infants* experience rapid growth. Human milk is preferred as their first food, with solid foods delayed until about 6 months of age when their metabolic processes have matured. *Toddlers, preschoolers,* and *school-age children* experience a slowed and irregular growth. During this period their energy demands are less, but they require a well-balanced diet for continued growth and health. Social and cultural factors influence their developing food habits.

Adolescents experience a large growth spurt before reaching adulthood. This rapid growth involves both physical and sexual maturing. Boys usually obtain their increased caloric and nutrient demands because they eat larger amounts of food. Girls more frequently feel social and peer pressure to restrict their food for weight control, causing some to develop severe eating disorders. This pressure may also prevent them from forming the nutritional reserves necessary for future childbearing.

❖ REVIEW QUESTIONS

1. Describe major factors responsible for the differences in the nutritional and feeding needs of preterm and full-term infants.
2. Why is breast-feeding the preferred method for feeding infants? Compare commercial formulas available for bottle-fed babies.
3. Outline a general schedule for a new mother to use as a guide for adding solid foods to her baby's diet during the first year of life.
4. Compare the growth and development changes in toddlers, preschoolers, and school-age children. What factors influence their nutritional needs and eating habits?
5. Describe factors that influence the changing nutritional needs and eating habits of adolescents. Who is usually at greater nutritional risk during this period—boys or girls? Why? What suggestions do you have for reducing this nutritional risk at this vulnerable age?

❖ SELF-TEST QUESTIONS

True-false
For each item you answer "false," write the correct statement.
1. A good way to avoid overweight infants and toddlers is to use nonfat milk in their diets.
2. A variety of carbohydrate foods in the child's diet helps provide all the essential amino acids for growth.
3. Hypervitaminosis C is possible during the growth period when an excess amount of the vitamin is given to infants.
4. The rooting and sucking reflexes must be learned by the newborn infant before he can obtain milk from the breast.
5. The toddler needs at least a quart of milk a day to meet increased growth needs.

Multiple choice
1. Fat is needed in the child's diet to supply:
   (1) Energy
   (2) Fat-soluble vitamins
   (3) Water-soluble vitamins
   (4) Essential amino acids
   (5) Essential fatty acids
      a. (1), (2), and (5)
      b. All of these
      c. (3) and (5)
      d. (1) and (4)
2. An iron deficiency in childhood is associated with the disease:
   a. Scurvy
   b. Rickets
   c. Anemia
   d. Pellagra

3. Growth and development of the school-age child are characterized by:
   a. A rapid increase in physical growth with increased food requirements
   b. More rapid growth of girls in the latter part of the period
   c. Body changes associated with sexual maturity
   d. Increased dependence on parental standards or habits

❖ SUGGESTIONS FOR FURTHER STUDY

Nutrition for growth

Select a child in one of the stages of growth from infancy through adolescence. Interview the mother and the child, depending on age, concerning the food and feeding/eating practices used. Analyze your findings, using general guides in your textbook for each age group, as well as RDA standards and food value table.

According to your findings, plan with the mother and child, depending on age, a satisfying food plan that would provide both nutritional and psychosocial support for the child's growth and development.

Snack foods for growing children

Prepare a discussion for a group of parents of toddlers and preschool children. Develop snack ideas with recipes and suggestions for use. Demonstrate the preparation of a number of these snacks and have a taste- testing panel of the products with the parents. If children are present, have them taste and respond to the products. Write a brief report of your project and discuss it with your class.

References

1. Anderson JJB: Dietary calcium and bone mass through the lifecycle, Nutr Today 25(2):9, 1990.
2. Kitchen WH and others: Health and hospital readmissions of very-low-birth-weight and normal-birth-weight children, Am J Dis Child 144:213, Feb 1990.
3. McCleary K: Eating disorders: daddy dearest, Am Health 5(1):86, 1986.
4. Johnson CL: A descriptive survey of dieting and bulimic behavior in a female high school population. In: Understanding anorexia nervosa and bulimia, Columbus, Ohio, 1983, Ross Laboratories.

Further Reading

Satter EM: Child of mine: Feeding with love and good sense, Palo Alto, Calif, 1986, Bull Publishing Co.

Satter EM: How to get your kid to eat . . . but not too much, from birth to adolescence, Palo Alto, Calif, 1987, Bull Publishing Co.

This experienced author, a nutritionist-therapist-mother, has given us two excellent compact paperbacks packed with information and practical guides for parents to help them support their children in developing healthy food habits.

American Academy of Pediatrics, American Dietetic Association, and Food Marketing Institute: Healthy start: Foods to grow on, Chicago, 1991, American Dietetic Association.

This set of four consumer nutrition brochures, designed to help parents develop healthy eating habits for their children ages 2 to 6, contains a variety of practical feeding tips: (1) Right from the start: ABCs of good nutrition for young children; (2) What's to eat? Healthy foods for hungry children; (3) Feeding kids right isn't always easy: Tips for preventing food hassles; and (4) Growing up healthy: Fat, cholesterol, and more. These colorful guides may be ordered from the American Dietetic Association (P.O. Box 97215, Chicago, IL, 60678) in packets of 25 for use in the classroom or the community.

12

❖

Adulthood: nutrition for aging and the aged

KEY CONCEPTS

Aging is an individual *process based on genetic heritage and life experiences.*

Aging is a total life *process — biologic, nutritional, social, economic, psychologic, and spiritual.*

*T*he rapid growth and development of the adolescent years bring us to physical maturity as adults. Physical growth in the sense of increasing size levels off, but it continues in the constant cell growth and reproduction necessary to maintain our bodies. Other aspects of growth and development — mental, social, psychologic, and spiritual — continue in individual ways for a lifetime.

Food and nutrition continue to provide essential support during the adult aging process in adulthood. Life expectancy is lengthening, and thus health promotion and disease prevention are even more important as we seek to ensure quality of life to our extended years.

In this chapter we see that as a group adults include many individuals in many different life situations. Each person is unique, and each one experiences adult years in terms of physical and psychosocial events and imprints of all his yesterdays. Each one faces challenges, opportunities, and problems as she grows older. In varying degrees, each person has health concerns. In this chapter we see how nutrition relates to the human aging process. We see ways that positive nutrition and good food can help these still growing and developing adults lead healthier and happier lives.

AGING IN AMERICA

The process of human aging begins at birth and lasts a lifetime. Each stage has its unique potential for growth and fulfillment. The periods of adulthood—young, middle, and older—are no exception. Patterns of physical and psychosocial development change as persons mature and grow older.

Stages of adulthood

Young adults (18 to 40 years). With physical maturity young adults are increasingly independent. They form many new relationships, adopt new roles, and make many life choices concerning continued education, career, jobs, marriage, and family. Young adults experience considerable stress but also significant personal growth. These are years of career beginnings, of establishing one's own home, and of starting young children on their way through the same human life stages—all part of early personal struggles to make one's own way in the world. Sometimes health problems relate to these early stress periods.

Middle adults (40 to 60 years). Often the middle years present an opportunity to expand personal growth. In most cases children have grown and gone to make their own lives, and parents may have a sense of "it's my turn now." This is also a time of coming to terms with what life has offered, a "regrouping" of ideas, life directions, and activities. There is also a sort of regeneration of one's own life in the lives of young people following along the same way. In some middle adults early evidences of chronic disease appear. Wellness, health promotion, and reduction of disease risks are becoming the focus of health care.

Older adults (60 years and older). Adults vary widely in their personal and physical resources to deal with older age. They may have a sense of wholeness and completeness, or they may increasingly withdraw from life. If the outcome of their life experiences is positive, they arrive at older ages as rich persons—rich in wisdom of the years—and enjoy life and health (Fig. 12-1), enriching the lives of those around them. But some elderly people arrive at these years poorly equipped to deal with adjustments of aging and health problems that may arise.

Population changes

Age distribution. The American population is growing older. For the first time in U.S. history, the median age has passed 30. People over 65 years of age outnumber teenagers. Thanks to the postwar "baby boom," the fastest growing group in America today is aged 35 to 44 and now numbers about 28 million. Already there are about 26.3 million Americans aged 65 and over, and the second fastest growing group is aged 85 and over. Currently there is about a 15% increase in the 65- to 75-year-old population and a 33% increase in the 75-year-old and older group. The Census Bureau projects that by 2030, one person in every five will be over 65 years old.[1]

Life expectancy. In 1900, people in America could expect to live only to about age 47. Because of modern science and health care, the average life expectancy for all Americans today is about 77 years. When we reach 65, we can expect to live about 16 more years. At age 75, it is another 10. Many older adults are active and able to take care of themselves for longer than the general American myth and stereotype of *ageism* pictures. However, many of

❖ **FIG. 12-1**

Retired couple enjoying a
good breakfast.

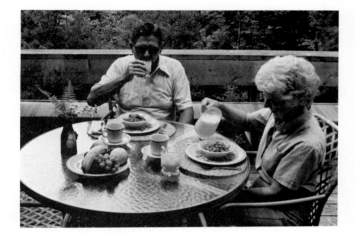

them are concerned as they grow older about the *quality* of their extended
years.

Socioeconomic and psychologic factors

Social and economic situations. Often more negative than positive, American social attitudes toward older people affect their position in American
society. Industry policies of early forced retirement and employment problems
as they grow older place many older people under increasing financial pressure.
Economic insecurity creates added stress and often leads to the need for food
assistance (Fig. 12-2). At the same time, a tighter economy and cutbacks in
such assistance programs have increased the number of people living below
the poverty level. The Physician Task Force on Hunger in America reports
that about 12 million children and 8 million adults, or about 9% of the
population, are hungry and malnourished.[2] Many of these people are older
adults. General U.S. living standards are high, but many "new poor" have
begun to suffer. Many elderly people, however, are able to live with extended
families or in a variety of group or self-help situations. Only one of every 20
elderly persons is in a health care facility, and only 10% of those over 65 are
incapacitated in any serious way. But older persons are often removed from
general activities of society, and they need such stimuli for as long as possible.

Psychologic factors. The greater part of the aging process in any area is
culturally determined. Unfortunately, in many ways our culture views old age
negatively. Social and financial pressures, along with a decreasing sense of
acceptance and productivity, cause many elderly persons to feel unwanted and
unworthy. All people need a sense of belonging, achievement, and self-esteem.
Instead many elderly people are often lonely, restless, unhappy, and uncertain.
Basic needs common to older persons are economic security, personal effectiveness, suitable housing, constructive and enjoyable activities, satisfying social
relationships, and spiritual values.

AGING PROCESS AND NUTRITIONAL NEEDS
General physiologic changes

Biologic changes. Human biologic growth and then decline extends over
the entire life span. Throughout the life process all experiences make their

❖ **FIG. 12-2**

Elderly disabled man
assisted by the Food Stamp
Program to obtain needed
food.

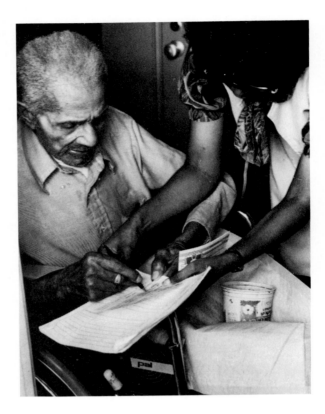

imprint on individual genetic heritage. Everyone ages in different ways, depending on individual makeup and resources. In general, however, during middle and older adulthood there is a gradual loss of functioning cells with reduced cell metabolism. As a result body organ systems gradually lose some capacity to do their jobs and maintain their reserves. The rate of this decline accelerates in later life. For example, by age 70 the kidneys and lungs lose about 10% of their former weight, the liver loses 18% of its weight, and skeletal muscle is reduced by 40%.

Effect on food patterns. Some of the physical changes of aging affect food patterns. For example, secretion of digestive juices and motility of gastrointestinal muscles gradually decrease. This causes decreased absorption and use of nutrients. Also decreased taste, smell, and vision affect appetite and persons eat less. Often older persons experience increased concern about body functions, more social stress, personal losses, and fewer social opportunities to maintain self-esteem. All of these concerns affect food intake. Much of what we see in older people and call "just aging" is really the result of poor nutrition.[3] The primary nutrition problem of older adults is lack of sufficient nourishment.

Individuality of the aging process. The biologic changes in aging are general. However, since each person is unique, older persons show a wide variety of individual responses to aging. They get old at different rates and in different ways, depending on their genetic heritage and their health and nutrition resources of past years. Each older adult has specific needs.

Nutritional needs

Kilocalories—energy. In general, because of gradual loss of functioning body cells and reduced physical activity, adults require less energy intake as they grow older. The RDA standard is based on estimates of 5% decreased metabolic activity in middle and older years. The recommended allowance for energy need is 1900 kcal/day for women over age 51 and 2300 kcal/day for men of the same age range. These are only general estimates. Individual physical and health status, as well as living situations, varies widely among older adults. In addition, our knowledge of energy and nutrient needs in elderly persons has many gaps. There is doubt, for example, about traditional standards of "ideal" weight based on weight-for-height tables. Ongoing review of these tables indicates that the weight ranges associated with longer lives are not necessarily the conventionally "desirable" weights given but levels 10% to 25% greater.[4] Thus the very thin older adult, rather than the individual of moderate weight, has a reduced life expectancy. The basic fuels needed to supply these energy needs are primarily carbohydrate with moderate fat.

1. Carbohydrate. About 50% to 55% of the total diet kcalories should come from carbohydrate foods with the majority being mostly complex carbohydrates such as starches. Easily absorbed sugars may also be used for energy. Carbohydrate metabolism usually is undisturbed in older age. The fasting blood glucose level is essentially unchanged in the aged. They can choose freely among carbohydrate foods, according to individual needs, desires, and physical responses.

2. Fat. Fats usually contribute about 30% of total kcalories. They provide a backup energy source, important fat-soluble vitamins, and essential fatty acids. A reasonable goal is to avoid large quantities of fat and emphasize the quality of the fat used. Fat digestion and absorption may be delayed in elderly persons, but these functions are not greatly disturbed. Sufficient fat for helping food taste better aids appetite and in some cases provides needed kcalories to prevent excessive weight loss.

Protein. The RDA standard recommends an adult protein intake of 0.8 g/kg of body weight, making a total protein need for the average weight man 63 g/day and for an average weight woman 50 g/day. There may be some increased protein need during illness, convalescence, or a wasting disease. In any case, protein needs are related to two basic factors: (1) the protein quality—the quantity and ratio of its amino acids, and (2) adequate total kcalories in the diet. Healthy adults do not need supplemental amino acid preparations, which are an expensive and inefficient source of available nitrogen.

Vitamins and minerals. A diet with a variety of foods should supply vitamins and minerals in amounts needed for healthy adults. Normal aging does not usually require increased amounts. Individual problems may arise from inadequate intake rather than increased need. However, several of these essential nutrients may need special attention in relation to two possible health problems in aging.

1. Osteoporosis. Vitamin D and calcium are essential nutrients for growth and maintenance of healthy bone tissue. Older adults may carry higher risk of developing the bone disease *osteoporosis* because they (1) use less calcium-rich food such as milk and other dairy products, (2) have loss of appetite and lack adequate body fat, (3) have less outdoor physical exercise, and (4) have a decreased capacity of the skin to produce vitamin D with exposure to sunlight.[5] The RDA calcium standard for all adults aged 25 and older is 5 μg/day (200 IU). The usual dietary intake in the United States as measured by a recent USDA survey is 1.25 to 1.75 μg/day (50 to 70 IU), so apparently vitamin D stores are enriched in most people by regular exposure to sunlight.[6]

2. *Anemia.* The poor diet of many older adults lacks sufficient iron to prevent iron-deficiency *anemia*. These individuals need attention and encouragement to help them eat more iron-rich foods.

The question of nutrient supplementation. There is no evidence that *healthy* adults in middle and older years require additional nutrient supplements. Nonetheless, use of supplements is widespread. Surveys show that about 40% of adult Americans take vitamin supplements regularly, with much higher use in Western states. The use of nutritional supplements by elderly adults is common, with 30% to 70% taking vitamins, usually on a self-prescribed basis.[7] Although such routine use may not be necessary, supplements are often required for persons in debilitated states, along with a nourishing diet, to help restore tissue strength and health.

CLINICAL NEEDS
Health promotion and disease prevention

Chronic disease risk reduction. The current emphasis in adult health care is on reducing individual risks of developing chronic disease as persons grow older. This approach has been used in development of the U.S. dietary guidelines, *Nutrition and Your Health: Dietary Guidelines for Americans*, issued jointly by the Department of Agriculture and the Department of Health and Human Services and related to the current national health objectives, *Healthy People 2000: National Health Promotion and Disease Prevention Objectives.*[1,8] These guidelines outline life-style changes that we can make to live healthier lives: (1) eat a variety of foods; (2) maintain healthy weight; (3) choose a diet low in fat, saturated fat, and cholesterol; (4) choose a diet with plenty of vegetables, fruits, and grain products; (5) use sugars only in moderation (6) use salt and sodium only in moderation; (7) if you drink alcoholic beverages, do so in moderation (see Box 1-1, p. 9). The guidelines emphasize individual needs and good eating habits based on moderation and variety.

Nutritional status. Many of the health problems of older adults are not the result of general aging alone but of states of malnutrition (Box 12-1). This undernourishment may develop for several reasons: (1) poor food habits, often from lack of appetite or loneliness and not wanting to eat alone, as well as lack of sufficient money to buy needed food; (2) oral problems, such as poor teeth or poorly fitting dentures; (3) general gastrointestinal problems, such as declining salivary secretions and dry mouth with diminished thirst and taste sensations, less hydrochloric acid secretion in the stomach, decreased enzyme and mucous secretion in the intestines, and general decline in gastrointestinal motility. Older adults may voice concerns about adequate dietary fiber. Individual medical complaints range from vague indigestion or "irritable colon" to specific diseases such as *peptic ulcer* or *diverticulitis*. (See Chapter 18.)

Weight management. Both excessive weight loss and excessive weight gain can be signs of malnutrition. Many of the same depressed living situations and emotional factors described earlier may also lead to excessive weight gain.

BOX 12-1

❖ ———————— CLINICAL APPLICATION ———————— ❖

Case Study: Situational Problem of an Elderly Woman

Mrs. Johnson, a 78-year-old widow, lives alone in a three-bedroom house in a large city. A year ago, a fall resulted in a broken hip, and she is now dependent on a walker for limited mobility. Her husband died suddenly 6 months ago, and almost all of her friends have died or are disabled. Her only child, a daughter, lives in a distant city and does not care to bear the burden of responsibility for her mother.

Mrs. Johnson's only income is a monthly Social Security check for $160. Her monthly property taxes, insurance payments, and utility bills amount to $130.

A recent medical examination revealed that Mrs. Johnson is severely anemic and that she has lost 20 pounds in the past 3 months. Her current weight is 82 pounds and she is 5 feet, 4 inches tall. She states that she has not been hungry, and her daily diet is repetitious: broth, a little cottage cheese and canned fruit, saltine crackers, and hot tea. She lacks energy, rarely leaves the house, and appears emaciated and generally distraught.

Questions for Analysis

1. Identify Mrs. Johnson's personal problems and describe how they might have influenced her eating habits. How has her physical problem influenced her food intake?
2. What nutritional improvements could she make in her diet (include food suggestions), and how are they related to her physical needs at this stage of her life?
3. What practical suggestions do you have for helping Mrs. Johnson cope with her physical and social environment? What resources, income sources, food, and companionship can you suggest? How do you think these suggestions would benefit her nutritional status and overall health?

Overeating or undereating becomes a compensation for the conditions encountered in older age. Poor food choices result, and physical activity is usually decreased.

Individual approach. In all cases, personal and realistic planning with every person is essential. Individual personalities and problems are unique, and individual needs vary widely. The malnourished older person needs much personal sensitive support to build improved eating habits (Box 12-2).

Chronic diseases of aging

Diet modifications. Chronic diseases of aging—such as heart disease, cancer, diabetes, renal disease—may occur in adult years, or at younger ages when family history for them exists. Diet modifications and nutritional support are an important part of therapy. Details of these modified diets are given beginning in Chapter 17. In any situation, individual needs and food plans continue to be essential for successful therapy.

Drugs. Because people are living longer, many with chronic diseases, older adults take as many as 8 to 12 different prescription drugs for multiple health problems, plus additional over-the-counter drugs. Many drug-nutrient-food interactions can occur.[9] Each person needs careful evaluation of all drugs used and instruction about how to take these medications in relation to food intake.[7] Many drugs affect appetite or absorption and use of nutrients, so they may contribute to malnutrition.

BOX 12-2

❖ ———————— CLINICAL APPLICATION ———————— ❖

Feeding Older Adults With Sensitivity

Many older adults have eating problems and may easily become malnourished. Each person is a unique individual with particular needs and requires sensitive support to meet both nutritional and personal requirements. A personal approach, providing assistance for eating when needed, can help meet these needs.

Basic guidelines
- **Analyze food habits carefully.** Learn personal attitudes, situations, and desires of the older person. Nutritional needs can be met with a variety of foods, so make suggestions in a practical, realistic, and supportive manner.
- **Never moralize.** Never say, "Eat this because it's good for you." This approach has little value for anyone, especially for a person struggling to maintain personal integrity and self-esteem in a youth-oriented, age-fearing culture that largely alienates its aged.
- **Encourage food variety.** Mix new foods with familiar "comfort foods." Often new tastes and seasonings encourage appetite and increase interest in eating. Many people think that a bland diet is best for all elderly persons. *It is not.* A decreased taste sensitivity in aging needs added attention to variety and seasoning. Smaller amounts of foods and more frequent meals may also encourage better nutrition.

Assisted feeding suggestions
- Make no negative remarks about the food served.
- Identify the food being served.
- Allow the person at least three bites of the same food before going on to another food, to allow time for the taste buds to become accustomed to the food.
- Allow sufficient time for the person to chew and swallow.
- If using a syringe to feed, never feed more than 30 ml (1 ounce) at a time to allow sufficient time for the person to swallow, and always remove the syringe from the mouth while he is swallowing.
- Give liquids throughout the meal, not just at the beginning and end.

COMMUNITY RESOURCES
Government programs for older Americans

Older Americans Act. The Administration on Aging of the U.S. Department of Health and Human Services administers programs for older adults under the Older Americans Act Amendments of 1987. Nutrition programs are promoted through Title III—Grants for State and Community Programs on Aging, Part C—Nutrition Services. These services include both congregate and home-delivered meals, with related nutrition education and food service components.

1. Congregate meals. This program provides older Americans, particularly those with low incomes, with low-cost, nutritionally sound meals in senior centers and other public or private community facilities. In these settings older adults can gather for a hot noon meal. They have access to both good food and social support.

2. Home-delivered meals. For those persons who are ill or disabled and cannot attend the congregate meals, meals are delivered by couriers to the home. This service meets nutritional needs and provides human contact and support. The couriers are usually volunteers concerned about the people and their needs. Often a courier is the only person the homebound individual may contact during the day.

U.S. Department of Agriculture (USDA). The U.S. Department of Agriculture (USDA) provides both research and services for older adults.

1. Research centers. Research centers for studies on aging are being established in various areas of the United States. For example, a new Human Nutrition Research Center on Aging has been built at Tufts University in Boston. It is the largest research facility in the U.S. specifically authorized by Congress to study the role of nutrition in aging. Current studies there involve protein needs in the aged, the nutritional status of elderly men and women, and the prevention and slowing of osteoporosis through nutritional support. Much more knowledge about the nutritional requirements of older adults is needed in order to provide better care.

2. Extension services. The USDA operates agricultural extension services in state "land grant" universitites, including food and nutrition education services. County home advisors aid communities with practical materials and counsel for elderly persons and community workers.

Public Health Service (PHS). The Public Health Service (PHS) is a major division of the U.S. Department of Health and Human Services. Skilled health professionals work in the community through local and state public health departments. Public health nutritionists are important members of this health care team. They provide nutrition counseling and education and help with various food assistance programs.

Professional organizations and resources

National groups. The American Geriatric Society and the Gerontological Society are national professional organizations of physicians, nurses, and other interested health workers.They publish journals and promote community and government efforts to meet needs of aging persons.

Community groups. Local medical societies, nursing organizations, and dietetic associations sponsor a variety of programs to help meet the needs of elderly people. Also, an increasing number of qualified nutritionists—registered dietitians—are in private practice in most communities and can supply a variety of individual and group services. Senior centers in local communities are also resources.

Volunteer organizations. Many activities of volunteer health organizations such as the Heart Association and the Diabetes Association relate to the needs of older persons.

SUMMARY

Meeting the nutritional needs of adults, especially older adults, is a challenge for several reasons. We lack research on which to base the determination of energy and nutrient needs as persons grow older. Current and past social, economic, and psychologic factors influence needs, and the biologic process of aging differs widely in individuals. Moreover, standards for older adults are based mainly on data available for younger adult populations or on requirements to counteract disease processes of aging, such as heart disease.

Much of the illness in older adults results from malnutrition, not from the effects of aging. Thus in working with older people, food habits must be analyzed carefully and approached with encouragement to make any positive changes. Individual supportive guidance and patience are required, using available nutrition resources as needed.

❖ REVIEW QUESTIONS

1. Identify three major biologic changes that occur with aging; give an example of each.
2. Identify and describe three major factors contributing to malnutrition in older adults. How do these factors influence the nutrition counseling process?
3. List and describe the resources of several agencies providing nutrition-related services for elderly persons.

❖ SELF-TEST QUESTIONS

True-false
For each item you answer "false," write the correct statement.

1. Old persons in American society are generally given much value and made to feel needed and productive.
2. In American health care much progress has been made in control of chronic disease in old age and related medical and social care practices in meeting the needs of the aged.
3. Beginning at about the age of 30, a gradual increase occurs in the performance capacity of most organ systems that lasts throughout adulthood.
4. We have an extensive research base of knowledge about nutritional needs of elderly persons and can state their specific energy and nutrient requirements.
5. The simplest basis for judging adequacy of kcalorie intake is the maintenance of normal weight.
6. The protein requirement increases with age.
7. Most elderly persons require additional supplements of vitamins and minerals.

Multiple choice

1. The basic biologic changes in old age include:
   a. An increase in number of cells
   b. A decreasing sense of self-worth
   c. An increased basal metabolic rate
   d. A gradual loss of functioning cells and reduced cell metabolism
2. Protein needs in adulthood are influenced by:
   (1) The biologic value of the dietary protein being used
   (2) Adequacy of the diet's energy value (kcalories)
   (3) The individual state of health
   (4) The nature of the dietary fats—the saturated/unsaturated ratio
       a. 1, 2, and 3   c. 3, 4, and 5
       b. 1, 3, and 4   d. All of these
3. Which of the following responses give examples of physiologic changes in aging?
   (1) Increased cell metabolism to meet increased aging needs
   (2) Decreased gastrointestinal motility
   (3) A gradual increase in the body's reserve capacity
   (4) Decreased digestive secretions
       a. 2 and 4   c. 1 and 2
       b. 1 and 3   d. 3 and 4
4. Which of the following actions would help elderly persons most in finding solutions to health problems?
   (1) Analyze the individual living situation and food habits carefully
   (2) Reinforce good habits, leave harmless ones alone, and suggest needed changes that are practical within the living situation

(3) Encourage possible variety in foods and seasonings
(4) Explore and use available community resources for assistance
    a. 1 and 4   c. 3 and 4
    b. 2 and 3   d. All of these

❖ SUGGESTIONS FOR ADDITIONAL STUDY

Nutritional analysis of an older adult's diet

Select an older adult and plan, if possible, a home visit, individually or in a small group of two or three students. In the home, interview the older person and observe food use and habits. For example, go with the person into the kitchen and show your interest in facilities for cooking and food storage. Note the food products on hand in the refrigerator (if there is one) and on shelves.

Analyze your findings in terms of kcalories (energy value) and four nutrients: protein, vitamin D, calcium, and iron. Also note the nature of the carbohydrates (complex, simple, fiber) and fats (animal or plant sources) used.

Plan with the person a suitable diet with suggestions to meet: (1) variety in foods and seasonings, (2) personal desires, (3) practical living situation, and (4) nutritional needs.

Go with the person to a nearby market, if possible, and suggest some tips for wise buying of food products. Return to the home and help prepare a meal or snack, discussing the values of various food items.

Follow up with a later visit, if possible, to provide additional support and encouragement to continue any needed improvement in food habits.

Community senior citizens center

Arrange for an informal interview with the center director to learn about the center activities and programs. Plan with the director a follow-up visit for one of the center activities. Discuss informally with persons there some of their programs and activities at the center. Bring your findings to class.

References

1. U.S. Department of Health and Human Services, Public Health Service, Healthy people 2000: National health promotion and disease prevention objectives, Washington, DC, 1990.
2. Brown JL: Hunger in the U.S., Sci Am 256(2):37, 1987.
3. Fanelli MT and Woteki CE: Nutrient intakes and health status of older Americans, Data from NHANES II. In Murphy C, Cain WS, and Hegstead DM: Nutrition and the chemical senses in aging, Ann NY Acad Sci 561:94, 1989.
4. Andres R: Mortality and obesity: the rationale for age-specific height-weight tables. In Andres R and others, editors: Principles of geriatric medicine, New York, 1985, McGraw-Hill.
5. Anderson JJB: Dietary calcium and bone mass through the lifecycle, Nutr Today 25(2):9, 1990.
6. National Research Council, Food and Nutrition Board: Recommended dietary allowances, ed 10, Washington, DC, National Academy Press.
7. Bayle L: "Brown bag" vitamin review for elders, J Nutr Ed 22(6):310B, 1990.
8. National Research Council, Food and Nutrition Board, Committee on Diet and Health: Diet and health, implications for reducing chronic disease risk, Washington, DC, 1989, National Academy Press.
9. Roe DA: Therapeutic effects of drug-nutrient interactions in the elderly, J Am Diet Assoc 85(2):174, 1985.

Further Reading

Anderson JJB: Dietary calcium and bone mass through the lifecycle, Nutr Today 25(2):9, 1990.

D'Urso-Fischer E and others: Reaching out to the elderly, Nutr Today 25(5):20, 1990.

These two articles from the journal *Nutrition Today* provide helpful background for working with older adults. The first author, an expert on osteoporosis, gives us a better understanding of this chronic disease in many older women. The second group of authors, nutrition specialists working with older adults, report their outreach programs for bringing diet, nutrition, and health information to different parts of the elderly population, each using unique and creative educational techniques.

13

❖

Community food supply and health

K E Y   C O N C E P T S

*Modern food production, processing, and marketing have both
positive and negative influences on food safety.*

Many organisms in contaminated food transmit disease.

*Poverty effectively prevents individuals and families from having
adequate access to their surrounding community food supply.*

$\mathcal{T}$he health of a community largely depends on the safety
of its available food and water supply. Our system of government control
agencies and regulations, along with local and state public health officials,
work diligently at maintaining a safe food supply. They generally succeed, but
not always. There are problems because our technologic advances are rapidly
changing our total environment. As always, such progress brings new problems.
Our concern here is the effect of this progress on our food supply and thus
our health.

In this chapter we explore factors that influence the safety of the food we
eat. Modern American food production, processing, and marketing have provided a bountiful food supply, but certain hazards have accompanied this
bounty. Potential health problems related to our food supply can also arise
from two other sources, food-borne disease and poverty.

FOOD SAFETY

The character of America's present food supply has radically changed over the years. These changes, which have swept the food-marketing system, are rooted in widespread social change and in scientific advance. The agricultural and food processing industries have developed various chemicals to increase and preserve our food supply. Critics, however, voice concerns about how these changes have affected food safety and the overall environment. Their concerns center on pesticides and food additives.

Agricultural pesticides

Reasons for use. Large American agricultural corporations, as well as individual farmers, use a number of chemicals to promote their crop yields. These materials have made possible the advances in food production required to feed a growing population. Farmers use these chemicals to control a wide variety of destructive insects, kill weeds, control plant diseases, stop fruit from dropping prematurely, cause leaves to fall and thus facilitate harvesting, make seeds sprout, keep seeds from rotting before they sprout, increase yield, and improve marketing quality.

Problems. Concerns and confusion continue about the use and effects of these chemicals. Problems have developed in four main areas: (1) pesticide residues on foods, (2) gradual leaching of the chemicals into ground water and surrounding wells, (3) increased exposure of farm workers to these strong chemicals, and (4) increased amount of chemicals required as insect tolerance for them develops. Over time use of these chemicals has created our "pesticide dilemma."[1,2] What do we do in the face of conflicting interests? Only recently have the opposing parties, chemical companies and the public interest groups, reached some agreement. They have hammered out beginning steps to reform existing government regulations controlling these chemicals.[3] Thousands of pesticides are in use, but only a small fraction have been fully tested for safety. Better technology also is needed for day-to-day testing of difficult-to-detect food residues. The Food and Drug Administration's routine screening assays in current use can detect only about 40% of all U.S. pesticides.[4]

Another basic problem focuses on the difficult task of risk assessment for specific pesticides in use, especially for children who are more vulnerable to larger amounts as well as for adults who are eating an increasing amount of fresh vegetables and fruits in their daily diets.[5,6] As an alternative to full dependence on pesticide use, an increasing number of farmers, especially in California, the major supplier of U.S. fruits and vegetables, are introducing organic farming, using this system of nonchemical control practices entirely or combining it with limited pesticide use in a farming system known as Integrated Pest Management.[7,8]

Food additives

Reasons for use. Over the past few decades, *food additives*, or chemicals intentionally added to foods, have become part of our food supply. Our present variety of food market items would be impossible without them. They have helped turn the corner grocery store into our giant supermarket chains. Scientific advances have created these processed food products, and our changing society has created the market for them. Our expanding population, greater work force, and more complex family life have increased our desire for more variety and convenience in foods, as well as for better safety and quality. Food additives help achieve these needs and serve many purposes. For example, additives (1) enrich foods with added nutrients; (2) produce uniform qualities such as color, flavor, aroma, texture, and general appearance; (3) standardize many functional factors such as thickening or stabilization (keeping parts from separating out); (4) preserve foods by preventing oxidation; and (5) control acidity or alkalinity to improve flavor, texture, and the cooked product. Table 13-1 lists some examples of these food additives. A number of micronutrients and antioxidants are used as additives in processed foods, not for increasing the nutrient content but for their technical effects either during the processing or in the final product.[9]

Problems. Although food additives have served many useful purposes, problems also have developed. Initial control of food safety began in 1938 with establishment of the Federal Food, Drug, and Cosmetic Act. Such control continued in 1960 with amendments regulating the use of food additives. These amendments created what has become know as the *GRAS list*, "Generally Recognized As Safe" additives. Rigid testing to determine their true safety, however, was lacking. Any additives developed after 1960 required this rigid testing before approval. Also, in the final hours of debate, Congress added another statement to the amendments. The Delany clause (a clause is a separate portion or distinct article of a document), named for the congressman who proposed it, banned food additives found to cause cancer "in man or animal." Problems multiplied with the GRAS list. As use of these "passed" additives increased, concern arose about long-term effects. Also, knowledge concerning toxicity testing had developed. As a result, in 1977 Congress directed the Food and Drug Administration (FDA) to test all the GRAS items. This has been a massive undertaking, however, and only with modern computers has the FDA been able to list how many thousands exist. This task is still in progress.

Control measures

Government agencies. Several government agencies help control the safety and quality of our food. Concerned sections in the U.S. Department of Health and Human Services are the FDA and the Public Health Service (PHS). The U.S. Department of Agriculture (USDA) controls use of pesticides in farming; related work is assigned to the Agricultural Research Service and the Consumer Marketing Service. The Federal Trade Commission and the National Bureau of Standards also protect the consumer. Of these various agencies, the main one controlling food safety is the FDA.

Food and Drug Administration. The FDA is a law enforcement agency charged by Congress to ensure, among other things, that our food supply is safe, pure, and wholesome. With a newly appointed commissioner at its head, who as both a physician and a lawyer is one of the most qualified directors in FDA history, the agency is speeding up the backlog of assessment work and strengthening the agency's credibility through tough enforcement.[10] The agency enforces federal food-safety regulations through various activities including: (1) food sanitation and quality control, (2) control of chemical contaminants

❖ **TABLE 13-1**   *Examples of food additives*

Function	Chemical compound	Common food uses
Acid, alkalis, buffers	Sodium bicarbonate	Baking powder
	Tartaric acid	Fruit sherbets
		Cheese spread
Antibiotics	Chlortetracycline	Dip for dressed poultry
Anticaking agents	Aluminum calcium silicate	Table salt
Antimycotics	Calcium propionate	Bread
	Sodium propionate	Bread
	Sorbic acid	Cheese
Antioxidants	Butylated hydroxyanisole (BHA)	Fats
	Butylated hydroxytoluene (BHT)	Fats
Bleaching agents	Benzoyl peroxide	Wheat flour
	Chlorine dioxide	
	Oxides of nitrogen	
Color preservative	Sodium benzoate	Green peas
		Maraschino cherries
Coloring agents	Annotto	Butter, margarine
	Carotene	
Emulsifiers	Lecithin	Bakery goods
	Monoglycerides and diglycerides	Dairy products
		Confections
	Propylene glycol alginate	
Flavoring agents	Amyl acetate	Soft drinks
	Benzaldehyde	Bakery goods
	Methyl salicylate	Candy; ice cream
	Essential oils; natural extractives	Canned meats
	Monosodium glutamate	
Nonnutritive sweeteners	Saccharin	Diet canned fruit
	Aspartame	Low-calorie soft drinks
Nutrient supplements	Potassium iodide	Iodized salt
	Vitamin C	Fruit juices
	Vitamin D	Milk
	Vitamin A	Margarine
	B vitamins, iron	Bread and cereal
Sequestrants	Sodium citrate	Dairy products
	Calcium pyrophosphoric acid	
Stabilizers and thickeners	Pectin	Jellies
	Vegetable gums (carob bean, carrageenan, guar)	Dairy desserts and chocolate milk
	Gelatin	Confections
	Agar-agar	"Low-calorie" salad dressings
Yeast foods and dough conditioners	Ammonium chloride	Bread, rolls
	Calcium sulfate	
	Calcium phosphate	

and pesticides, (3) control of food additives, (4) regulation of movement of foods across state lines, (5) nutrition and nutrition labeling of foods, (6) safety of public food service, and (7) safety of meat and milk. Its methods of enforcement are recall, seizure, injunction, and prosecution. The use of recalls is the most common method, followed by seizures of contaminated food.

Consumer education. The FDA's division of consumer education conducts an active program of protection through consumer education and general public information. Special attention is given to nutrition misinformation. Materials are prepared and distributed to individuals, students, and community groups. Consumer specialists work through all FDA district offices.

Research. Along with the USDA's Agricultural Research Service, FDA scientists continually evaluate foods and food components through their own research (Fig. 13-1). In the past, FDA views and policies have varied with administrators and sometimes left much to be desired. Nevertheless, broader views more in tune with today's needs seem to prevail now. Today people want to know more than just that a given food will not kill them. They want to know if it has any positive nutritional value. For a more health-conscious public and a changed marketplace, the FDA is developing nutrition guidelines for a variety of food products. These include new foods such as main dishes, meat substitutes, groups of foods having high malnutrition risks, fruit juices and fruit drinks, and snack foods. This is a broad jump from former attitudes involving a purely regulatory function. Such guidelines should go far in meeting our changing needs in these changing times.

Food labeling

Development of label regulations. In the mid-1960s, the FDA established "truth in packaging" regulations that dealt mainly with *food standards*. Today's labels have more *nutritional information* added, but exactly what food labels should include is still being debated. Both types of label information are important to consumers:

1. *Food standards.* The basic *standard of identity* requires that labels on foods not having an established reference standard must list all the ingredients in the order of amount found in the product. Other food standard information on labels relates to food quality, fill of container, and enrichment.

2. *Nutritional information.* Under regulations adopted in 1973, the FDA has been developing a labeling system that describes the food item's nutritional value to meet the consumer's increasing nutritional interest and concern. Some producers have added limited information on their own to meet this increasing market demand. Many persons are concerned that nutrition labeling is inadequate, but the real problem is what, how much, and in what form. Nutrients and food constituents that consumer groups believe should be listed on labels include the macronutrients (carbohydrate, protein, fat) and their total energy value (calories), key micronutrients (vitamins, minerals), sodium, cholesterol, and saturated fat. Some products also list nutrients in terms of percentages of the U.S. RDA per defined portion (Fig. 13-2).

Current status of new FDA label regulations. Over the past few years, the rapid increase in the variety of food products entering the U.S. marketplace and the changing patterns in American food habits have led many health-

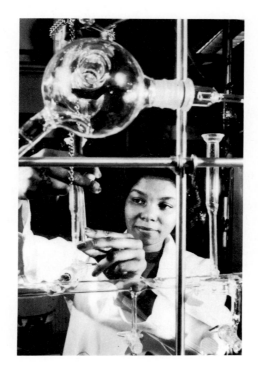

❖ FIG. 13-1

Research in food chemistry. A chemist in the U.S. Department of Agriculture's Agricultural Research Service makes an adjustment on a molecular still used in a project to aid in the manufacture of dry milk.

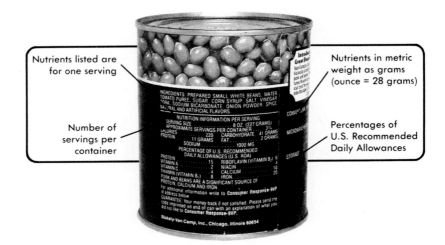

❖ FIG. 13-2

A nutrition label showing detailed nutrition information. (From Wardlaw G and Insel P: Perspectives in nutrition, St. Louis, 1990, Mosby−Year Book.)

conscious consumers and professionals alike to rely increasingly on nutrition labeling on foods to help them meet health goals. However, a number of labeling problems including lack of uniformity, misleading health claims, and indefinite terms such as "natural" and "light" have indicated a need to reorganize and coordinate the entire food labeling system.[11-13] This need has been reinforced by three recent landmark reports relating nutrition and diet to national health goals: *The Surgeon General's Report on Nutrition and Health*, the National Research Council's *Diet and Health*, and the Public Health Service's *Healthy People 2000*.[14-16] Based on these reports, the Institute of Medicine of the National Academy of Sciences established a Committee on the Nutrition Components of Food Labeling to study and report on the scientific issues and practical needs involved in food-labeling reform. The report of this committee was released on Sept. 26, 1990, and is now a component of the comment and rule-making process currently being conducted by FDA, the U.S. Departments of Agriculture and Health and Human Services, and the U.S. Congress to achieve the needed reforms.[17,18] Highlights of the committee's recommendations are summarized in Box 13-1.

FOOD-BORNE DISEASE
Costs of food-borne disease

Many disease-bearing organisms inhabit our environment and can contaminate our food and water. We have learned much about them in past years and have taken many steps to control their spread. Lapses in control still occur, however, resulting in high incidences of illness, death, and economic cost. This impact is probably greatest in developing countries of the world, for few facts are known about real costs, but lapses also occur in developed countries. For example, preliminary U.S. estimates of food-borne disease are 12.6 million cases/year costing $8.4 billion.[19] Microbiologic diseases, bacterial and viral, represent 84% of these U.S. costs, compared with 88% in Canada. The most economically important U.S. diseases are salmonellosis and staphylococcal poisoning, costing annually $4.0 billion and $1.5 billion, respectively. Other costly types of food-borne disease include listeriosis, trichinosis, *Clostridium perfringens* enteritis, and botulism. Botulism has a high annual cost per case of $322,200, but its total comparative impact is only $87 million because relatively few cases (270) occur.[19]

Food Sanitation

Food and its environment. Control of food-borne disease obviously focuses on strict sanitation measures and rigid personal hygiene. First, the food itself should be of qood quality and not defective or diseased. Second, its dry or cold storage should protect it from deterioration or decay. This is especially important for such newly developed products as refrigerated convenience foods, the fastest-growing segment of the convenience food market and potentially the most dangerous because they are not sterile.[20,21] All food preparation areas must be scrupulously clean, and foods must be washed or cleaned well. Cooking procedures and temperatures must be followed as directed. All utensils, dishes, and anything coming in contact with food must be clean. Leftover food must be stored and reused appropriately or discarded. Garbage

❖

BOX 13-1
Nutrition Labeling: Recommendations for the 1990s

There is no longer any doubt. The U.S. government is now committed to the long-awaited food-labeling reform mandated by a health-conscious public, a proliferation of new health-related food products marketplace, and concerned health professionals. It is apparent that nutrition "sells" to today's consumers.

As part of the comment and rule-making process now underway at the FDA and USDA, the report of the Institute of Medicine's Committee on the Nutrition Components of Food Labeling, National Academy of Sciences, has been released. It is based on a 1-year study requested by the U.S. Department of Health and Human Services (DHHS) and the USDA. In the following four areas of concern, the study committee recommends:

Foods covered by nutrition labeling
- That nutrition labeling be made mandatory on most packaged foods.
- That nutrition labeling be provided at the point of purchase for produce, seafood, meats, and poultry.
- That restaurants make information on the nutrient content of menu items available to customers on request.

Label presentation
- That FDA and USDA set standardized serving sizes.
- That more complete ingredient listings be provided on all foods.
- That a modified regulatory scheme be established for the development and approval of lower-fat alternative foods that currently have standards of identity. Further, the committee recommends the steps that should be followed to evaluate new label formats before selection of a final format.

Educating consumers
- That a well-designed nutrition labeling program be fashioned as one part of a comprehensive education program, concurrent with the adoption of new regulations on nutrition labeling content and format, to assist consumers in making wise dietary choices.

Congress wants to develop legislative proposals to clarify the legal basis for anticipated reforms. The food industry, health professionals, and consumer groups want to promote nutrition labeling changes that reflect current dietary guidelines and related product development. These committee recommendations provide a helpful basis for all concerned.

References
Earl R and Wellman NS: Position of the American Dietetic Association: Nutrition and health information on food labels, J Am Diet Assoc 90:583, 1990.

National Research Council: Diet and health: Implications for reducing chronic disease, Washington, DC, 1989, National Academy Press.

Porter DV and Earl RO, editors: Nutrition labeling: Issues and directions for the 1990s. Report of the Committee on the Nutrition Components of Food Labeling, Food and Nutrition Board, Institute of Medicine, Washington, DC, 1990, National Academy Press.

must be contained and disposed of in a sanitary manner. We know about all these measures, but we do not always practice them.

Food handlers. All persons handling food, especially those working with public food services, should follow strict rules of personal hygiene. Simple handwashing, for example, is imperative, along with clean clothing and aprons. Basic rules of hygiene should apply to all persons handling food, whether they work in food processing and packaging plants, process and package foods in markets, or prepare and serve food in restaurants. In addition persons with infectious disease obviously should not work near food, although it sometimes occurs.

Food contamination

Bacterial food infections. Bacterial food infections result from eating food contaminated by large colonies of different types of bacteria. Specific diseases result from specific bacteria. Three such examples are *salmonellosis, shigellosis,* and *listeriosis.*

1. Salmonellosis is caused by the bacteria *Salmonella,* named for the American veterinarian-pathologist Daniel Salmon (1850-1914), who first isolated and identified species commonly causing human food-borne infections—*S. typhi* and *S. paratyphi.* These organisms grow readily in common foods such as milk, custards, egg dishes, salad dressings, and sandwich fillings. Seafood, especially shellfish such as oysters and clams, from polluted waters may also be a source of infection. Unsanitary handling of foods and utensils can spread the bacteria. Resulting cases of gastroenteritis may vary in intensity from mild diarrhea to severe attacks. Practices of immunization, pasteurization, and sanitary regulations involving community water and food supplies as well as food handlers help to control such outbreaks. Because incubation and multiplication of the bacteria take time after the food is eaten, symptoms of food infection develop relatively slowly, usually 12 to 24 hours after ingestion.

2. Shigellosis is caused by the bacteria *Shigella,* named for the Japanese physician Kiyoshi Shiga (1870-1957), who first discovered a main species of the organism—*S. dysenteriae*—during a dysentery epidemic in Japan in 1898. Shigellosis is usually confined to the large intestine and may vary from a mild transient intestinal disturbance in adults to fatal dysentery in young children. The bacteria grow easily in foods, especially in milk, a common vehicle of transmission to infants and children. The boiling of water or the pasteurization of milk kills the organisms, but the food or milk may easily be reinfected through unsanitary handling by a carrier. The disease is spread in much the same way as salmonella is transmitted—by feces, fingers, flies, milk, and food and by articles handled by unsanitary carriers.

3. Listeriosis is caused by the bacteria *Listeria,* named for the English surgeon Baron Joseph Lister (1827-1912) who first applied knowledge of bacterial infection to principles of antiseptic surgery in a benchmark 1867 publication, leading to "clean" operations and the development of modern surgery. It has only been within the past 10 years, however, that knowledge of its role in directly causing food-borne disease in humans, both occasional illness and disease epidemics, has increased and the major species causing human illness— *L. monocytogenes*—identified.[22] Before 1981 *Listeria* was thought to be only

an animal disease organism transmitted to humans by direct contact with infected animals. Now we know that these organisms occur very widely in the environment. In high-risk individuals such as elderly persons, pregnant women, infants, or patients with suppressed immune systems the organisms can produce rare but often fatal illness, with severe symptoms such as diarrhea, flulike fever and headache, pneumonia, sepsis, meningitis, and endocarditis. Food-borne disease has been traced to a variety of foods including soft cheese, poultry, seafood, raw milk, commerically broken and refrigerated raw liquid whole eggs, and meat products such as pate.[23-27]

Bacterial food poisoning. Food poisoning is caused by the ingestion of bacterial toxins that have been produced in the food by the growth of specific kinds of bacteria before the food is eaten. The powerful toxin is ingested directly and symptoms of the food poisoning therefore develop rapidly, usually within 1 to 6 hours after the food is eaten. Two types of bacterial food poisoning are most commonly responsible, *staphylococcal* and *clostridial.*

1. Staphyloccal food poisoning, named for the shape of the causative organism, mainly *Staphylcoccus aureus*—round bacteria forming in masses of cells (Gr. *staphyle*-bunch of grapes; *kokkos*-berry), is by far the most common form of bacterial food poisoning observed in the United States. Powerful preformed toxins in the contaminated food produces illness rapidly within 1 to 6 hours after ingestion.[28] The symptoms appear suddenly—severe cramping and abdominal pain with nausea, vomiting, and diarrhea, usually accompanied by sweating, headache, and fever. There may be prostration and shock. However, recovery is fairly rapid and the symptoms subside within 24 hours (see Box 13-2). The amount of toxin ingested and the susceptibility of the individual

---

BOX 13-2

❖ ———————— **CLINICAL APPLICATION** ———————— ❖

Case Study: A Community Food Poisoning Incident

John and Eva Wesson, a middle-aged couple, agreed that their lodge dinner had been the best they had ever had, especially the dessert—custard-filled cream puffs, John's favorite. He had eaten two, despite Eva's protests at the time. Maybe that was why he began to feel ill shortly after they arrived home. Eva's stomach felt a little upset too, so they both took some antacid pills, thinking their "stomach ache" was from eating more rich food than usual. They went to bed early.

By 11 PM, however, Eva woke up alarmed. John was vomiting and having diarrhea and increasingly severe stomach cramps. He complained of a headache. His pajamas were wet with sweat. He had a fever and appeared to be in shock. Eva herself began to have similar pains and symptoms, although not as severe as John's.

The phone rang. It was one of their friends who had also been at the lodge dinner. She and her husband were also experiencing the same reactions.

Now Eva was really frightened. John had recently begun to have some heart trouble and she thought this attack was related. By now he was prostrate, unable to move. Eva immediately called their physician, who arranged for John to be taken to the hospital. After treatment in the emergency room for shock, followed by observational care and rest the following day, John's symptoms had subsided and he was allowed to

Continued.

BOX 13-2

❖ ─────── CLINICAL APPLICATION, cont'd ─────── ❖

go home. The doctor advised them to eat lightly for a few days and get more rest, and said in the meantime he would investigate the cause. They learned during the next few days that almost all of their lodge friends who had been at the dinner had had an experience similar to theirs.

The doctor contacted the public health department to report the incident. His was one of several similar calls, a public health officer said, and the department was already investigating.

The following week the officer returned the doctor's call to report his findings. The cream puffs served that evening by the restaurant had been purchased from a local bakery. At the bakery the health officials had located a worker with an infected cut on his little finger, a small thing, the worker said. He couldn't understand what all the fuss was about.

The health officials also located the delivery truck driver, who had started out at midmorning to make his rounds and take the cream puffs to the restaurant. On questioning the driver, however, they learned that the truck had "broken down" during the afternoon deliveries before he reached the restaurant. He said he remembered because he had been irritated by a 3-hour wait at the garage while the truck was being fixed. But he still got the order to the restaurant in time for the dinner, he said, so what was the problem?

At the restaurant the chef said that everyone was so busy with the dinner that when the cream puffs finally arrived, no one had time to give much notice to them. They had decided that there was no point in putting the cream puffs in the refrigerator at the time, since they were to be served in a very short while.

When John and Eva's doctor called them afterward to report the story, John and Eva decided they would not eat at that restaurant again. By then John had already lost his taste for cream puffs.

Questions for Analysis

1. Why is control of the community's food supply an important responsibility of the health department?
2. What disease agents may be carried by food or water?
3. What was the agent causing John and Eva's illness? Was this a food infection or a food poisoning? How do you know?

   While the investigation was ongoing and before John and Eva learned the real cause of their illness, John thought it must have been caused by "those things farmers and food processers put into food these days. I've been reading about those things in the paper. It's a wonder we're not sick all the time."
4. What substances did John mean? Can you give some examples?
5. Why are these materials used for growing and processing food?
6. What controls do we have for their use?
7. What are some ways in which food is protected from its point of production to our tables? How can food be preserved for later use?
8. What agency controls food safety and quality? How does it do so? What are food standards? What are the current labeling regulations for food products?

eating it determine the degree of severity. The source of the contamination is usually a staphylococcal infection on the hand of a worker preparing the food. Often it is only a minor infection, considered harmless or even unnoticed by the food handler. Foods that are particularly effective culture beds for staphylococci and their toxins include custard- or cream-filled bakery goods, processed meats, ham, tongue, cheese, ice cream, potato salad, sauces, chicken and ham salads, and combination dishes such as spaghetti and casseroles. The toxin causes no change in normal appearance, odor, or taste of the food, so the victim is not warned. A careful food history helps determine the source of the poisoning. If possible, portions of the food are obtained for bacterial examination. Few bacteria may be found, for heating kills the organisms but does not destroy toxin produced.

2. Clostridial food poisoning, named for the spore-forming rod-shaped bacteria Clostridium (Gr. *kloster*, spindle), mainly C. *perfringes* and C. *botulinum*, that are also capable of forming powerful toxins in infected foods. The C. *perfringes* spores are widespread in the environment in soil, water, dust, refuse—everywhere. The organism multiplies in cooked meat and meat dishes and develops its toxin in foods held for extended periods at warming temperatures or at room temperature. A number of outbreaks from food eaten in restaurants, college dining rooms, and school cafeterias have been reported. In each case, cooked meat was improperly handled in preparation and refrigeration. Control rests principally on careful preparation and adequate cooking of meats, prompt service, and immediate refrigeration at sufficiently low temperatures. The bacteria C. *botulinum* causes far more serious, often fatal food poisoning—*botulism*—from ingestion of food containing its powerful toxin. Depending on the dose of toxin taken and the individual response, the illness may vary from mild discomfort to death within 24 hours. Mortality rates are high. Nausea, vomiting, weakness, and dizziness are initial complaints. Progressively, the toxin irritates motor nerve cells and blocks transmission of neural impulses at the nerve terminals, causing gradual paralysis. Sudden respiratory paralysis with airway obstruction is the major cause of death. C. *botulinum* spores are widespread in soil throughout the world and may be carried on harvested food to the canning process. Like all clostridia, this species is anaerobic (develops in the absence of air) or nearly so. The relatively air-free can and the canning temperatures (above 27° C [80° F]) provide good conditions for toxin production. The development of high standards in the commercial canning industry has eliminated this source of *botulism*, but cases still result each year, mainly from eating carelessly home-canned foods. Since boiling for 10 minutes destroys the toxin (not the spore), all home-canned food, no matter how well-preserved it is considered to be, should be boiled at least 10 minutes before eating. In the United States, the states of Alaska and Washington have the highest incidence of botulism. Alaska has the greater number of cases because of native habits of eating uncooked or partially cooked meat that has been fermented, dried, or frozen.[29]

Table 13-2 summarizes these bacterial sources of food contamination.

Viruses. Illnesses produced by viral contamination of food are few in comparison to those produced by bacterial contamination of food. These include upper respiratory infections, such as colds and influenza, and viral infectious hepatitis. Explosive epidemics of infectious hepatitis have occurred in schools,

❖ **TABLE 13-2**   *Selected examples of bacterial food-borne disease*

Food-borne disease	Causative organisms Genus Species	Food source	Symptoms and course
Bacterial food infections			
Salmonellosis	Salmonella *S. typhi* *S. paratyphi*	Milk, custards, egg dishes, salad dress-ings, sand-wich fillings, polluted shellfish	Mild to severe diarrhea, cramps, vomiting. Ap-pears 12-24 hours or more after eating; lasts 1-7 days.
Shigellosis	Shigella *S. dysenter-iae*	Milk and milk products, seafood, and salads	Mild diarrhea to fatal dysentary (especially in young children). Appears 7-36 hours after eating; lasts 3-14 days.
Listeriosis	Listeria *L. monocy-togenes*	Soft cheese, poultry, sea-food, raw milk, meat products (paté)	Severe diarrhea, fever, headache, pneumona, meningitis, endocardi-tis. Symptoms begin after 3-21 days.
Bacterial food poisoning (enterotoxins)			
Staphylococcal	Staphylococcus *S. aureus*	Custards, cream fill-ings, pro-cessed meats, ham, cheese, ice cream, potato salad, sauces, cas-seroles	Severe abdominal pain, cramps, vomiting, diarrhea, sweating, headache, fever, pros-tration. Appears sud-denly 1-6 hours after eating; symptoms sub-side generally within 24 hours.
Clostridial Perfringes enteritis	Clostridium *C. perfringes*	Cooked meat, meat dishes held at warm or room temperature	Mild diarrhea, vomit-ting. Appears 8-24 hours after eating; lasts a day or less.
Botulism	*C. botulinum*	Improperly homecanned foods; smoked and salted fish, ham, sau-sage, shellfish	Symptoms range from mild discomfort to death within 24 hours; initial nausea, vomiting, weakness, dizziness, progressing to motor and some-times fatal breathing paralysis.

towns, and other communities after fecal contamination of water, milk, or food. Contaminated shellfish from polluted waters have caused several outbreaks. Again, stringent control of community water and food supplies, as well as personal hygiene and sanitary practices of food handlers, are essential for prevention of disease.

Parasites. Two types of worms are of serious concern in relation to food: (1) roundworms, such as the *trichina (Trichinella spiralis)* worm found in pork, and (2) flatworms, such as the common *tapeworms* of beef and pork. Two control measures are essential: (1) laws controlling hog and cattle food sources and pastures to prevent transmission of the parasites to the meat produced for market; and (2) avoidance of rare beef or underdone pork as an added personal precaution.

Environmental food contaminants. Heavy metals such as lead and mercury may also contaminate food and water as well as the air and environmental objects. Children are especially vulnerable to lead poisoning, particularly children of poor families sheltered in urban hotels or other impoverished areas with peeling lead paint.[30] Paint remains the most important source of lead for children. It is estimated currently that 30 million homes in the United States have leaded-paint surfaces, and young children live in 3 million homes that have peeling, deteriorated leaded surfaces.[31,32] They face exposure by eating paint chips or by breathing air-borne paint dust particles from abrasive paint removal before remodeling, a situation that lingers for some time in the house after the remodeling is completed. Drinking water remains a major lead source in high-risk households whose water comes through lead service pipes or through plumbing joints that have been sealed with leaded solder.[33] However, new U.S. Environmental Protection Agency (EPA) rules for public drinking water will lower still further the controlled lead exposure levels (see Box 13-3). A recently discovered food source is lead pigment used to label soft plastic food wrappings for items such as bread, not only when the wrapping is turned inside out and reused to store food but also when it is thrown away and the lead becomes part of the environmental waste.[34] Children suffering these elevated lead exposures develop brain damage with subsequent learning deficits from what has been called "this silent, relentless destroyer of brain cells."[31]

Mercury poisoning was first reported in 1953 from massive exposure of a local population in Japan to seafood taken from water contaminated by waste discharge from a local plastics factory. Over a third of the affected individuals died, many suffered neurologic problems such as mental confusion, convulsions, and coma, and many infants and children suffered permanent brain damage. A similar incident occurred again in Japan in 1964. During the winter of 1971-1972 another mercury poisoning disaster occurred in Iraq when barley and wheat grain treated with methylmercury as a fungicide had been purchased from Mexico. The grain sacks carried a written warning, but only in Spanish. Now the FDA limits possible mercury contamination of food by close inspection of seafood and pesticide residues on crops.

FOOD NEEDS AND COSTS
Hunger and malnutrition

World malnutrition. We are made increasingly aware through the daily news that malnutrition, even famine and death, exists in many countries of

❖

BOX 13-3
Lead in Children's Diets

Lead poisoning has been a major public health problem for centuries. New studies have shown that lead not only poisons our air and soil, but also contaminates the food we eat, the dust in our homes, and the water that millions of us drink. Most disturbing of all, however, is its danger to our children, especially during the first 6 years of life.

In the United States more than 250,000 children, most of them between the ages of 2 and 3 years, are found to have absorbed excessive amounts of lead each year. Most health workers have assumed that these children obtained most of the excess lead from lead-based paint chips or contaminated dirt or dust. However, researchers have found that 55% to 85% of this daily lead intake is contributed by food and water. About 25% of the lead in food comes from canned vegetables, fruits, and juices, especially acidic foods that extract any lead present in cans. The lead pigment used to print labels on soft plastic food packaging can also be a source, especially if families reuse the bag for food storage.

Increased research has shown that even low levels of lead can have damaging effects on both children and adults, leading the Environmental Protection Agency (EPA) to issue new rules to reduce levels of lead in U.S. drinking water. These new rules, to be phased in over 1992-1993, will establish a monitoring system by which tap water lead values must not exceed 15 parts per billion (ppb), lowering the existing standards of 50 ppb for drinking water.

The brain-damaging effects of lead poisoning in young children are associated with anemia, fatigue, and poor attention span and learning ability. The new federal definition of lead toxicity is now 10 μg/dl, putting at least 17% of all children, even 50% of children in poverty, at neurotoxic risk with blood levels above this newly defined level. Recognizing this increasing danger of childhood lead poisoning, the Department of Health and Human Services has begun a plan of prevention, reduced exposure, and national surveillance to eradicate this serious problem. These measures are not new, but this degree of federal commitment is—and none too soon to meet this increasing threat to the living environment and health of every child.

References
Needleman HL: Childhood lead poisoning: a disease for the history texts, Am J Pub Health 81(6):685, 1991.

Centers for Disease Control, Department of Health and Human Services: Strategic plan for the elimination of childhood lead poisoning, Washington, DC, Feb 1991.

Report: New lead rules for water, Science News 139(20):308, 1991.

the world. Also, hunger and disease go hand in hand. Many environmental problems influence malnutrition. It is not merely a problem of agriculture, of soil erosion and drought, but also of sanitation, culture, social problems, and economic and political structure. Close to U.S. borders, for example, peoples of Mexico, Central and South America are plagued by social conditions such as economic depression, revolution, inequity, and desperate poverty. The interaction of some of these factors that lead relentlessly to malnutrition are shown in Fig. 13-3.

American malnutrition. Hunger, however, does not stop at the U.S. border. In the United States, one of the wealthiest countries on earth, many studies document widespread hunger and malnutrition among the poor. In any society, at both governmental and personal levels, food availability and use involves

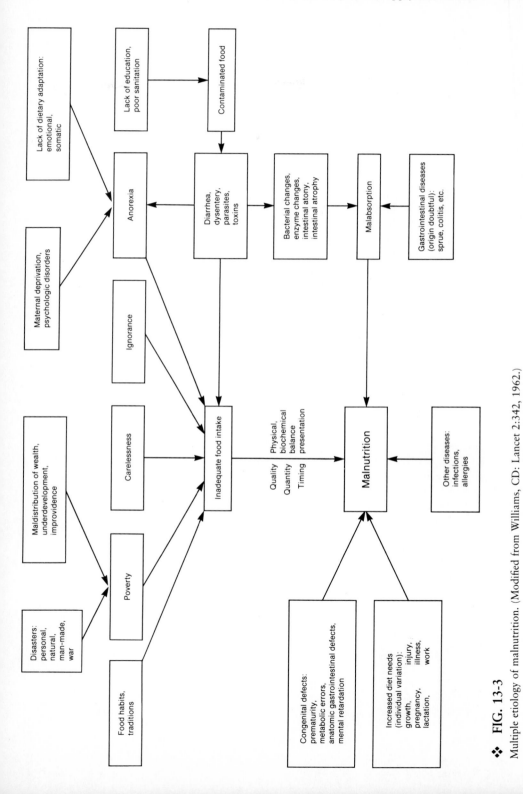

❖ **FIG. 13-3**

Multiple etiology of malnutrition. (Modified from Williams, CD: Lancet 2:342, 1962.)

both money and politics. Various factors are involved, such as land management practices, water distribution, long-term use of questionable pesticides, food production and distribution policies, and food assistance programs for individuals and families in need. Often a "culture of poverty" develops among the poor, reinforced by society's values and attitudes.

Food assistance programs

In situations of economic stress, individuals and families need financial help. Currently, a depressed economy and federal cutbacks in food assistance programs have increased the number of persons in the United States who experience hunger each day. You may need to discuss available food assistance programs and make appropriate referrals.

Commodity distribution program. Under this act, the federal government purchases market surpluses of food items to support prices of agricultural products. These items include both perishable goods and price-supported basic and nonperishable commodities. This accumulation of food stocks led to the present program as a means of distributing the stored products to persons in need (Fig. 13-4).

Food Stamp program. The Food Stamp program began in the late depression years of the 1930s and was developed further in the 1960s and 1970s. It has helped many poor persons purchase needed food, although federal cuts in the 1980s have curtailed its help to many persons in need. Under this program the person or "household" is issued coupons, or "food stamps." These coupons are supposed to be sufficient to cover the household's food needs for 1 month. Households must have a monthly income below the program's eligibility pov-

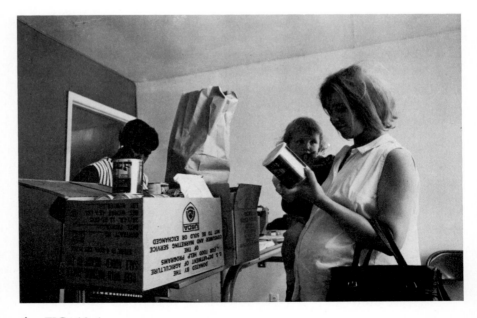

❖ **FIG. 13-4**

Pregnant mother and her child participating in the supplemental Commodities Distribution Program.

erty limit in order to qualify. This limit is quite low. Usually persons who qualify simply do not make enough money to buy needed food.

Special supplemental food program for women, infants, and children. This program (WIC) provides nutritious foods to low-income women who are pregnant or breast-feeding and to their infants and children under age 5, as well as those shown to be at nutritional risk. The food is either distributed free or purchased by free vouchers. The vouchers are good for such foods as milk, eggs, cheese, juice, fortified cereals, and infant formulas. These foods supplement the diet with rich sources of protein, iron, and certain vitamins that help reduce risk factors such as poor growth patterns, low birth weight or prematurity, toxemia, miscarriages, and anemia.

National school lunch and breakfast programs. These programs enable schools to provide nutritious lunches and breakfasts to students. Poor children eat free or reduced-rate meals, often their main food intake of the day. Other students pay somewhat less than the full cost of the meal. The lunches are required to fulfill approximately one third of the child's RDA standard for energy and nutrients.

Older Americans program. Under this act, two types of food programs benefit the growing number of elderly citizens in the United States. Regardless of their income, all persons over 60 can eat hot noon meals at some community center under the Congregate Meals Programs, or they can receive meals at home under the Home Delivered Meals Program if they are ill or disabled. The act specifies that economically and socially needy persons be given priority. Both programs accept voluntary contributions for meals.

Food buying and handling practices

For many American families, the problem is buying food wisely with their limited food dollars. Shopping for food often is no easy task, especially when each marketed item in a supermarket's overabundant supply shouts, "Buy me!" Food marketing is big business and producers compete for prize placement and shelf space. A large supermarket may stock 8000 or more different food items, and more are being added daily. A single food item may be marketed a dozen different ways at as many different prices. In diet counseling, clients and families typically express their greatest need for help in food buying. Four wise shopping and handling practices will help provide healthy foods as well as control food costs.

1. Plan ahead. Use market guides in newspapers, plan general menus, and keep a checklist of kitchen supplies. Make out a list ahead of time according to location of items in a regularly used market (Fig. 13-5). Such planning controls "impulse buying" and extra trips.

2. Buy wisely. Know the market, market items, packaging, labels, grades, brands, portion yields, measures, and food values in various market units. Read labels carefully. Watch for sale items. Buy in quantity only if it results in real savings and the food can be adequately stored or used. Be cautious in selecting so-called convenience foods. The time saved may not be worth the added cost. Also, for fresh foods and good buys, try alternative food sources such as farmers' markets, consumer co-ops, and gardens.

3. Store food safely. Control food waste and prevent illness from food spoilage or contamination. Conserve food by storing items according to their

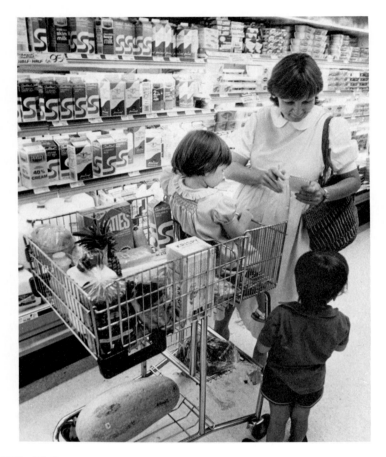

❖ FIG. 13-5
Wise food buying using a prepared market list can help shoppers avoid costly "impulse buying."

nature and use. Use dry storage, covered containers, and refrigeration as needed. Keep opened and partly used food items at the front of the shelf for early use. Avoid plate waste by preparing only the amount needed. Use leftovers in creative ways.

4. *Cook food well.* Use cooking processes that retain maximum food value. Prepare food with imagination and good sense. Give zest and appeal to dishes with a variety of seasonings, combinations, and serving arrangements. No matter how much persons may know about nutrition and health, they usually eat because they are hungry and the food looks and tastes good, not necessarily because it is healthy.

SUMMARY

Common public concerns about the safety of the community food supply focus on the use of many chemicals as pesticides and food additives. These substances have produced an abundant food supply but also have brought dangers as well and thus require control. The main government agency established to maintain this control is the FDA. It conducts activities related to such areas as food safety, food labeling, food standards, consumer education, and research.

Food-borne disease may be caused by many organisms, such as bacteria, viruses, and parasites that can contaminate food. Rigorous public health measures control sanitation of food areas and personal hygiene of food handlers. The same standards should apply to home food preparation and storage.

Families in economic stress need counseling concerning financial assistance. Various U.S. food assistance programs help families in need, and referrals can be made to appropriate agencies. Families also may need help in wise buying and handling of food.

❖ REVIEW QUESTIONS

1. What is the basis of concern about food additives and pesticide residues?
2. Describe ways that various organisms may contaminate food. What standards of food preparation and handling should be used to keep food safe?
3. List and describe food assistance programs available to help low-income families. What other local resources are available in your community?
4. List and discuss the "wise food buying and handling practices" described in this chapter. How many of these practices do you follow in selecting, storing, and preparing foods?

❖ SELF-TEST QUESTIONS

True-false

For each item you answer "false," write the correct statement.

1. In the United States, surveys reveal little or no real malnutrition.
2. The politics of a region or country is not involved in the nutritional status of the people.
3. The number of new processed food items using food additives has been declining in recent years because of public pressure and concern.
4. The use of pesticides on farm crops and food additives in processed foods is under the control of the USDA and FDA.
5. Food poisoning is caused by viral contamination of food.
6. The Commodity Distribution Program buys agricultural food surpluses to support market prices of food and distributes these goods to needy persons.
7. The number of poor persons assisted by the Food Stamp Program has been increasing due to expanded federal support.
8. The Older Americans Program provides group meals for all persons over 60 years of age, regardless of their income.

Multiple choice

1. Food additives are used in processed food items to:
   (1) Preserve food and lengthen its market life
   (2) Enrich food with added nutrients
   (3) Improve flavor, texture, and appearance
   (4) Enhance or improve some physical property of the food
   (5) Create a new market product to meet industry competition and increase company profits
   a. 1, 4, and 5
   b. 2 and 3
   c. 1 and 5
   d. All of these

2. The use of food additives in food products is controlled by:
   a. U.S. Public Health Service
   b. U.S. Department of Agriculture
   c. Food and Drug Administration
   d. Federal Trade Commission

❖ SUGGESTIONS FOR ADDITIONAL STUDY

Food Market Survey: Food Labeling

Visit a local community food market and survey the variety of food products. Find as many new processed food items as you can, at least 10. Read the labels carefully and study the nature and use of each item.

1. List the food items you located. Describe each in terms of its nature, packaging, and use.
2. What does the label on each item tell you about the relative amounts of ingredients and how the food was processed? List the food additives used and determine the purpose of as many as you can. Call your nearest FDA district office for information or write to the federal FDA office in Washington, DC for information on food additives.
3. What nutrition information did you find on each label?
4. How would you evaluate these processed food items?

Market Survey of Comparative Food Costs

Visit a local community food market and compare the different forms of 10 food items—for example, fresh, canned, frozed, processed. List the different forms you found for each food item with the unit price for each form.

1. What form was the least expensive in each case?
2. In view of your findings, what suggestions can you give for economical food buying?
3. What factors influence the cost of food items?

References

1. Blair D: Uncertainties in pesticide risk estimation and consumer concern, Nutr Today 24(6):13, 1989.
2. Thonney PF and Bisogni CA: Residues of agricultural chemicals on fruits and vegetables: pesticide use and regulatory issues, Nutr Today 24(6):6, 1989.
3. Sun M: Antagonists agree on pesticide law reform, Science 232:16, 1986.
4. Walker T: Better assay for pesticides tainting food, Science News 139(19):293, 1991.
5. Roberts L: Pesticides and kids, Science 243:1280, 1989.
6. Green C: A new look for supermarket produce sections, National Food Review 11(4):1, 1988.
7. Newsome R: Organically grown foods: an Institute of Food Technology Scientific Perspective, Food Technology 44:26, June 1990.
8. Expert Panel on Food Safety and Nutrition, Institute of Food Technology, Scientific Status Summary: Quality of fruits and vegetables, Food Technology 44:106, June 1990.
9. Waslien CI and Rehwoldt RE: Micronutrients and antioxidants in processed foods—analysis of data from 1987 Food Additives Survey, Nutr Today 25(4):36, 1990.
10. Gibbon A: Can David Kessler revive the FDA? Science 252:200, Apr 12, 1991.
11. McNutt K: Choices—will food labeling legislation help consumers? Food Engineering 61:62, Sept 1989.
12. Pennington JAT and others: Descriptive terms for fat labeling, J Nutr Ed 22:51, Jan/Feb 1990.
13. Earl R and Wellman NS: Position of The American Dietetic Association: Nutrition and health information on food labels, J Am Diet Assoc 90(4):583, 1990.
14. US Department of Health and Human Services, Public Health Service: The Surgeon General's Report on Nutrition and Health, Washington, DC, 1988, US Government Printing Office.

15. National Research Council, Food and Nutrition Board: Diet and health: Implications for reducing chronic disease risk, Washington, DC, 1989, National Academy Press.
16. US Department of Health and Human Services, Public Health Service: Healthy people 2000: national health promotion and disease prevention objectives, Washington, DC, 1990, US Government Printing Office.
17. Porter DV and Earl R, editors: Nutrition labeling: issues and directions for the 1990s. Report of the Committee on the Nutrient Components of Food Labeling, Food and Nutrition Board, Institute of Medicine, Washington, DC, 1990, National Academy Press.
18. Earl R, Porter DV, and Wellman NS: Report summary: Nutrition labeling: issues and directions for the 1990s, J Am Diet Assoc 90(11):1599, 1990.
19. Todd ECD: Preliminary estimates of costs of foodborne disease in the United States, J Food Protection 52:595, Aug 1989.
20. Corlett DA Jr: Microbiological safety considerations in refrigerated convenience foods, Cereal Foods World 34:980, Dec 1989.
21. Convenience foods: the second revolution, Food Engineering 61:69, Sept 1989.
22. Donelly, CW: *Listeria*—an emerging foodborne pathogen, Nutr Today 25(5):7, 1990.
23. Linnan MJ and others: Epidemic listeriosis associated with Mexican-style cheese, N Engl J Med 319:823, 1988.
24. Farber JM-Sanders GW, and Johnston MA: A survey of various foods for the presence of *Listeria* species, J Food Protection 52:456, 1989.
25. Pearson LJ, and Marth EH: *Listeria monocytogenes*—threat to a safe food supply: a review, J Dairy Sci 73:912, 1990.
26. Leasor SB and Foegeding PM: *Listeria* species in commercially broken raw liquid whole eggs, J Food Protection 52:777, Nov 1989.
27. Morris IJ and Ribeiro CD: *Listeria monocytogenes* and paté, Lancet 2:1285, 1989.
28. Halpin-Dohnalek MI: *Staphylococcal aureus*: production of extracellular compounds and behavior in foods—a review, J Food Protection 52:267, Apr 1989.
29. Lancaster MJ: Botulism: north to Alaska, Am J Nursing 90:60, Jan 1990.
30. Alperstein G, Rapport C, and Flanigan JM: Health of homeless children in New York City, Am J Pub Health 78(9):1232, 1988.
31. Needleman HL: Childhood lead poisoning: a disease for the history texts, Am J Pub Health 81(6):685, 1991.
32. Centers for Disease Control, US Department of Health and Human Services: Strategic plan for the elimination of childhood lead poisoning, Washington, DC, 1991, US Goverment Printing Office.
33. Report: New lead rules for water, Science News 139(20):308, 1991.
34. Weisel C and others: Soft plastic bread wrapping: lead content and reuse by families, Am J Pub Health 81(6):756, 1991.

Further Reading

Blair D: Uncertainties in pesticide risk estimation and consumer concern, Nutr Today 24(6):13, Nov/Dec 1989.

Crane NT and others: Nutrition labeling of foods: a global perspective, Nutr Today 25(4):28, 1990.

These two articles from *Nutrition Today* describe two issues of current nutrition concern; pesticide residues on food and nutrition and health labeling of food products, in the usual helpful format of this excellent journal.

14

❖

Food habits and cultural patterns

KEY CONCEPTS

Personal food habits develop as part of one's social and cultural heritage as well as changing life-style and life situation.

Short term food patterns, or "fads," stem from food misinformation that appeals to some human need.

The force of social change brings changes in food patterns.

*W*hy do people eat what they eat? We know that food is necessary to sustain life and health. We also know that people eat certain foods for many other reasons, least of all perhaps for "good health and nutrition," although this concern is currently increasing. As we have seen in Chapter 13, the broader food environment from which persons have to choose is often influenced by factors such as politics and poverty, limiting personal control and choice.

We attach many meanings to food. All of our food habits are intimately related to our whole way of life: our values, our beliefs, our life situation. Sometimes, however, these food beliefs come from food misinformation and "fads" rather than sound nutrition knowledge.

In this chapter we examine some of these personal and cultural influences on our food choices. We shall see how our food habits develop and why they are difficult to change. They *are* changing, however, because our society and our way of life are changing — and changing rapidly.

CULTURAL DEVELOPMENT OF FOOD HABITS

Food habits, like any other form of human behavior, do not develop in a vacuum. They grow from many personal, cultural, social, economic, and psychologic influences. For each of us, these factors are interwoven.

Strength of personal culture

Culture involves much more than the major and historic aspects of a person's communal life, such as language, religion, politics, and technology. It also develops from all the habits of everyday living and family relationships, such as preparing and serving food, caring for children, feeding them, and lulling them to sleep. We learn these things as we grow up. In a gradual process of conscious and unconscious learning, our culture's values, attitudes, habits, and practices become a deep part of our lives. Although as adults we may revise parts of this heritage or even reject some aspects, it remains within us to influence our lives and pass on to following generations.

Food in a culture

Food habits are among the oldest and most deeply rooted aspects of many cultures. Cultural background largely determines what is eaten as well as when and how it is eaten. Of course, much variation exists. All types of customs, whether rational or irrational, beneficial or injurious, are found in every part of the world. Whatever the situation, however, food habits are primarily based on food availability, economics, and personal food meanings and beliefs. Many foods in any culture take on symbolic meanings related to major life experiences from birth through death, to religion, to politics, and to general social organization. From ancient times ceremonies and religious rites involving food have surrounded certain events and seasons. Food gathering, preparing, and serving have followed specific customs, many of which remain today.

Some traditional cultural food patterns

In the past, the United States has been called a "melting pot" of ethnic and racial groups. In more recent years, however, it has become clear that this image is no longer appropriate. We have come to recognize and even celebrate our diversity as a basis for national strength.[1] This recognition is especially strong in the diversity of our cultural food patterns.

Many different cultural food patterns are part of American family and community life. They have contributed special dishes or modes of cooking to American eating habits. In turn, many of these subcultural food habits have been Americanized. Traditional foods are used more regularly by older members of the family, with younger persons in the family using them mainly on special occasions or holiday. Nevertheless, these traditional foods have strong meanings and serve to bind families and cultural communities in close fellowship. A few representative cultural food patterns of five types are briefly reviewed here. In each, individual tastes and geographic patterns vary.

Religious dietary laws

Jewish. Observance of Jewish food laws differs among the three basic groups within Judaism: (1) Orthodox, strict observance; (2) Conservative, less strict; and (3) Reform, less ceremonial emphasis and minimum general use. The basic body of dietary laws is called the *Rules of Kashruth*. Foods selected and prepared according to these rules are called *kosher*, from the Hebrew word meaning "fit, proper." Originally these laws had special ritual significance. Present Jewish dietary laws apply this significance to laws governing the slaughter, preparation, and serving of meat, to the combining of meat and milk, to fish, and to eggs. Various food restrictions exist.

1. *Meat*. No pork is used. Forequarters of other meats are allowed, as well as all commonly used forms of poultry. All forms of meat used are rigidly cleansed of all blood.

2. *Meat and milk*. No combining of meat and milk is allowed. Orthodox homes maintain two sets of dishes, one for serving meat and the other for meals using dairy products.

3. *Fish*. Only fish with fins and scales are allowed. These may be eaten with either meat or dairy meals. No shellfish or eels may be used.

4. *Eggs*. No egg with a blood spot may be eaten. Eggs may be used with either meat or dairy meals.

Influence of festivals. Many of the traditional Jewish foods relate to festivals of the Jewish calendar that commemorate significant events in Jewish history. Often special Sabbath foods are used. A few representative foods include:

- **Bagels** Doughnut-shaped, hard yeast rolls.
- **Blintzes** Thin filled and rolled pancakes.
- **Borscht (borsch)** Soup of meat stock, beaten egg or sour cream, beets, cabbage, or spinach. Served hot or cold.
- **Challah** Sabbath loaf of white bread, shaped as a twist or coil, used at the beginning of the meal after the kiddush, the blessing over wine.
- **Gefüllte (gefilte) fish** From a German word meaning "stuffed fish," usually the first course of Sabbath evening meal, made of fish fillet, chopped and seasoned and stuffed back into the skin or rolled into balls.
- **Kasha** Buckwheat groats (hulled kernels), used as a cooked cereal or as a potato substitute with gravy.
- **Knishes** Pastry filled with ground meat or cheese.
- **Lox** Smoked, salted salmon.
- **Matzo** Flat unleavened bread.
- **Strudel** Thin pastry filled with fruit and nuts, rolled, and baked.

Moslem. Moslem dietary laws are based on restrictions or prohibitions on some foods and promotion of others, derived from Islamic teachings in the Koran. The laws are binding and must be followed at all times, even during pregnancy, hospitalization, or travel. They are also binding to visitors in the host Moslem country. The general rule is that "all foods are permitted" unless specifically conditioned or prohibited.[2]

1. *Milk products*. Permitted at all times.

2. *Fruits and vegetables*. Except if fermented or poisonous.

3. *Breads and cereals*. Unless contaminated or harmful.

4. *Meats*. Seafood including fish, shellfish, eels, and sea animals, and land animals except swine; pork is strictly prohibited.

5. *Alcohol*. Strictly prohibited.

Any food combinations are used as long as no prohibited items are included. Milk and meat may be eaten together, in contrast to Jewish kosher laws. The

❖

BOX 14-1

Id Al-Fitr, The Post-Ramadan Festival

Traditionally in Moslem countries at the conclusion of Ramadan, Islam's holy month of prayer and fasting, wealthy merchants and princes hold public feasts for the needy. This is the festival of Id al-Fitr.

Over the years, many delicacies have been served to symbolize the joy of return from fasting, and the heightened sense of unity, brotherhood, and charity that the fasting experience has brought to the people. Among the foods served are chicken or veal, sautéed with eggplant and onions, them simmered slowly in pomegranate juice and spiced with turmeric and cardamon seeds. The highlight of the meal usually is kharuf mahshi, a whole lamb (symbol of sacrifice) stuffed with a rich dressing made of dried fruits, cracked wheat, pine nuts, almonds, and onions, and seasoned with ginger and coriander. The stuffed lamb is baked in hot ashes for many hours, so that it is tender enough to be pulled apart and eaten with the fingers.

At the conclusion of the meal, rich pastries and candies are served. These may be flavored with spices or flower petals. Some of the sweets are taken home and savored as long as possible as a reminder of the festival.

Koran mentions certain foods as being of special value: figs, olives, dates, honey, milk, and buttermilk. Prohibited foods in the Moslem dietary laws may be eaten when no other sources of food are available.

Influence of festivals. Among the Moslem people, a 30-day period of daylight fasting is required during **Ramadan**, the ninth month of the Islamic lunar calendar, thus rotating through all seasons. The fourth pillar of Islam commanded by the Koran is fasting. Ramadan was chosen for the sacred fast because it is the month in which Mohammed received the first of the revelations that were subsequently compiled to form the Koran and also the month in which his followers first drove their enemies from Mecca in AD 624. During the month of Ramadan, Moslems throughout the world observe daily fasting, taking no food or drink from dawn to sunset. Nights, however, are often spent in special feasts. First, an appetizer is taken, such as dates or a fruit drink, followed by the family's "evening breakfast," the *iftar.* At the end of Ramadan a traditional feast lasting up to three days climaxes the observance. Special dishes mark this occasion. There are delicacies such as thin pancakes dipped in powdered sugar, savory buns, and dried fruits (see Box 14-1).

Spanish and Native American influences

Mexican. Food habits of early Spanish settlers and Indian nations form the basis of present food patterns of persons of Mexican heritage who now live in the United States, chiefly in the Southwest. Three foods are basic to this pattern: dried beans, chili peppers, and corn. Variations and additions may be found in different places or among those of different income levels. Relatively small amounts of meat are used, and eggs are eaten occasionally. Some fruit, such as oranges, apples, and bananas, are used, depending on availability. For centuries corn has been the basic grain used as bread in the form of tortillas, flat cakes baked on a hot surface or griddle. Some wheat is now being used in making tortillas; rice and oat are added cereals. Coffee is a main beverage. Major seasonings are chili peppers, onions, and garlic; the basic fat is lard

Puerto Rican. The Puerto Rican people share a common heritage with the Mexicans, so much of their food pattern is similar. They add tropical fruits and vegetables, however, many of which are available in their neighborhood markets in the United States. A main type of food is *viandas*, starchy vegetables and fruits such as plantain and green bananas. Two other staples of the diet are rice and beans. Milk, meat, yellow and green vegetables, and other fruits are used in limited quantities, but dried codfish is a staple food. Coffee is a main beverage. The main cooking fat is usually lard.

Native American. The Native American population, Indian and Alaskan Natives, is composed mainly of more than 500 federally recognized diverse groups living on reservations, in small rural communities, or in metropolitan areas.[3,4] Despite their individual diversity, the various groups share a spiritual attachment to the land and a determination to retain their culture. Food has great religious and social significance, and is an integral part not only of celebrations and ceremonies but also of everyday hospitality, which includes a serious obligation for serving food. Foods may be prepared and used in different ways from region to region and vary according to what can be grown locally, harvested or hunted on the land or fished from its rivers, or is available in food markets. Among the Native American groups of the southwest United States, the food pattern of the Navajo people, whose reservation extends over a 25,000-square-mile area at the junction of three states—New Mexico, Arizona, and Utah, may serve as an example.[3]

Historically, the Navajos learned farming from the early Pueblo people, establishing corn and other crops as staples. Later they learned herding from the Spaniards, making sheep and goats available for food and wool.[5] Some families also raised chickens, pigs, and cattle. Currently, Navajo food habits combine traditional dietary staples with modern food products available from supermarkets and fast-food restaurants. Meat is eaten daily—fresh mutton, beef, pork, chicken, or smoked or processed meat. Other staples include: bread—tortillas or fry bread, blue corn bread, and cornmeal mush; beverages—coffee, soft drinks and other fruit-flavored sweet ades; eggs; vegetables—corn, potatoes, green beans, tomatoes; some fresh or canned fruit.[3] Frying is a common method of food preparation; lard and shortening are main cooking fats. Some researchers express concern about an increased use of modern convenience or snack foods high in fat, sugar, calories, and sodium, especially among children and teenagers.[6]

Southern United States influences

African Americans. The black populations, especially in the Southern states, have contributed a rich heritage to American food patterns, particularly to Southern cooking as a whole. Like their moving original music of spirituals, blues, gospel, and jazz, Southern black food patterns were born of hard times, and developed through a creative ability to turn any basic staples at hand into memorable food.[7] Although regional differences occur as with any basic food pattern, surveys indicate representative use of foods from basic food groups[8]:

1. *Breads/cereals.* Traditional breads include hot breads such as biscuits, spoonbread (a soufflelike dish of cornmeal mush with beaten eggs), cornmeal muffins, and skillet cornbread. Commonly used cereals are cooked cereals such

as cornmeal mush, hominy grits (ground corn), and oatmeal. In general, more cooked cereal is used than ready-to-eat dry cereals.

2. *Eggs/dairy products.* Eggs are used and some cheese, but little milk, probably due to the greater prevalence of lactose intolerance among blacks than among whites.

3. *Vegetables.* A frequent type of vegetable is leafy greens: turnip greens, collards, mustard greens, and spinach, usually cooked with bacon or salt pork. Cabbage is used boiled or chopped raw with a salad dressing (cole slaw). Other vegetables used include okra (coated with cornmeal and fried), sweet potatoes (baked whole or sliced and "candied" with added sugar), green beans, tomatoes, potatoes, corn, butterbeans (limas), and dried beans such as black-eyed peas or red beans cooked with smoked ham hocks and served over rice. The black-eyed peas over rice is a dish called Hopping John, traditionally served on New Year's Day to bring good luck for the new year.

4. *Fruits.* Commonly used fruits include apples, peaches, berries, oranges, bananas, and juices.

5. *Meat.* Pork is a common meat, including fresh cuts and ribs, sausage, and smoked ham. Some beef is used, mainly ground for meat loaf or hamburgers. Poultry is used frequently, mainly fried chicken, and baked holiday turkey. Organ meats such as liver, heart, intestines (chitterlings), or poultry giblets (gizzard and heart) are used. When it is available fish includes catfish, some flounder, and shellfish such as crab and shrimp. Frying is a common method of cooking; fats used are lard, shortening, or vegetable oils.

6. *Desserts.* Favorites include pies—pecan, sweet potato, pumpkin, and deep-dish peach or berry cobblers; cakes such as coconut and chocolate; and bread pudding to use left over bread.

7. *Beverages.* Coffee, apple cider, fruit juices, lemonade, iced tea, carbonated soft drinks, and buttermilk—a better-tolerated cultured form of milk.

French Americans. The Cajun people of the southwestern costal waterways in southern Louisiana have contributed a unique cuisine and food pattern to America's rich and varied fare. It provides a model for learning about rapidly expanding forms of American ethnic food.[9] The Cajuns are descendants of the early French colonists of Acadia, a peninsula on the eastern coast of Canada now known as Nova Scotia. In the prerevolutionary wars between France and Britian, both countries contended for the area of Acadia. However, after Britian finally won control of all of Canada, fear of an Acadian revolt led to a forcible deportation of the French colonists in 1755. After a long and difficult journey down the Atlantic coast, then westward along the Gulf of Mexico, a group of the impoverished Acadians finally settled along the bayou country of what is now Louisiana. To support themselves, they developed their unique food pattern from seafood at hand and what they could grow and harvest. Over time they blended their own French culinary background with the Creole cookery they found in their new homeland around New Orleans, which had descended from classical French cuisine combined with other European, American Indian, and African cooking.[9]

Thus the unique Cajun food pattern of the southern Unites States represents an ethnic blending of cultures using basic foods available in the area. Cajun foods are strong-flavored and spicy, with the abundant seafood as a base, usually cooked as a stew and served over rice. The well-known hot chili sauce, made of crushed and fermented red chili peppers blended with spices and vinegar and sold world wide under the trade name Tabasco sauce, is still made by generations of a Cajun family on Avery Island on the coastal waterway of southern Louisiana. The most popular shellfish native to the region is the crawfish, now grown commercially in the fertile rice paddies of the bayou areas. Other seafood used include catfish, red snapper, shrimp, blue crab, and oysters. Cajun dishes usually start with a *roux* made from heated oil and flour mixed with liquid to form a sauce base, to which vegetables, then meat or seafood, and seasonings are added to form a stew. Vegetables used include onions, bell peppers, parsley, shallots, and tomatoes; seasonings are cayenne (red) pepper, hot pepper sauce (tabasco), crushed black pepper, white pepper, bay leaves, thyme, and filé powder. Filé powder is made from ground sassafras leaves and serves both to season and to thicken the dish being made. Some typical Cajun dishes include seafood or chicken gumbo, jambalaya (dish of Creole origin, combining rice, chicken, ham, pork, sausage, broth, vegetables, and seasonings), red beans and rice, blackened catfish or red snapper (blackened with pepper and seasonings and seared in a hot pan), barbecued shrimp, breaded catfish with Creole sauce, and boiled crawfish.[10] Breads and starches include French bread, hush puppies (fried cornbread-mixture balls), cornbread muffins, cush-cush (cornmeal mush cooked with milk), grits, rice, and yams. Vegetables include okra, squash, onions, bell peppers, and tomatoes. Desserts include ambrosia (fresh fruits such as oranges and bananas with grated coconut), sweet potato pie, pecan pie, berry pie, bread pudding, or pecan pralines.

Eastern-Oriental food patterns

Chinese. Chinese cooks believe that refrigeration diminishes natural flavors. Therefore they select the freshest foods possible, hold them the shortest time possible, then cook them quickly at a high temperature in a *wok* with only small amounts of fat and liquid. This basic round-bottom pan allows control of heat in a quick stir-frying method that preserves natural flavor, color, and texture. Vegetables cooked just before serving are still crisp and flavorful when served. Meat is used in small amounts in combined dishes rather than as a single main entree. Little milk is used but eggs and soybean products such as tofu add other protein sources. Foods that have been dried, salted, pickled, spiced, candied, or canned may be added as garnishes or relishes to mask some flavors or textures or to enhance others. Fruits are usually eaten fresh. Rice is the staple grain used at most meals. The traditional beverage is unsweetened green tea. Seasonings include soy sauce, ginger, almonds, and sesame seed. Peanut oil is a main cooking fat.

Japanese. In some ways, Japanese food patterns are similar to those of the Chinese. Rice is a basic grain at meals, soy sauce is used for seasoning, and tea is the main beverage. The Japanese diet contains more seafood, especially raw fish items called *sushi*. Many varieties of fish and shellfish are used. Vegetables are usually steamed, and pickled vegetables are also used. Fresh fruit is eaten in season, a tray of fruit being a regular course at main meals.

Southeast Asian. Since 1971, in the wake of the war in Vietnam, more than 340,000 Southeast Asians have come to the United States as refugees

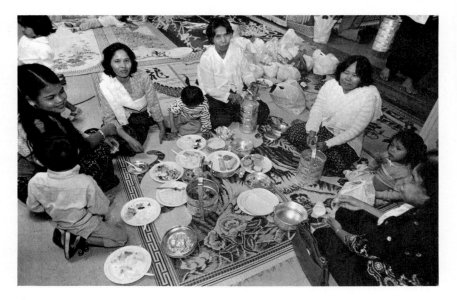

❖ **FIG. 14-1**
A Cambodian family enjoys a festival meal.

(Fig. 14-1).[11] The largest group are Vietnamese; others have come from the adjacent war-torn countries of Laos and Cambodia. They have settled mainly in California, with other groups in Florida, Texas, Illinois, and Pennsylvania. Their basic food patterns are similar. They are making an impact on American diet and agriculture, and Asian grocery stores stock many traditional Indo-Chinese food items.[12] Rice, both long-grain and glutinous, forms the basis of the Indonesian food pattern, and is eaten at most meals. The Vietnamese usually eat rice plain in a separate rice bowl and not mixed with other foods, whereas other Southeast Asians may eat rice in mixed dishes. Soups are also commonly used at meals. Many fresh fruits and vegetables are used along with fresh herbs and other seasonings such as chives, spring onions, chili peppers, ginger root, coriander, turmeric, and fish sauce. Many kinds of seafood, fish and shellfish are used, as well as chicken, duck, pork, and beef.[13] Stir-frying in a wok-type pan with a small amount of lard or peanut oil is a common method of cooking. A variety of vegetables and seasonings are used, with small amounts of seafood or meat added. Since coming to the United States, the Indonesians have made some diet changes that reflect American influence. These include use of more eggs, beef and pork, but less seafood, more candy and other sweet snacks, bread, fast foods, soft drinks, butter and margarine, and coffee.[14,15]

Mediterranean influences

Italian food patterns. The sharing of food is an important part of Italian life. Meals are associated with warmth and fellowship, and special occasions are shared with families and friends. Bread and pasta are basic foods. Milk, seldom used alone, is typically mixed with coffee in equal portions. Cheese is a favorite food, with many popular varieties. Meats, poultry, and fish are used in many ways, and the varied Italian sausages and cold cuts are famous. Vegetables are used alone, in mixed main dishes or soups, in sauces, and in salads. Seasonings include herbs and spices, garlic, wine, olive oil, tomato puree, and salt pork. Main dishes are prepared by initially browning vegetables and seasonings in olive oil; adding meat or fish for browning as well; covering with such liquids as wine, broth, or tomato sauce; and simmering slowly on low heat for several hours. Fresh fruit is often the dessert or a snack.

Greek. Everyday meals are simple, but Greek holiday meals are occasions for serving many delicacies. Bread is always the center of every meal, with other foods considered accompaniments. Milk is seldom used as a beverage, but rather as the cultured form of yogurt. Cheese is a favorite food, especially *feta*, a special white cheese made from sheep's milk and preserved in brine. Lamb is a favorite meat, but others, especially fish, are used also. Eggs are sometimes a main dish, never a breakfast food. Many vegetables are used, often as a main entree, cooked with broth, tomato sauce, onions, olive oil, and parsley. A typical salad of thinly sliced raw vegetables and feta cheese, dressed with olive oil and vinegar, is often served with meals. Rice is a main grain in many dishes. Fruit is an everyday dessert, but rich pastries, such as *baklava* are served on special occasions.

SOCIAL, PSYCHOLOGIC, AND ECONOMIC INFLUENCES ON FOOD HABITS
Social influences

Social structure. Human group behavior reveals many activities, processes, and structures that make up social life. In any society, social groups are formed largely by such factors as economic status, education, residence, occupation, or family. Values and habits vary in different groups. Subgroups also develop on the basis of region, religion, age, sex, social class, health concerns, special interests, ethnic backgrounds, politics, or other common concerns. All of our various group affiliations influence our basic habit patterns, including our food attitudes and habits.

Food and social factors. In our social relationships, food is a symbol of acceptance, warmth, and friendliness. People tend to accept food or food advice more readily from friends or acquaintances or from persons they view as trusted authorities. These influences are especially strong in our family relationships. Food habits that are closely associated with family sentiments stay with us throughout life. Throughout adulthood certain foods trigger a flood of childhood memories and are valued for reasons totally apart from any nutritional value.

Psychologic influences

Understanding diet patterns. We begin to understand diet patterns better when we also see psychologic influences involved. Food has many personal meanings and relationships to personal needs. Our social relationships in turn affect our individual behavior. Many of these psychologic factors are rooted in childhood experiences with food in the family. For example, when a child is hurt or disappointed, parents may offer a sweet food to help the child feel better. Then, when we feel hurt as adults, we turn to those sweets to help us feel good again. Now we are learning that this food behavior may actually have some physiologic components as well. Certain foods, especially sweets and other pleasurable tastes, apparently stimulate "feel good" body chemicals in the brain, called *endorphins*, that give us a mild "high" or help relieve pain.[16]

Food and psychosocial development. Throughout our lives, because food has such a fundamental relationship to our physical survival, it also relates closely to our psychosocial development as individuals. From infancy to old age, our emotional maturity grows along with our physical development. At each stage of human growth, food habits are part of both physical and psychosocial development. For example, when 2-year-old toddlers are struggling with their necessary first steps toward eventual independence from parents, they learn that they can control their parents through food and often become picky eaters, refusing to eat any new foods. Psychologists now believe that another normal developmental factor is involved, which they call *food neophobia*, or fear of unfamiliar foods. This universal trait may be an instinct from our evolutionary past that protected children from eating harmful foods when they were just becoming independent from their mothers.[17]

Economic influences

Family income and food habits. Except perhaps for the small group of very wealthy, most American families live under socioeconomic pressures, especially in periods of recession and inflation. The problems of middle-income families differ in relative terms, but it is the low-income families, especially those in poverty situations, that suffer extreme needs. They often lack adequate housing and they have little or no access to educational opportunities. As a result, they are poorly prepared for jobs and often make only a day-to-day living at low-paying work or are unemployed. Nearly one in every eight Americans lives in a family with an income below the federal poverty level, and one in every four children under the age of 6 years are members of such families.[18] It is unserstandable that people with low incomes bear the greater burden of unnecessary illness and malnutrition, and have death rates twice the rates for people with adequate incomes.[19]

Food assistance programs. Many low-income families are being helped to better health by better food habits developed through community projects conducted by the U.S. federal extension service with extension services in the states working at the county level. These county extension agents, home economists, and their aides from the community help families to use better food buying practices, acquire skills in food preparation, and improve eating habits. Meals are better balanced, better use is made of government-donated commodity foods, and federal food stamps are spent more wisely. Some of these economical ways of handling food, and available food-assistance programs were discussed in the previous chapter on the community food supply and health.

FOOD MISINFORMATION AND FADS

The word *fad* is a shortened form of an old word "faddle" (retained today in the phrase "fiddle-faddle"), meaning "to play with." A fad is something one "plays with" for awhile. A fad is any popular fashion or pursuit, without substantial basis, that its followers embrace with fervor. Food fads are scientifically unsubstantiated beliefs about certain foods, that may persist for a time in a given community or society. The word *fallacy* (L. *fallacia*, a trick to deceive) means a deceptive, misleading, or false notion or belief. Food fallacies, then, are false or misleading beliefs that underlie food fads. The word *quack*, as used in this sense, is a shortened form of "quacksalver," a term invented centuries ago by the Dutch to describe the pseudophysician or pseudoprofessor who sold worthless salves, "magic" elixirs, and cure-all tonics. He proclaimed his wares, like a barker, in a patter that skeptical people compared to the quacking of a duck. In medicine, nutrition, and allied health fields, a quack is a fraudulent pretender who claims to have skill, knowledge, or qualifications he does not possess. The motive for such quackery is usually money, and the quack uses some cruel hoax to feed on the physical and emotional needs of his victims. The food quack exists because food faddists exist.

Unscientific statements about food often mislead consumers and contribute to poor food habits. False information may come from folklore or fraud. We need to make wise food choices and recognize misinformation as such, based on sound scientific knowledge from responsible authorities.

Food fads

Types of claims. Food faddists make exaggerated claims for certain types of food. These claims fall into four basic groups.

1. Food cures. Certain foods will cure specific conditions.

2. Harmful foods. Certain foods are harmful and should be omitted from the diet.

3. Food combinations. Special food combinations restore health and are effective in reducing weight.

4. "Natural" foods. Only so-called natural foods can meet body needs and prevent disease.

Basic error. Look at these claims carefully. On the surface they seem to be simple statements about food and health. Further observation, however, reveals that each one focuses on foods per se, not on the specific chemical components in food, the *nutrients*, which are the actual physiologic agents of life and health. Certain individuals may be allergic to specific foods and obviously should avoid them. Also, certain foods may supply relatively large amounts of certain nutrients and are therefore good sources of those nutrients. The *nutrients*, however, not the specific foods, have specific functions in the body. Each of these nutrients is found in a wide variety of different foods. Remember, persons require specific nutrients, never specific foods.

Dangers. Why should the health worker be concerned about food fads and their effect on food habits? What harm do they cause? Generally food fads involve four possible dangers.

1. Dangers to health. Responsibility for care of one's health is fundamental. Self-diagnosis and self-treatment can be dangerous, however, especially when such action follows questionable sources. By following such a course, persons with real illness may fail to seek appropriate medical care. Many ill and anxious people have been misled by fraudulent claims of cures and have postponed effective therapy.

2. *Cost.* Some foods and supplements used by faddists are harmless, but many are expensive. Money spent for useless items is wasted. When dollars are scarce, the family may neglect to buy foods that will fill its basic needs and instead purchase a "guaranteed cure."

3. *Lack of sound knowledge.* Misinformation hinders the development of individuals and society and ignores lines opened up by scientific progress. Certain superstitions that are perpetuated can counteract sound health teaching.

4. *Distrust of food market.* Our food environment is changing and we do need to be watchful. Blanket rejection of *all* modern food production, however, is unwarranted. We must develop intelligent concerns and rational approaches to meet nutritional needs. A wise course is to select a variety of primary foods "closer to the source," or have minimal processing, then add a few carefully selected processed items for specific uses. We can evaluate each food product on its own merits in terms of individual needs: nutrient contribution, personal values, safety, and cost.

Vulnerable groups

Food fads appeal especially to certain groups of people with particular needs and concerns.

Elderly persons. Fear of aging changes leads many middle-aged and older adults to grasp at exaggerated claims that some product will restore vigor. Persons in pain living with chronic illness reach out for the "special supplement" that promises a sure cure. Desperately ill and lonely persons are easy prey for a cruel hoax.

Young persons. Figure-conscious girls and muscle-minded boys may respond to crash programs and claims that offer the "perfect body." Many who are lonely or have exaggerated ideas of glamour hope to achieve peer group acceptance by these means.

Obese persons. Obesity is one of the most disturbing personal concerns and frustrating health problems in America today. Obese persons face a constant bewildering barrage of propaganda pushing diets, pills, candies, wafers, formulas, and devices. Many are likely to follow fads.

Athletes and coaches. This group is a prime target for those who push miracle supplements. Always looking for the added something to give them the "competitive edge," athletes tend to fall prey to nutrition myths and hoaxes.

Entertainers. Persons in the public eye are often taken in by false claims that certain foods, drugs, or dietary combinations will maintain the physical appearance and strength on which their careers depend.

Others. The vulnerability of the groups above is obvious, but many other people in the general population follow the appeal of various food fads. Misinformation hinders the efforts of health professions and many concerned consumers to raise community nutrition standards.

What is the answer?

What can be done to counter food habits associated with food fads, misinformation, or even outright deception? What can health workers do? What *should* they do? Certainly an attitude of "do as I say, not as I do" will achieve nothing. You cannot counsel or teach others until you have first examined your own habits. Helpful instruction is based on personal conviction, practice, and enthusiasm. Then you can use the following positive teaching approaches.

Use reliable sources. Sound background knowledge is essential: (1) know the product being pushed and the persons behind it, (2) know how human physiology really works, and (3) know the scientific method of problem solving, that is, collect the facts, identify the real problem, determine a reasonable solution or action, carry it out, and evaluate the results.

Recognize human needs. Consider the emotional needs that food and food rituals help fulfill. Everyone has such needs; they are part of life. Use these needs in a positive way in your nutrition teaching. Even if a person is using food as an emotional "crutch," their emotional need is very real. We must never "break crutches" without offering a better and wiser way of support.

Be alert to teaching opportunities. Use any opportunity that arises to present sound nutrition and health information, formally or informally. Learn available resources: local or state university agricultural extension services, volunteer agencies, clinic and hospital facilities, public health departments, and professional health organizations. Develop communication skills, avoid monotony, and use a well-disciplined imagination. Otherwise, your message will not convince consumers of the falsehoods behind the attractive skills of the food faddist or bogus "nutritionist" credentialed by a "mail-order school" or best-seller "diet book."

Think scientifically. You can teach even very young children to use the problem-solving approach to everyday situations. Children are naturally curious. With their eternal *why*, they often seek evidence to support statements they hear. You must teach them and others the value of three basic questions: "What do you mean?" "How do you know?" and "What is your evidence?"

Know responsible authorities. The Food and Drug Administration (FDA) has the legal responsibility of controlling the quality and safety of food and drug products marketed in the United States. This is a tremendous task, however, and requires public help. Other governmental, professional, and private organizations can provide additional resources.

CHANGES IN AMERICAN FOOD HABITS
Personal food choices

Basic determinants. As we have seen, universal factors determining personal food choices clearly arise from physical, social, and physiologic needs. Table 14-1 summarizes some of these factors. Changing our own eating patterns is difficult enough; helping our clients to make needed changes for positive health reasons is even more difficult. Such teaching requires sensitive and flexible understanding of the complex factors involved.

Factors influencing change. Ethnic patterns and regional cultural habits are strong influences in our lives. They establish our early food habits and make changing those habits difficult. On the other hand, our changing society puts us in conflict with the old and the new. Some of these newer factors influence changes in our food habits.

1. Income. A generally improved economic situation as a society provides sufficient income in most cases to give us more choice and time.

❖ **TABLE 14-1** *Factors determining food choices*

Physical factors	Social factors	Physiologic factors
Food supply available	Advertising	Allergy
Food technology	Culture	Disability
Geography, agriculture, distribution	Education, nutrition and general	Health-disease status
		Heredity
Personal economics, income	Political and economic policies	Personal food acceptance
		Needs, energy, or nutrients
Sanitation, housing	Religion and social class, role	Therapeutic diets
Season, climate		
Storage and cooking facilities	Social problems, poverty, or alcoholism	

2. Technology. An expanding science and technology increases the number and variety of food items available.

3. Environment. Our rapidly changing environment results in concerns about our food and health.

4. Vision. Our expanding mass media, especially television, stimulates many options for new items and changes our expectations and desires. The current market target for television advertisements is younger children, who then influence the family's buying habits.

Changing American food patterns

The all-American family stereotype of parents and two children eating three meals a day with a ban on snacking is no longer the norm. We have made far-reaching changes in our way of living and subsequently in our food habits.

Households. American households have increased in number and changed in their nature. Most new households are groups of unrelated persons or persons living alone, an increase of about 75%, with family households increasing only about 15%. By the year 2000, the average size of American households is expected to decline from 2.69 persons reported in 1985 to 2.48 during the current decade, with husband-wife households decreasing from 58% to 53% of all households.[1] These changes reflect our rapidly changing society.

Working women. The number of women in the work force continues to increase rapidly and is not likely to reverse. This trend is not restricted to any one social, economic, or ethnic group. Women of all racial and ethnic groups will be the major entrants into the U.S. labor market, making up 47% of the total work force by 2000, compared to 45% in 1988.[1] This is a widespread change in society. Working parents rely increasingly on food items and cooking methods that save time, space, and labor.

Family meals. Family meals as we have known them in the past have changed. Breakfasts and lunches are seldom eaten in a family settings. Half the American people between the ages of 22 and 40, as well as many children, skip breakfast regularly, and 25% skip lunch. About 25% of American households do not have a sit-down dinner as often as five nights a week.

Meals and snacks. Our habits have changed dramatically as to when we eat and whether we eat with our families or not. Midmorning and midafternoon

❖

BOX 14-2

Snacking: An All-Amercian Food Habit

The snack market in the United States continues to grow. Consumer spending for all foods has increased, with a greater portion of that increase being spent for snacks, mainly salty snacks, cookies, and crackers. Other popular snacks include soft drinks, candies, gum, fresh fruit, bakery items, milk, and chips.

Snacking is said to "ruin your appetite," and we certainly consume too many soft drinks. But is snacking all bad? Not necessarily. Surveys have shown a direct association between more complete nutrition and an increase in snacking. Those who snack more show higher nutrient percentages in the "adequate" range of the RDAs. Many people snack on foods that are not "empty extras" but essential contributions to total nutritional adequacy. These items include fruit, cheese, eggs, bread, and crackers.

Snacking, or "grazing" as some persons do with more frequent nibbling, is clearly a significant component of food behavior. Rather than rule against the practice, we need to promote snack foods that enhance nutritional well-being.

---

breaks at work usually involve food or beverage. Evening television snacks plus a midnight refrigerator raid are common. Nutrition hardliners of the old school may denounce this snacking behavior, but they are out of step. Americans are moving toward a concept of "balanced days" instead of "balanced meals." They are increasing the number of times a day they eat to as many as 11 "eating occasions," a pattern recently termed *grazing*. This is not necessarily bad, depending on the nature of the periodic snacking or more constant "grazing." In fact, studies indicate that frequent small meals are better for the body than three larger ones a day, especially when healthy snacking and grazing contribute to needed nutrient and energy intake (see Box 14-2).

Health and fitness. The interest of Americans in health and fitness is increasing. It has affected food buying in several ways, with more nutrition awareness, weight concern, and interest in gourmet or specialty foods. Whole new lines of so-called light foods are popular.

Economical buying. More and more Americans are making diet changes to save money. They are seeking bargains and cutting back on expensive "convenience foods." They are buying in larger packages and in bulk and doing less "store- hopping," staying with one that maintains fairer overall prices. They are less loyal to brand names and buy more generic products. They are using food labels both for unit pricing and for "calorie counting."

Fast foods. At one time or another, at least 90% of all Americans eat in a fast-food restaurant, averaging about one in 12 meals and spending $200 a year per person.[20] From a modest beginning by McDonald's in 1955 in Des Plaines, Illinois, fast-food business has grown into a multibillion-dollar enterprise, now capturing 40% of the money spent on meals away from home. As family income rises, so does the consumption of fast foods, especially among the middle class.

All of these social changes have radically changed our American food marketplace. Our food habits reflect this changing market and society.

SUMMARY

We all grow up and live our lives in a social setting. We each inherit a culture and live in our particular social structure, complete with its food habits and attitudes about eating. We need to understand the effects on health associated with major social and economic shifts. We also need to understand current social forces to best help persons make new dietary changes that will benefit their health. We must meet concerns about food misinformation.

America is changing several of its food patterns. We increasingly rely on new food forms in our fast complex life. More women are working, households are getting smaller, more people are living alone, and our meal patterns are different. We search for less fancy, lower-cost food items, and also creative cooking. In general we are more nutrition and health conscious. Fast-food outlets and snacking are social habits here to stay.

❖ REVIEW QUESTIONS

1. What is the meaning of culture? How does it affect our food patterns?
2. What are social and psychologic factors that influence our food habits? Give examples of personal meanings related to food.
3. Why does the public tend to accept nutrition misinformation and fads so easily? What groups of people are more susceptible? Select one such group and give some effective approaches you might use in reaching them.
4. Name current trends in American food habits and discuss their implications for nutrition and health.

❖ SELF-TEST QUESTIONS

True-false

For each item answered "false," write the correct statement:
1. Food habits result from instinctive behavioral responses throughout life.
2. American social class structure is largely determined by occupation, income and education, and residence.
3. Life-style changes as society's values change.
4. From the time of birth, eating is a social act, built on social relationships.
5. Food fads are usually long lasting and seldom change.
6. Special food combinations are effective as weight-reducing diets and have special therapeutic effects.

Multiple choice
1. A healthy body requires:
   a. Specific foods to control specific functions
   b. Certain food combinations to achieve specific physiologic effects
   c. Natural foods to prevent disease
   d. Specific nutrients in various foods to perform specific body functions
2. Food habits in a given culture are largely based on:
   (1) Food availability
   (2) Genetic differences in food tastes
   (3) Food economics, market practices, and food distribution
   (4) Symbolic meanings attached to certain foods
        a. 1, 2, and 3   c. 1 and 3 only
        b. 1, 3, and 4   d. All of these

3. In the Jewish food pattern, the word *kosher* refers to food prepared by:
   (1) Ritual slaughter of allowed animals for maximum blood drainage
   (2) Avoiding meat and milk combinations in the same meal
   (3) Special seasoning to avoid salt use
   (4) Special cooking of food combinations to ensure purity and digestibility
       a. 1 and 3   c. 1 and 2
       b. 2 and 4   d. 3 and 4
   (4) Special cooking of food combinations to ensure purity and digestibility
       a. 1 and 3   c. 1 and 2
       b. 2 and 4   d. 3 and 4

4. The basic grain used in the Mexican food pattern is:
       a. Rice   c. Wheat
       b. Corn   d. Oat

5. Stir-frying is a basic cooking method used in the food pattern of:
       a. Mexican Americans   c. Chinese
       b. Jews   d. Greeks

❖ SUGGESTIONS FOR FURTHER STUDY

True-false

Cultural food pattern survey

Select a person of a different cultural background from your own. Interview this person concerning food habits. Inquire about food items most commonly used and general methods of preparing them. Then ask about the basic meal pattern for a day. If possible, visit a market carrying these foods and seasonings and survey the items there. Also arrange to have a home or restuarant meal of this cultural food pattern. Compare your findings with the discussion in your textbook and other resources, and with other cultural patterns in your class discussion.

True-false

Food fad survey

Select a person (or persons) in one of the vulnerable groups discussed in relation to food misinformation and fads. Interview them about any food or supplement practices or misinformation they may have encountered and how they feel about these practices or any suggestions they may have regarding them. Summarize your findings and list any approaches you can think of to help correct these beliefs or practices. Review your report with those of others presented in your follow-up class discussion.

References

1. US Department of Health and Human Services, Public Health Service: Healthy people 2000, national health promotion and disease prevention objectives, Washington, DC, 1990, US Government Printing Office.
2. Twaigery S and Spillman D: An introduction to Moslem dietary laws, Food Technology 43:88, Feb 1989.
3. Pelican S and Bachman-Carter K: Navajo food practices, customs, and holidays, Chicago, 1991, American Dietetic Association.
4. Jackson MY: Federal nutrition services for American Indians and Alaska native elders, J Am Diet Assoc 90(4):568, 1990.
5. US Department of Commerce, Bureau of the Census: We, the first Americans, Washington, DC, 1988, US Government Printing Office.
6. Koehler KM, Harris MB, and Davis SM: Core, secondary, and peripheral foods in the diets of Hispanic, Navajo, and Jemez Indian children, J Am Diet Assoc 89(4): 538, 1989.
7. Egerton J: Roots of Southern food. In Southern Living 1990 annual recipes, Birmingham, 1990, Oxmoor House, Inc.
8. Borrud, LG, and others: Food group contributions to nutrient intake in whites, blacks, and Mexican Americans in Texas, J Am Diet Assoc 89(8):1061, Aug 1989.
9. Broussard-Marin L and Hynak-Hankinson MT: Ethnic food, the use of Cajun cuisine as a model, J Am Diet Assoc 89(8):1117, 1989.
10. Southern Living 1990 annual recipes, Birmingham, 1990, Oxmoor House, Inc.

11. US Bureau of the Census, Department of Commerce: Statistical abstracts of the United States, Washington, DC, 1986, US Government Printing Office.

12. Vietmeyer N: Exotic edibles are altering America's diet and agriculture, Smithsonian 16(9):34, 1985.

13. Ziegler, VS, Sucher, KP, and Downes, NJ: Southeast Asia renal exchange list, J Am Diet Assoc 89(1):85, 1989.

14. Tong A: Food habits of Vietnamese immigrants, Family Econ Rev 2:28, 1986.

15. Crane NT and Green NR: Food habits and food preferences of Vietnamese refugees living in northern Florida, J Am Diet Assoc 76(6):591, 1980.

16. Neimark J: Appetite—is delicious additive, Am Health V(6):122, 1986.

17. Shell ER: Fighting "food neophobia": win the food wars—without really trying, Am Health V(7):68, 1986.

18. National Center for Children in Poverty: A statistical profile of our poorest young citizens, New York, 1990, The Center.

19. Amler RW and Dull HB: Closing the gap: the burden of unnecessary illness, New York, 1987, Oxford University Press.

20. Shields JE and Young E: Fat in fast foods—evaluating changes, Nutr Today 25(2):32, 1990.

Further reading

Samolsky S, Dunker K, and Hynak-Hankinson MT: Feeding the Hispanic hospital patient: cultural considerations, J Am Diet Assoc 90(12):1707, 1990.

This article summarizes national trends in eating habits and health problems of Mexican and Puerto Rican Americans, the largest Hispanic subgroups, and provides guidelines for feeding them in culturally acceptable ways when they are hospitalized.

Sucher KP and Kittler PG: Nutrition isn't color blind, J Am Diet Assoc 91(3):297, 1991.

This article emphasizes respect for cultural values and personal preferences as a precondition for successful health promotion in an American society of increasing ethnic diversity.

15

❖

Weight management

K E Y   C O N C E P T S

America's obsession with thinness carries social and physiologic costs.

Underlying causes of obesity are a complex of psychosocial, physiologic, and genetic factors.

Realistic weight management focuses on the person and health promotion.

*O*n any given day, at least one out of every four Americans is on a weight reduction diet. Use of these "diets" seems to increase daily, with a new "diet book" constantly appearing in the public press. Despite this obsession and weight loss being big business, however, as a people we are actually getting heavier. The average American has gained about 2.25 kg (5 pounds) over the past decade or so. Why has this occurred?

Much of the answer lies in our changing life-style. Our growing technology is producing a more sedentary society. In general, we are becoming less and less physically active, although the current upswing in exercise offers hope. The other part of the answer is the sad fact that all of these popular "diets" do not work. Only about 5% of these dieters manage to maintain their weight at the new lower level after such a diet. There must be a better way.

In this chapter we examine the problem of weight management. We seek a more positive and realistic "health model" that recognizes personal needs as well as sound weight goals.

THE PROBLEM OF OBESITY AND WEIGHT CONTROL
Body weight and body fat

Definitions. Obesity is not "simple," although we have often called it that in general practice. It develops from many interwoven factors, both personal and physical, and is difficult to define. *Obesity*, as used in the traditional medical sense, is a clinical term for excess body weight generally applied to persons who are 20% or more above a desired weight for height. But we must always remember that every person is individual, and *normal* values in healthy persons vary over a wide range. Also, until recently we had overlooked the important factor of *age* in setting a reasonable body weight for adults. With advancing age, body weight usually increases until about age 50 for men and age 70 for women, then declines.[1] It is extreme thinness that carries more overall health risk than does moderate overweight as persons grow older.

Often the terms *overweight* and *obesity* are used interchangeably. Actually, however, they have different meanings. The word "overweight" simply means a body weight that is above a population weight-for-height standard. On the other hand, the word "obesity" is a more specific term. It is from a Latin word meaning "excess fat," so it refers to the degree of *fatness*—the relative amount of fat in the total body composition, which is the real health problem. For example, a football player in peak condition can be extremely "overweight" according to standard weight-height charts (Fig. 15-1). That is, he can weigh considerably more than the average man of the same height, but much of his weight is lean muscle mass, not excess fat.

Body composition. We would be more correct, therefore, to talk in terms of *fatness* and *leanness*, or body composition, rather than *overweight*. Health professionals now try to measure body fatness in working with overweight or obese persons. They use calipers to measure skinfold widths at specific body sites, because most of the body fat is deposited in layers just under the skin. Underwater weighing is used in athletic programs or research studies. In this way obesity can be better defined in terms of body fat content. The standard body fat content for healthy men, estimated from underwater body weighing, ranges from about 14% to 28% of total body weight; for women it is somewhat higher, 15% to 30%. Obesity occurs when the percentage of body fat exceeds these estimates.

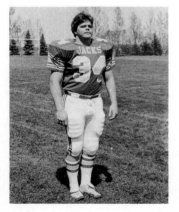

❖ **FIG. 15-1**

According to standard weight-height charts, a football player would be considered overweight. These charts should be used with discretion.

Measures of weight maintenance goals

General guide. A general rule of thumb has been passed along to determine weight goals:

Males—106 pounds for the first 5 feet, then add 6 pounds/inch, plus or minus 10 pounds.

Females—100 pounds for the first 5 feet, then add 5 pounds/inch, plus or minus 10 pounds.

This guide is seldom used now because it produces unrealistically low weights, especially for women, and does not account for age differences.

Standard weight-height tables. These tables are tools or general guides, and they should be regarded as such. Individual needs as a whole must be considered. Most of the standard tables are based on the Metropolitan Life Insurance Company's "ideal" weight-for-height charts. However, these charts have been developed from life expectancy information gathered since the 1930s. Many people have questioned how well they represent our total current population.[2] Also, studies show that health risks are as great, if not greater, in very thin low-weight persons as for extremely obese ones. Within each age group, extremely thin as well as extremely fat persons have higher mortality rates. It seems that we should try to be neither excessively overweight nor excessively underweight, and that the multitude of health problems attributed to *moderate* amounts of overweight are unfounded.

Ideal weight. Thus the term *ideal weight* is not very useful. It may give you a "ballpark" figure, but not much more. You should be wary of this term for two important reasons.

1. Individual variation. The basic problem with "ideal weight" is that it varies with different people at different times under different circumstances. Any person's ideal weight depends on many factors including age, body shape, metabolic rate, genetic makeup, sex, and physical activity. Persons need varying amounts of weight and can carry different amounts in good health. Specific individual situations govern needs.

2. Necessity of body fat. In our zeal to lose weight, we may forget that some body fat is essential to survival. Human starvation shows this. These victims die of fat loss, not protein depletion. For mere survival, males require 3% body fat, and females require 12%. Menstruation begins when the female body reaches a certain size or, more precisely, when the young girl's body fat reaches this critical part of body weight, about 20%. This is the amount needed for ovulation and thus any eventual pregnancy.

Obesity and health

Weight extremes. Clearly massive or *morbid* obesity is a health hazard in itself. It places severe strain on all the body systems. Both extremes of weight, fatness and thinness, pose medical problems.

Overweight and health problems. The major problem affecting most Americans, however, is the degree of general overweight that is a risk to positive health. Current studies indicate that direct relationships between overweight and disease have been demonstrated in two conditions: adult noninsulin dependent diabetes mellitus (NIDDM) and hypertension, which in turn through these risk factors may contribute to cardiovascular disease. Health risks certainly exist in *extreme* obesity. Unless a person is at least 30% *overfat*, however, the relation of weight to mortality is questionable.

Indirect relationship to disease. As studies show, general obesity *is* related directly to NIDDM and hypertension. These two conditions are also risk factors in coronary heart disease, a much larger health problem. General obesity thus is an indirect factor in heart disease. Losing excessive weight is associated with improvement of hypertension and diabetes. In obese persons with NIDDM or hypertension, weight loss can bring significant reductions in elevated blood glucose or blood pressure. These improvements in turn reduce risks related to heart disease.

Causes of obesity

Basic energy balance. How does a person become overweight? The underlying energy imbalance, more energy intake as food than energy output as basal metabolic needs and physical activity, is the basic cause. The excess intake is stored in the body. About 3500 kcal is the equivalent of 1 pound of body fat (Table 15-1). This is part of the answer. We also know from experience, however, that some overweight persons really eat only moderate amounts of food, and that some persons with average weight eat much more but never seem to gain. Because many individual differences exist, more factors must be involved.

Genetic and family factors. Genetic inheritance probably influences a person's chance of becoming fat more than any other factor. Family food patterns reinforce this genetic base.

1. Genetic control. A genetic base regulates differences in body fat and sex differences in weight. Ongoing study has indicated that an internal genetic control regulates the amount of body fat an individual carries.[3,4] A person will then eat to regain or lose whatever amount of fat the body is naturally "set" or "programmed" for, according to the weight below or above this internally regulated point. Thus persons who have lost body fat below their programmed level, either by strenuous "dieting" or lack of food, will eat to regain to their genetic fat point when food is available again. Similarly, persons with lower programmed fat levels, who have gained excess body fat above their genetic level by eating more, although their body metabolism remains unchanged by pushing food, will lose this excess fat when they resume their regular food intake.[5,6] It seems that the only way to help lower a higher genetic setting for

---

❖ **TABLE 15-1**   *Kilocalorie adjustment required for weight loss*

To lose 454 g (1 lb) a week—500 fewer kcal daily
          Basis of estimation
          1 lb body fat   = 454 g
          1 g pure fat   = 9 kcal
          1 g body fat   = 7.7 kcal (some water in fat cells)
          454 g × 9 kcal/g   = 4086 kcal/454 g fat (pure fat)
          454 g × 7.7 kcal/g = 3496 kcal/454 g body fat (or 3500 kcal)
          500 kcal × 7 days = 3500 kcal = 454 g body fat

body fat is through an increase in regular exercise.

2. *Family reinforcement.* The individual's genetic predisposition for increased body fat is then reinforced by family food patterns. Within families, if one parent is obese, a child has a 40% chance of becoming obese. This chance is 80% if both parents are obese. It is only about 10% if neither parent is obese. In addition to genetic influence, families also exert social pressure and teach children habits and attitudes toward food.

Physiologic factors. The amount of body fat a person carries, whether through inheritance or eating habits, is related to the number and size of fat cells in the body. Critical periods for developing obesity occur during early growth periods when cells are multiplying rapidly in childhood and adolescence. Once the body has added extra fat cells for more fuel storage, they remain and can store varying amounts of fat. Middle-aged and older adults may store more fat when they get less and less exercise. Women store more fat during pregnancy and after menopause because hormones are involved.

Psychosocial factors. Many persons respond to emotional stress by eating, especially those foods they regard as "comfort" foods. Also, social pressures, especially on women, to maintain our cultural "ideal" thin-body type contributes to eating disorders and social discrimination against obese persons.

Individual differences and extreme practices

Individual energy balance levels. As we have seen, several factors influence a person's individual point of energy balance. Some persons do have more genetic-based metabolic efficiency. They just "burn" food more readily than others do. Also, remember that when you calculate a person's energy balance, a worthwhile general factor to determine, your figures indicate only an *approximate* value. Reported food values represent averages of many samples of that food tested. Many factors also influence how much energy a person is "burning up," including basal metabolic rate (BMR), body size, lean body mass, age, sex, and physical activity. These calculations, however, do provide useful general information and indicate areas of individual needs and goals.

Extreme practices. Individual differences in energy needs, along with social pressures, lead many overweight persons to use extreme measures to lose weight, often at risk to their health.

1. *Fad diets.* A constant array of "diets" floods the market, putting more money in producers' pockets than removing real pounds from users' bodies. To the extent that they work at all, temporary loss comes from the reduced kcalorie intake, not from the proclaimed "magic mixture." Also, many diets are nutritionally inadequate and can be dangerous at extreme, very-low-caloric levels. At best, more recent very-low-calorie programs have failed in the critical period after initial rapid weight loss to help clients maintain the new weight when refeeding begins.[7]

2. *Fasting.* This drastic approach is also dangerous. Such starvation produces acidosis, low blood pressure, electrolyte loss, tissue protein loss, and decreased BMR. Sometimes sufficient loss of heart muscle occurs to cause death.

3. *Clothing and body wraps.* Special "sauna suits" or body wrapping are claimed to help weight loss in special spots of the body or to clear up so-called cellulite tissue, which simply does not exist. The word "cellulite" was coined

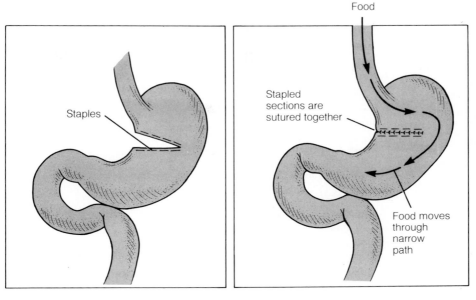

❖ **FIG. 15-2**

Gastroplasty is a type of restrictive gastric surgical procedure used for treatment of severe obesity.

by a European beauty operator years ago and has no basis in scientific fact. Also, any spot reducing is achieved only by special exercises designed to use the particular muscles in that area in repeated workouts; the fat is certainly not sweated or pressed out as claimed. Some persons endure the mummylike body wrapping in an attempt to reduce body size. The resulting small weight loss is caused only by temporary water loss. The only way to lose weight is to burn up more kilocalories than are consumed.

4. *Drugs.* Various amphetamine compounds, commonly called "speed," were once popular in the medical treatment of obesity. However, they are no longer used because of their danger to health. Typical over-the-counter drugs used now include *phenylpropylamine (PPA)*, a stimulant similar to amphetamine. PPA has been linked to increased blood pressure and damage to blood vessels in the brain, which can lead to central nervous system disorders such as confusion, stroke, hallucination, and psychotic behavior. No diuretics or hormones, such as thyroid hormone or steroids, should ever be used to affect body weight or leanness without strict medical indication and supervision.

5. *Surgery.* Surgical techniques are usually reserved for medical treatment of extreme morbid obesity. A former surgical procedure, the ileal bypass, is no longer done because it caused many malabsorption and malnutrition problems. Also, problems have followed other previous procedures such as wiring the jaws shut to prevent normal eating or insertion of a free-floating "gastric bubble" to give a feeling of fullness and reduce food intake, so they are not being used at present.[8] Current surgical procedures include various forms of gastric stapling, such as the *gastroplasty* (illustrated in Fig 15-2). These types of surgical intervention are designed to reduce the space for food in the stomach

and thus limit appetite and eating. They require a skilled team of specialists, careful patient selection and preparation, and continuous follow-up over time in partnership with the patient and family.[9] A more limited type of cosmetic surgery, developed in the 1980s and still in current vogue, is a form of local fat removal, *lipectomy*, commonly called "liposuction." It is used to remove fat deposits under the skin in places of cosmetic or figure concern such as the hips or thigh areas. A thin tube is inserted through a small incision in the skin and a desired amount of the fat deposit is suctioned away. However, this procedure is quite painful and carries risks such as infection, large disfiguring skin depressions, or blood clots that can lead to dangerous circulatory problems, even kidney failure. Any surgical procedure carries some risk and may cause other problems as side effects.

SOUND WEIGHT MANAGEMENT PROGRAM
Essential characteristics

Experience in many clinics and community programs has shown that there are no shortcuts to successful weight control. It requires hard work and strong individual motivation. Weight management must be a personalized program focused on changed food and exercise behaviors, and in stress-relaxation habits. It must build a healthy life-style and have supportive individual, family, or group follow-up.[10]

Behavior modification

Basic principles. Food behavior is rooted in many human experiences, associations, environmental situations. Often addictive forms of eating responses and conditioning are produced. Behavior-oriented therapies are designed to help the obese person change food and eating patterns that contribute to the excessive weight. By understanding present behaviors, changing associations with the undesirable habit patterns, and reconditioning them into new desirable behavior patterns, overweight persons can plan constructive actions to meet their personal health goals. This behavioral approach must begin, therefore, with a detailed examination of each present undesirable eating behavior in its three basic aspects: (1) *Cues or antecedents*—What happens before and stimulates the behavior? (2) *Response*—What happens during the eating behavior following the "cue"? (3) *Consequences*—What happens after the eating behavior response that serves to reinforce it?

Basic strategies and actions. A program of personal behavior modification for weight management is directed toward (1) control of eating behavior—the when, why, where, how, and how much, and (2) promotion of physical activity to increase energy output. Three progressive actions follow in planning individual strategies.

1. *Define problem behavior.* Define *specifically* the problem behavior and the desired behavior outcome. This process clearly establishes specific goals and contributing objectives.

2. *Record and analyze baseline behavior.* Record present eating and exercise behavior and analyze it carefully in terms of setting and persons involved. What types of habit patterns emerge? How often do they occur? What conditions seem to "trigger" the behavior? What consequent events seem to main-

tain the habits—time and pace, place, persons, social responses, hunger before and after, emotional mood, other factors?

3. *Plan behavior management strategy.* Set up controls of the external environment involving situational forces related to each of the three behavior areas involved: what goes before, how you respond, and what results. Then break these identified links to old undesirable behaviors and recondition them to your desired new eating and exercise behaviors. Think of as many creative ways as possible for reconditioning some of you own food and exercise behaviors you may wish to change. Box 15-1 provides a few examples.

Dietary principles

The central dietary approach in a weight management program that holds hope of achieving a degree of *lasting* success must be based on five characteristics.

1. *Realistic goals.* Goals must be realistic in terms of overall loss and rate of loss, no more than 1 to 2 pounds (450 to 900 g)/week.

2. *Kilocalories reduced according to need.* The diet must be low enough in kcalories in relation to individual output of energy to produce a gradual weight loss of 1 to 2 pounds/week.

3. *Nutritional adequacy.* The diet must be nutritionally adequate. Lower caloric levels may need supplementation. The ratio of energy nutrients—carbohydrate, fat, and protein—should have an appropriate balance based on a wide variety of food sources.

4. *Culturally desirable.* The food plan must be similar enough to the personal cultural eating pattern of the individual to form the basis for *permanent* re-education of eating habits. It must be a good, personal lifetime plan.

5. *Kilocalorie readjustment to maintain weight.* When the desired weight level is reached, the kcalorie level is adjusted according to maintenance needs. The changed basic habits of eating provide the continuing means of weight control.

Basic energy balance components

The two sides of energy balance are *energy intake* in the form of food and *energy output* in the form of metabolic work and physical activity. For successful weight reduction, both of these basic components must be changed.

Energy input: food behaviors. The energy value of the food intake must be reduced. To accomplish this, note the usual amount of food served and eaten. Then use smaller portions, attractively served. Eat *slowly*. Savor the food taste and texture. Reduce seasonings such as fat, sugar, and salt. Increase the fiber content. Choose a variety of foods from a basic food guide, such as the food exchange lists (see Appendix), in the amounts suggested in Table 15-2. These guides can serve as a focus for sound nutrition education. Emphasize whole primary foods and use few processed ones. Plan a fairly even distribution of food throughout the day. Some practical suggestions are given in Box 15-2.

Energy output: exercise behaviors. Energy output in physical activity must be increased. Plan a regular daily exercise schedule. Start with simple walking for about a half hour each day. Build to a brisk pace. Add some form of aerobic

BOX 15-1

❖ ──────── **CLINICAL APPLICATION** ──────── ❖

Breaking Old Links: Strategies for Changing Food Behavior

Old habits die hard. They are never easy to change, but in the case of undesirable eating behaviors that contribute to excess body fatness and harm health, it's worth the effort. Here are some behavioral suggestions.

Deal first with behavioral cues.

Eliminate as many cues for the problem behavior as possible. Avoid situations and contacts associated with problem foods, put temptation out of reach, make the problem behavior as difficult as possible. Freeze leftovers, remove problem food items from kitchen or store in hard-to-reach places, take another route home than by the familiar bakery or candy shop.

Suppress those cues that can't be entirely eliminated. Control social situations that maintain the behavior, reward the alternate desired behavior, have a trusted person monitor eating patterns, minimize contact with excessive food, use smaller plates to make smaller food portions appear larger, control "poor me" moods with positive nonfood "treat" activities or physical activity.

Strengthen cues for desirable behaviors. Collect information and guides for a wide array of appropriate food choices and amounts. Use food behavior aids such as records, diary, or journal. Spread appropriate foods in desirable food meal/snack pattern. Make desirable food behavior as attractive and good-tasting as possible.

Deal next with actual food behavior in response to cues.

Slow the pace of eating. Take one bite at a time and place utensil on the plate between bites. Chew each bite slowly. Sip beverage. Consciously plan between-eating bits of conversation with meal companions. Delay starting the meal when first seated. Visualize eating in slow motion. Enhance the social aspect of eating.

Savor the food. Eat slowly, sensing taste and smell and texture of the food. Develop and practice these sensory feelings to the extent that they can be described and brought back to mind afterward. Look for food seasonings and combinations that will enhance this process and bring positive feelings to mind about the food experience.

Deal finally with the follow-up behavior that results.

Decelerate the problem behavior. Slow down its frequency. Respond only neutrally when it occurs rather than with negative self-talk or thoughts. Give social reinforcement to the decreasing number of times the problem behavior is occurring. Focus on the ultimate consequences of the undesirable behavior in health problems.

Accelerate the desired behavior. Update the progress records or personal journal daily. Respond positively to all desired behavior. Provide some sort of material reinforcement for positive behavior. Provide social reinforcement for all constructive efforts to modify behavior.

Such a program requires effort and motivation and work. Evaluate progress toward desired behavior goals continuously. Then plan maintenance support activities, individual or group, during an extended follow-up period.

You can do it! Become involved. Engage—make it so.

❖ **TABLE 15-2** *Weight reduction food plans using the exchange system of dietary control* (total kilocalorie distribution: 50% carbohydrate, 20% protein, 30% fat)*

Food exchange groups	1000 kcal	1200 kcal	1500 kcal	1800 kcal
Total number exchanges/day				
Milk (nonfat)	2	2	2	2
Vegetable	3	3	4	4
Fruit	3	3	4	4
Starch/bread	4	5	7	9
Meat (lean or medium fat)	3	4	5	7
Fat	4	4	5	5
Meal pattern of food exchanges				
Breakfast				
Fruit	1	1	1	1
Meat			1	1
Starch/bread	1	1	2	2
Fat	1	1	1	1
Milk	½	½	½	½
Lunch/supper				
Meat	1	1	1	2
Vegetables	1	1	2	2
Starch/bread	1	2	2	3
Fat	1	1	2	2
Fruit	1	1	1	1
Milk	½	½	½	½
Dinner				
Meat	2	2	2	3
Vegetables	2	2	2	2
Starch/bread	1	1	2	3
Fat	2	2	2	2
Fruit			1	1
Milk	½	½	½	½
Snack (afternoon or evening)				
Milk	½	½	½	½
Meat		1	1	1
Starch/bread	1	1	1	1
Fruit	1	1	1	1

*See food exchange lists in the Appendix.

exercise, such as swimming or running, or develop a set of body exercises (see Box 15-3). An exercise class may be helpful.

Principles of a sound food plan

On the basis of a careful diet history (p. 260), a sound personalized food plan can be developed with the client. It should involve each of the following principles of nutritional balance.

Energy balance. In general, a decrease of 1000 kcalories daily is needed to lose about 2 pounds/week; 500 kcalories to lose 1 pound/week (see Table 15-1). An average sound diet for women is about 1200 kcal/day; for larger

---

BOX 15-2

❖ ———————— CLINICAL APPLICATION ———————— ❖

Practical Suggestions to Dieters

Goals. Be realistic. Don't set your goals too high. Adapt your rate of loss to 450 to 900 g (1 to 2 pounds). If visible tools are helpful motivation techniques, use them.

Kilocalories. Don't be an obsessive "calorie counter." Simply become familiar with food exchanges in your diet list, learn the general values of some of your home dishes, then modify recipes or make occasional substitutes.

Plateaus. Anticipate plateaus. They happen to everyone. They are related to water accumulation as fat is lost. During these periods increase exercise to help get started again.

Binges. Don't be discouraged when you break down and have a dietary binge. This happens to most persons. Simply keep them infrequent, and when possible, plan ahead for special occasions. Adjust the following day's diet or remainder of the same day accordingly.

Special diet foods. There is no need to purchase special "low-calorie" foods. Learn to read labels carefully. Most special diet foods are expensive foods and many are not much lower in kilocalories than regular foods.

Home meals. Try to avoid a separate menu for yourself. Adapt your needs to the family meal, adjusting seasoning or method of preparing family dishes to lower kilocalories, especially by reducing or omitting fat.

Eating away from home. Watch portions. When a guest, limit extras such as sauces and dressings and trim meat well. In restaurants select singly prepared items rather than combination dishes. Avoid items with heavy sauces or fat seasoning and fried foods. Select fruit or sherbet as dessert rather than pastries.

Appetite control. Avoid dependence on appetite-depressant medications. Usually they are only crutches. Try nibbling on food items from the free food list or save meal items such as fruit or bread exchanges for use between meals.

Meal pattern. Eat three or more meals a day. If you are used to three meals, then leave it at that. If you are helped by snacks between meals, then plan part of your day's allowance to account for them. The main thing is that you don't take all of your kilocalories at one time. Avoid the all-too-common pattern of no breakfast, little or no lunch, and a huge dinner.

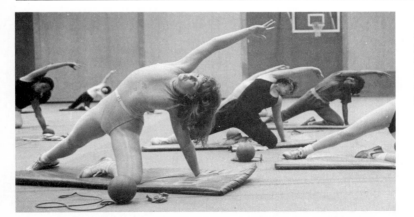

❖ **FIG. 15-3**
An exercise class provides regular support for an effective weight management plan.

❖

BOX 15-3
Benefits of Aerobic Exercise in Weight Management

The goal of weight management is to reduce excess body fat tissue and, in most cases, to build *lean body mass (LBM)*. However, both tissues are lost when a person tries to reach a weight goal by reducing food intake alone.

Optimal body composition can be achieved by combining food restriction with aerobic exercise. This type of exercise consists of activities that are sustained long enough to draw on the body's fat reserve for fuel while increasing oxygen intake (thus, the name *aerobic*). Lean body tissue burns fats in the presence of oxygen. Thus aerobic activity is best suited for achieving the ideal high LBM/low fatty tissue balance in the body.

The benefits of aerobic exercise to the overweight person in a weight management program include:

- Lowered genetic setting for body fat
- Suppressed appetite
- Reduced total body fat
- Higher basal metabolic rate
- Increased circulatory and respiratory function
- Increased energy expenditure
- Retention of tissue protein and building of LBM levels

Sometimes persons complain of disappointment in a slow rate of weight loss, difficulty in controlling appetite, and consistent "flabbiness" despite continuing diet management. These persons may welcome the suggestion of aerobic activity to help meet these needs. A brisk daily walk, jumping rope, swimming, bicycling, jogging, running, or some other activity may be sustained long enough for it to have an aerobic effect. Note carefully the physical stress this activity may place on individuals who have not exercised for some time or who have medical problems related to exertion. These persons should have a medical checkup before beginning such a program on their own or joining a local gymnasium or other community fitness center.

women and for men it would be about 1500 to 1800 kcal/day. Some persons may wish to determine their total energy needs are as a basis for diet-planning (see Table 15-3).

Nutrient balance. Basic energy nutrients are outlined in the diet to achieve the following nutrient balance:

Carbohydrate—about 50% of the total kcalories, with emphasis on complex forms such as starch with fiber, and a limit on simple sugars

Protein—about 20% of the total kcalories, with emphasis on lean food and small portions

Fat—about 30% of the total kcalories, with emphasis on low animal fats, scant total use, and alternate non-fat seasonings

This nutrient balance approximates the recommendations of the U.S. dietary guidelines for healthy Americans (p. 9). This can serve as a good general guide for long-term habits.

Distribution balance. Spread the food evenly through the day to meet energy needs. If you have certain "problem times" of the day, plan simple snacks for those periods.

❖ **TABLE 15-3**   *General approximations for daily adult basal and activity energy needs*

Daily energy needs (basis for calculations)		Male (70 kg) kcal	Female (58 kg) kcal
Basal energy needs			
1 kcal/kg/hr		70 × 24 = 1680	58 kg × 24 hr = 1392
Activity energy needs			
Sedentary	+20% basal	1680 + 336 = 2016	1392 + 278 = 1670
Very light	+30% basal	1680 + 504 = 2484	1392 + 418 = 1810
Moderate	+40% basal	1680 + 672 = 2352	1392 + 557 = 1949
Heavy	+50% basal	1680 + 840 = 2520	1392 + 696 = 2088

Food guide. The revised food exchange lists (Appendix) follow the general U.S. dietary guidelines for healthy Americans. Table 15-2 provides some examples of basic food plans for weight reduction. This basic food exchange system is a good general reference guide for comparative food values and portions, variety in food choices, and basic meal planning. Food items can be combined into desired dishes. Alternate nonfat seasonings can be used, such as herbs, spices, onion, garlic, lemon and lime juice, vinegar, wine, broth, mustard, and other condiments.

Preventive approach. Finally, the most positive work with weight management seems be aimed at *prevention*. Current studies indicate that the U.S. population of children and adolescents are getting fatter and the fatter members are becoming more obese, with a major culprit being inactivity, mainly hours of television viewing.[11] Support for young parents and children before the obese condition develops will help prevent many problems later in adulthood. This support and guidance should include early nutrition counseling and education, helping to build positive health habits, especially in positive eating behaviors and increased exercise behaviors of active play and physical activities.

THE PROBLEM OF UNDERWEIGHT
General causes and treatment

Extremes in underweight, just as in overweight, can bring serious health problems (p. 175). Although general underweight is a less common problem in the American population than is overweight, it does occur. It is usually associated with poor living conditions or long-term disease. A person who is more than 10% below the average weight for height and age is considered underweight; 20% or more is cause for concern. Serious results may occur in these persons, especially young children. Resistance to infection is lowered, general health is poor, and strength is reduced.

Causes. Underweight is associated with conditions that cause general malnutrition, including those listed here.

1. Wasting disease. Long-term wasting disease with chronic infection and fever that raise the basal metabolic rate (BMR).

2. Poor food intake. Diminished food intake resulting from (a) psychologic factors that cause a person to refuse to eat, (b) loss of appetite, or (c) personal poverty and limited available food supply.

3. *Malabsorption.* Poor nutrient absorption resulting from (a) long-lasting diarrhea, (b) a diseased gastrointestinal tract, or (c) excessive use of laxatives.

4. *Hormonal imbalance.* Hyperthyroidism or any other abnormalities may increase the caloric needs of the body.

5. *Energy imbalance.* This can result from greatly increased physical activity without a corresponding increase in food.

6. *Poor living situation.* An unhealthy home environment can result in irregular and inadequate meals, where eating is considered unimportant and an indifferent attitude toward food exists.

Dietary treatment. Underweight persons require special nutritional care to rebuild their body tissues and regain their health. Any food plan will need to be adapted for each person's unique situation, whether it involves personal needs, living situation, economic needs, and any underlying disease. The dietary goal, according to each person's tolerance, is to increase both energy and nutrient intake, with adherence to the following: (1) high-caloric diet, at least 50% above standard requirement; (2) high protein, to rebuild tissues; (3) high carbohydrate, to provide primary energy source in easily digested form; (4) moderate fat, to add kcalories but not exceed tolerance limits; and (5) good sources of all the vitamins and minerals, including supplements when individual deficiencies require them. Good food of wide variety attractively served helps to revive appetite and increase the desire to eat more. Nourishing meals and snacks are spread throughout the day and should often include favorite foods. A basic aim is to help build good food habits, so that the improved nutritional status and weight can be maintained once it is regained. Residents in long-term care facilities are especially vulnerable to weight-loss problems and have special needs (see Box 15-4). This rehabilitation process requires much creative counseling with each individual and family, with practical guides and support. In some cases, tube feeding or vein feeding (total parenteral nutrition, TPN) may be necessary (p. 353).

Extreme self-imposed eating disorders

Sometimes family and personal tensions as well as social pressures for thinness cause adolescent girls and young women to develop serious eating disorders. No matter what they weigh, they always see themselves as fat and develop a deep-seated fear of food and fatness.[12] Two forms of these extreme eating disorders are *anorexia nervosa* and *bulimia.*

Anorexia nervosa. This complex psychologic problem results in self-imposed starvation. The young girl, usually a high achiever who pushes herself constantly toward perfection, sees food and her body as ways in which she can be in control. Her distorted body image—she sees herself as fat even when she is really emaciated (Fig. 15-4)—keeps her in a state of near panic. She plans her days around ways of avoiding food. It becomes a full-time obsession, and she grows more and more depressed, irritable, and anxious.

Bulimia. In a sense, a bulimic is a "failed anorexic" individual. The young woman with bulimia also suffers from similar obsessions about her body and food. She also learns, however, that she can control her food and weight by "binge-purge" cycles. Compulsive binging on huge amounts of food is followed by induced vomiting. Some victims have even developed a callus on the finger that regularly rubs against the teeth when pushed into the throat to cause

BOX 15-4

❖ ─────────────── **CLINICAL APPLICATION** ─────────────── ❖

Problems of Weight Loss Among Older Adults in Long-Term Care Facilities

The American population of adults age 65 and older is increasing rapidly. By the year 2000 this older population is expected to number more than 36 million. The most rapid population increase over the next decade will be among those 85 years of age and older. Many of these elderly persons will require long-term care in nursing homes.

One of the problems encountered with these elderly residents is low body weight and rapid unintentional weight loss. It can become a serious health problem, a sensitive indicator of malnutrition, contributing to illness and death. Because weight loss is such a strong predictor of morbidity and mortality in these clinical settings, early and continuing observation to assess needs is important, especially in relation to factors that contribute to this weight loss.

In general, the weight loss can be caused by physical effects related to metabolic changes of aging or disease, or by factors that alter the amount and type of food eaten. Physical disease such as cancer can cause extreme weight loss from metabolic abnormalities, taste changes and loss of appetite, and nausea and vomiting. Other diseases underlying weight loss may be gastrointestinal problems, uncontrolled diabetes, and cardiovascular disorders such as congestive heart failure, pulmonary disease, infection, or alcoholism. Psychologic factors or psychiatric disorders may also contribute to malnutrition and weight loss through depression, memory loss, disorientation, apathy, or appetite disturbance. Some altered mental states may be caused by nutritional deficiencies, such as low levels of folate and the B-complex vitamins as well as protein-calorie malnutrition. These conditions can be corrected by specific nutritional support.

Additional physiologic, psychologic, and social factors may influence food intake and body weight and contribute to malnutrition in elderly persons:

Body composition changes. Height and body weight gradually decline. Body weight peaks between the ages of 34 and 54 in men and between ages 55 and 65 in women, decreasing thereafter. Body fat losses are generally not significant. The greatest cause of weight loss is a decline in body water, due in part to weakening of the normal thirst mechanism. Thus a feeling of thirst cannot be depended on to ensure adequate water intake, and water must be offered and encouraged frequently. Also, more constant attention to fluid intake helps with the prevalent problem of *xerostomia* (dry mouth) in older adults, due to inadequate salivary secretions to help with eating, thus contributing to malnutrition. Lean body mass also declines with age, resulting in lower basal metabolic rate, decreased physical activity, and energy requirements. Thus any possible increase in physical activity and in use of nutrient-dense foods is encouraged.

Taste changes. Taste cell regeneration slows with age, but the extent and effect on food intake varies widely. The sense of smell also declines with age and may affect taste. Increased use of appropriate seasoning and flavoring in food preparation is needed.

BOX 15-4

❖ ———————— CLINICAL APPLICATION, cont'd ———————— ❖

Dentition. About 50% of all Americans have lost their teeth by the age of 65. Many have dentures, but chewing problems are often present. About half of the nursing home populations studied report chewing, biting, and swallowing problems that interfere with eating and adequate food intake. Assessment of specific need and dental care solutions help correct eating problems.

Gastrointestinal problems. Delayed gastric emptying may contribute to distention and lack of appetite. A decrease of gastric secretions, including hydrochloric acid, may hinder absorption of vitamin B_{12}, folate, and iron, contributing to anemia and loss of appetite. Constipation is a common complaint, often leading to laxative abuse and resulting in interference with nutrient absorption from the chronic diarrhea. Increase in dietary fiber and liquids can help provide a better natural approach to establishing normal bowel action.

Drug/nutrient interactions. Elderly persons frequently take a number of prescribed and over-the-counter drugs. Some of them directly cause anorexia, nausea, and vomiting. Others are indirect causes by inducing nutrient malabsorption, which leads to deficiencies that in turn produce anorexia and weight loss. Drug therapy for elderly patients should have constant medical-nutritional-nursing monitoring to provide for appropriate use.

Functional disabilities. Eating problems can prevent or alter the capacity of elderly persons to take in a sufficient amount of food. These may vary from more difficult functional disabilities that interfere with putting food into the mouth and swallowing, problems that often require a trained therapist, to dependence on feeding assistance which sensitive nursing care can supply.

Social problems. Socioeconomic problems are often involved with care of the elderly. A specially trained geriatric social worker may help work to find possible financial assistance sources. Also, a sense of social isolation can lead to decreased food intake. Family support is needed, as well as sensitive contacts with nursing home staff and residents and involvment as much as possible in group activities.

Health workers in geriatric settings need continuing education and sensitizing to the potential dangers of low body weight and weight loss. Aged persons with acute and chronic illnesses and functional disabilities are at greatest risk for nutrition-related problems. They need continuing nutrition assessment and monitoring of body weight. Some of the restrictions of "special diets" should be relaxed or discontinued when risk of malnutrition is evident, with the goal of increasing nutrient intake and making eating as enjoyable as possible.

References

Fischer J and Johnson MA: Low body weight and weight loss in the aged, J Am Diet Assoc 90(12):1697, 1990.

Rhodus NL and Brown J: The association of xerostomia and inadequate intake in older adults, J Am Diet Assoc 90(12):1688, 1990.

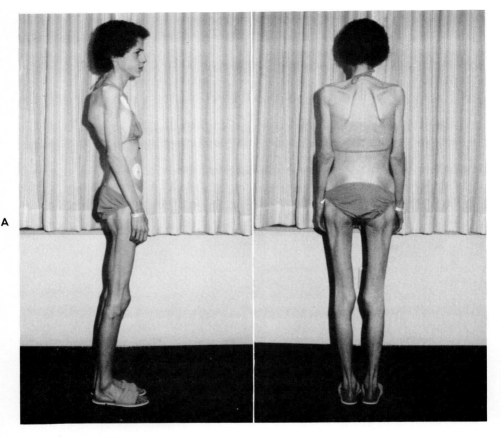

❖ FIG. 15-4

A, Anorectic woman before treatment. **B,** Same patient after *gradual* refeeding, nutritional managment, and psychologic therapy. Courtesy Sycamore Hospital, a division of Kettering Medical Center, Dayton, Ohio.

gagging and vomiting. Oral and dental problems from the purging behavior include oral mucosal irritation, decreased salivary secretions and dry mouth (xerostomia), and irreversible enamel erosion.[13] Many also use laxatives and diuretics to "purge" their bodies further.

    Treatment. These psychologic disorders require team therapy of skilled professionals, including physicians, psychologists, and nutritionists.[12] Even with the best of care, similar to alcoholism treatment, recovery is slow, a day at a time, and "cure" is a word not often used. Continuing support groups are important and national organizations provide resources.

SUMMARY

In the traditional medical model, obesity has been viewed as an illness and a health hazard. Extreme or morbid obesity is just that. Newer approaches view moderate overweight differently, however, in terms of the important aspect of fatness and leanness, or body composition, and propose a more person-centered positive health model for its care (Box 15-5). The American obsession with

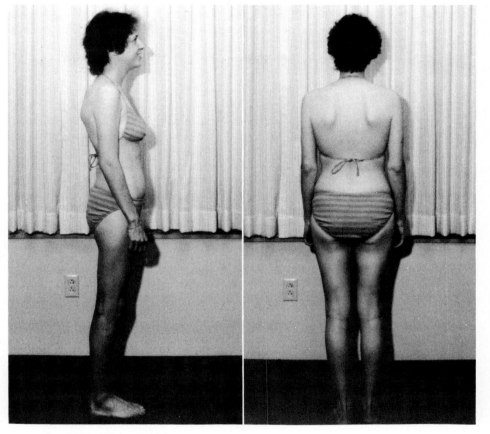

B

❖ **FIG. 15-4, cont'd**

BOX 15-5

❖❖ ——————— **CLINICAL APPLICATION** ——————— ❖❖

John's Energy Balance and Weight Management Plan

John is a college student leading a more or less sedentary life because of classes and study. However, he is interested in wrestling and wants very much to make the team. To do so, he must lose some of his excess weight.

He begins to look carefully at his energy balance picture: weight, 180 pounds at present; average food intake each day, approximately 3000 kcal. Next he plans a means of losing weight by reversing his energy balance.

Questions for Analysis

1. What does John decide his present daily total energy (kilocalories) must be?
2. How does this total energy need compare with his food energy intake?
3. To lose about 2 pounds/week, how much should he reduce the caloric value of his daily diet?
4. Besides reducing his diet kilocalories, what else could John do to help reverse his energy balance and improve his body condition?

thinness has created new weight management problems: eating disorders that result in self-starvation. These psychologic disorders require professional team therapy, including medical, psychologic, and nutritional care.

Planning a weight management program, either for the overweight or underweight person, involves the metabolic and energy needs of the individual. Personal food choices and habits, as well as fatty tissue needs during different stages of the life cycle, must be considered. Important aspects of such a weight reduction program include changing food behaviors and increasing physical activity. A sound program is based on reduced kcalories for a gradual weight loss and nutrient balance to meet the health standards of the U.S. dietary goals, with meals distributed throughout the day for energy needs.

The ideal plan begins with prevention, stressing formation of positive food habit in early childhood to prevent major problems later in life.

❖ REVIEW QUESTIONS

1. Why is the term "ideal weight" difficult to define? Explain some of the problems in determining this measure. What role does it play in weight management?
2. What does set-point mean in relation to individual weight? How does it relate to diet and exercise in a personal weight management program?
3. Describe the components of a positive health model for weight management. What are the basic principles of a sound food plan for such a program?
4. Describe factors influencing the development of an underweight malnourished condition. Explain the dietary treatment required.
5. Describe the two major eating disorders associated with a growing obsession with thinness. What social and psychologic factors contribute? What is the treatment?

❖ SELF-TEST QUESTIONS

True-false

For each item you answer "false," write the correct statement.

1. Development of childhood obesity results from genetics and family food practices that produce a decreased ratio of fat cells to lean cells.
2. Decreasing the energy expended in physical activity is a means of weight control.
3. During adolescence the boy usually has a higher deposit of subcutaneous fat tissue than the girl.
4. A reasonable weight reduction diet for an adult has an energy value of about 1200 to 1500 kcal, depending on individual size and need.
5. Between meal snacks should not be used on a weight reduction diet.

Multiple choice

1. Overweight is a direct risk factor in which of the following conditions?
   (1) Heart disease
   (2) Surgery
   (3) Noninsulin dependent diabetes mellitus (NIDDM)
   (4) Liver disease
   (5) Hypertension

   a. 1, 3, and 5   c. 3, 4, and 5
   b. 1 and 5   d. 3 and 5

2. A reduction of 1000 kcal in an obese person's daily diet would enable him to lose weight at which of the following rates?
   a. 1 pound/week   c. 3 pounds/week
   b. 2 pounds/week   d. 4 pounds/week
3. Which two of the following food portions have the lower caloric value and may be used as needed in a weight control diet?
   (1) Lean meat, 4-ounce dinner portion
   (2) Medium-sized baked potato
   (3) 1 slice of bread
   (4) 1 glass (8 ounce) of whole milk
       a. 1 and 4   c. 1 and 3
       b. 2 and 3   d. 2 and 4

❖ SUGGESTIONS FOR FURTHER STUDY

Individual project: personal energy balance

Determine your own personal energy balance by making the following comparison between your energy output or requirements and your energy intake in food (refer to Table 15-3).

Energy output

1. Record your weight in pounds (lb) and convert it to kilograms (kg).
2. Calculate your approximate basal energy needs.
3. Estimate your general activity level (Table 15-3) and calculate your approximate activity energy needs.
4. What is your approximate total energy output need in kilocalories?
5. Do you need more energy for activity or for basal metabolism? Does this answer surprise you?

Energy intake

1. Record your usual food intake for one day. Be sure to list portion sizes and method of seasoning and preparation.
2. Use the food value tables in the Appendix to calculate the total approximate caloric value of your day's food.
3. Compare your total energy input (food) with your total energy output (energy needs). What do you find is your present energy balance state? Compare your present body weight with the standard weight-height tables (Appendix). By your calculated energy balance state, where do you stand? What plan do you suggest to maintain or change your present energy balance?

Weight control products and programs

Organize project groups in your class. Assign several group members to visit various pharmacies, markets, and health food stores to survey products advertised for weight control. Read the labels carefully. Evaluate the claims made for each product. Check the cost. Talk with the clerk about the product's value. Ask questions such as "Do you think this would help me lose weight? How does it work? Do you sell many of these items?" etc. Note any customers' reactions. Check any diet books displayed. Purchase a few if possible for class evaluation.

Assign other group members to investigate various community weight control programs. If possible interview someone working in the program and someone participating in it as a customer. Compare individual responses and attitudes. How do the programs operate and what do they cost?

Have a follow-up discussion of all your findings in your class. Compare the products and programs investigated. Evaluate them in terms of the principles of sound weight reduction you have learned.

References

1. US Department of Agriculture and US Department of Health, Life Sciences Research Office, Federation of American Societies for Experimental Biology: Nutrition monitoring in the US—an update report, Washington, DC, 1989, US Government Printing Office.
2. Weigley ES: Average? Ideal? Desirable? A brief overview of height-weight tables in the United States, J Am Diet Assoc 84(4):406, 1984.
3. Gurin J: What's your natural weight? Am Health 3(3):43, 1984.
4. Bennett W and Gurin J: The dieter's dilemma, New York, 1982, Basic Books, Inc.
5. Keesey RE and Corbett SW: Metabolic defense of the body weight set-point. In Stunkard AJ and Stellar E, editors: Eating and its disorders, New York, 1984, Raven Press.
6. USDA Study Report: Metabolism does not change to prevent weight gain during overfeeding, J Am Diet Assoc 90(11):1556, 1990.
7. Sikand G and others: Two-year follow-up of patients treated with a very-low-calorie diet and exercise training, J Am Diet Assoc 88(4):487, 1988.
8. Morrow SR and Mona LK: Effect of gastric balloons on nutrient intake and weight loss in obese subjects, J Am Diet Assoc 90(5):717, 1990.
9. Forse A, Benotti PN, and Blackburn GL: Morbid obesity: weighing the treatment options—surgical intervention, Nutr Today 24(5):10, 1989.
10. Hart J and others: The importance of family support in a behavior modification weight loss program, J Am Diet Assoc 90(9):1270, 1990.
11. Gortmaker SL, Dietz WH, and Chueng LWY: Inactivity, diet, and the fattening of America, J Am Diet Assoc 90(9):1247, 1990.
12. Woodside DB and Garfinkel PE: National Institute of Nutrition review: An overview of the eating disorders anorexia nervosa and bulimia nervosa, Nutr Today 24(3):27, 1989.
13. Howat PM, Varner LM, and Wampole RL: The effectiveness of a dental/dietitian team in the assessment of bulimic dental health, J Am Diet Assoc 90(8):1099, 1990.

Further reading

Czajka-Narins DM and Parham ES: Fear of fat: attitudes toward obesity, Nutr Today 25(1):26, 1990.

This article presents a good review, with many reported studies, of the negative attitudes and deep prejudices toward obese persons held by many Americans and constantly voiced by the mass media. This steadily growing cultural bias, especially toward women, causes both psychologic and physiologic damage from lowered self-esteem, eating disorders, constant "yo-yo dieting," and more frequent resort to undesirable methods of weight control such as fasting or self-induced vomiting.

Paulsen BK: ADA Report, Position of the American Dietetic Association: very-low-calorie weight loss diets, J Am Diet Assoc 90(5):722, 1990.

This brief report states the ADA position on use of very-low-calorie diets based on semifasting use of liquid formulas for rapid weight loss followed by retraining of eating habits. Although such diets may benefit some persons, they have health risks and frequently fail as more weight is regained.

16

❖

Nutrition and physical fitness

K E Y   C O N C E P T S

*Healthy muscle structure and function depend on appropriate energy
fuels and tissue-building material, along with oxygen and water.*

*Different levels of physical activity and athletic
performance draw on different body fuel sources.*

A sedentary life-style contributes to health problems.

*A healthy personal exercise program combines
both general and aerobic activities.*

$\mathcal{P}$ublic interest in physical fitness has been growing recently, sparked by the modern approach of preventive medicine and positive
health promotion. This approach has been stimulated by the effort to prevent
or control various chronic diseases in our aging population.

In this chapter we see that nutrition and physical fitness are essential interrelated parts of positive health promotion. Both reduce risks associated with
chronic diseases. Both are important therapies in dealing with already developed
chronic conditions. For both recreational desires and health demands, we need
to provide our clients and patients with sound guidelines for physical fitness.
We must also practice them ourselves.

PHYSICAL ACTIVITY AND ENERGY SOURCES
The growing physical fitness movement

Over the past few years, surveys have indicated that about half of all Americans have been exercising regularly. These initial results identified a major trend away from a previously more sedentary life-style. Follow-up surveys show that the number of active Americans has continued to grow. Currently more than two out of every three Americans follow some type of regular physical activity. It seems that physical fitness is no longer just a fad or a trend.

The longer people follow some form of regular exercise, the more committed they become. The new fashion for walking and "soft" workouts has enabled more people to participate, such as those who cannot enter marathons or do "go-for-the-burn" aerobics. Many of these persons are older adults who have health problems that moderate exercise helps control. They find that regular exercise not only helps their health problem, but also helps them feel more in control of their lives.

Muscle action and body fuels

Muscle structure and function. Millions of special cells and fibers make up our skeletal muscle mass. These coordinated structures make possible all our physical activity. They are stimulated and controlled by nerve endings to produce smooth muscle contraction and relaxation.

Fuel sources. All of this action requires fuel to burn for energy. These fuel sources are our basic energy nutrients, primarily carbohydrate and some fat. Their metabolic products—glucose, glycogen, and fatty acids—provide ready fuels for immediate, short-term, and long-term energy needs. A good diet to meet these needs is essential, whatever our level of physical activity.

Fluids and oxygen

Fluids. More water is necessary for increased exercise. With continued exercise, the body temperature rises due to the release of heat as part of the energy produced. To control this temperature rise, the body sends as much heat as possible to the skin, where it is released in sweat. Over time, and especially in hot weather, this excessive sweating can lead to *dehydration*.[1] This is a serious complication.

Oxygen. The constant supply of oxygen necessary for life becomes even more important during exercise. A person's ability to deliver this vital oxygen to the tissues for energy production determines how much exercise can be done. This **aerobic capacity** depends on (1) the fitness of the lungs, heart, and blood vessels; and (2) the body composition.[2]

1. Body fitness. Physical fitness may be defined in terms of aerobic capacity. This is the body's ability to deliver and use oxygen in sufficient quantities to meet the demands of increasing levels of exercise. Aerobic capacity varies with body size, so it is measured by amount of oxygen consumed per kilogram body weight per minute. The lungs, heart, and blood vessels deliver this necessary oxygen to the cells. Thus their fitness is essential.

2. Body composition. The body tissues that use more oxygen make up the *lean body mass*, mainly muscle mass. These are the active metabolic tissues of the body. A person's aerobic capacity depends on the percentage of body fat and lean body mass. Body composition (p. 221) is determined by the relative amounts of these two components of body weight.

DIET AND EXERCISE
General nutrient needs

Nutrient stores. For the athlete as well as the active person, proper diet choices are essential for the winning performance, daily energy needs, and nutrient reserves.[3] When nutrient reserves become depleted during continued exercise, the body burns its fuel stores to meet increasing energy demands and requires replenishing. With prolonged exercise, nutrient levels fall too low to sustain the body's continued demands. Fatigue follows and exhaustion may result. Carbohydrate and fat are basic fuels to maintain these energy reserves, and very little is drawn from protein. These general needs apply to all individuals, although children have special growth needs.

Carbohydrate. The major nutrient for energy support in exercise is carbohydrate. This carbohydrate body energy reserve comes from two sources: (1) circulating *blood glucose*, and (2) *glycogen* stored in muscle cells and the liver. Thus, for the active person, carbohydrate should contribute about 55% to 60% of the daily diet's kcalories. Complex carbohydrates, or starches, are preferred to simple sugars. On the whole, the more complex starches break down more slowly and help maintain blood sugar levels more evenly, avoiding decreases in blood sugar levels. Also, starches are more readily converted to glycogen to maintain this store of constant primary fuel. Simple sugars, on the other hand, are less efficient at maintaining the body's glycogen stores. They are mainly converted to fat and stored as such. Simple sugars also trigger a sharper insulin response, contributing to the dangers of follow-up **hypoglycemia**. Many studies have shown that low-carbohydrate diets hinder exercise performance. Athletes especially experience fatigue, dehydration, and hypoglycemia. Well-conditioned athletes sometimes use a glycogen-loading procedure to build up glycogen stores for endurance events of 1 hour or more (see Box 16-1). In addition, complex carbohydrates supply needed fiber, vitamins, and minerals.

Fat. In the presence of oxygen, *fatty acids* serve as a fuel source from stored fat tissue. It is important to recognize that fat as a fuel source is not drawn from the diet directly but from body fat stores. There is no basis for increased levels of fat in the diet. No basis exists for increased levels of fat in the diet. There is a need for some dietary fat, however, to supply *linoleic acid*, the body's essential fatty acid. Although some fat in the diet of an active person is necessary, a moderate amount is sufficient. The total fat should not exceed about 25% to 30% of the diet's total daily kcalories.

Protein. Some amino acid breakdown may occur during exercise, but protein is usually discounted as a fuel source. It makes an insignificant contribution to energy. No more than the usual adult RDA standard is needed to meet general needs during exercise. This amounts to about 10% to 15% of the total day's kcalories from protein. Actually most Americans eat about twice this amount, putting a taxing load on the kidneys. This can contribute to dehydration because the excess nitrogen must be excreted. High-protein diets can also lead to increased calcium loss in the urine.

Vitamins and minerals. Vitamins and minerals cannot be used as fuel. They are not oxidized or used up in the energy production process. They are essential in this process but only as co-enzyme partners (p. 63). Increased exercise does not require increased vitamins or minerals. In general, exercise increases the body's efficient use of vitamins and minerals.[4] Since athletes require more

❖

BOX 16-1

Carbohydrate Loading for Endurance

Glycogen is the body storage form of carbohydrate, designed to provide an immediate source of backup fuel and protect blood glucose levels during sleep hours of fasting. It is restored with each day's food intake. However, during heavy exercise normal glycogen stores are quickly used up and the person reaches the point of exhaustion. In athletics, this is a no-win situation.

During the 1960s, trainers and coaches began to explore ways of avoiding this state of exhaustion in their players during endurance events. They reasoned that if they gave heavy exercise and a low-carbohydrate diet for three days, to use up the stored glycogen, then only light exercise and a high-carbohydrate diet for the next three, the athletes' glycogen stores would become supersaturated and enable them to perform at a higher level. When they tested this practice, tests proved the increase in muscle glycogen stores. The athletes' performance was nearly twice the former work load.

This practice in athletics has become known as "glycogen loading" and is specifically designed for endurance sports. Today a modified depletion-taper process, as shown in Table 16-3, is used to prevent possible injury to muscle tissue. It can thus be used more frequently than the initial schedule and, in the long run, is more productive.

References

Sherman M and Lamb D: Nutrition and prolonged exercise. In Lamb D and Murray R (eds): Perspectives in exercise science and sports medicine: prolonged exercise, Indian-apolis, 1988, Benchmark Press.

Wright ED: Carbohydrate nutrition and exercise, Clin Nutr 7(1):18, 1988.

---

energy, their larger intake of good food also increases their dietary intake of vitamins and minerals. However, female and adolescent athletes need to focus special attention on iron and may require therapeutic iron supplements if blood iron levels are consistently low.

Exercise and energy

Kilocalories. Physical activity requires kcalories. Table 16-1 gives some examples of kilocalories expended in general activities. (Also see Table 15-3 for energy expenditure by a very active person compared to that of an inactive individual.) Exercise raises the kcalorie need and helps regulate appetite to meet these needs. At moderate exercise levels, persons have actually been shown to eat less than inactive persons do. Exercise is the only way to regulate the individual's internal genetic *set-point*, regulating how much body fat the person will carry naturally (p. 223). This body fat set-point is raised (that is, more body fat is stored) when the susceptible individual becomes inactive. It is lowered when that person exercises regularly.

Nutrient ratios. The active person, even the athlete, requires no more protein or fat than the inactive person does. Carbohydrate is the preferred fuel. It is the critical food for the active person, not only prior to an exercise period but also during the recovery period afterward. The complex carbohydrate forms (starches) not only sustain energy needs but also supply added fiber,

❖ **TABLE 16-1** *Approximate energy expenditure per hour for an adult weighing 70 kg (154 pounds) and performing different activities*

Activity	Kcalories per hour
Sleeping	65
Lying still, awake	75
Sitting at rest	100
Standing relaxed	105
Dressing and undressing	120
Rapid typing	140
Light exercise	170
Walking slowly (2.5 mph)	200
Active exercise	290
Intensive exercise	450
Swimming	500
Running (5.5 mph)	580
Very intense exercise	600
Walking very fast (5.2 mph)	640
Walking up stairs	1110

vitamins, and minerals. Thus the recommended ratio of energy nutrients for support of physical activity may be summarized as follows:

Carbohydrate: 55% to 60% of total kcalories

Fat: 30% of total kcalories

Protein: 10% to 15% of total kcalories

Athletic performance

Misinformation. Athletes and their coaches are particularly susceptible to magic claims and myths about foods and dietary supplements. All athletes, particularly those involved in very competitive sports, search constantly for the "competitive edge" over their opponents. Knowing this, manufacturers sometimes make distorted or false claims for products. In addition, the world of athletics holds numerous superstitions and myths about food and nutrients.

- Athletes need protein for extra energy.
- Extra protein builds bigger and stronger muscles.
- Muscle tissue breaks down during exercise and protein supplements are needed to replace it.
- Vitamin supplements enable the athlete to use more energy.
- Vitamins and minerals are burned up in workouts and training sessions.
- Electrolyte solutions are important during exercise to replace sweat loss.
- A pregame meal of steak and eggs ensures maximum performance.
- Sugar is needed before and during performance to maintain energy levels.
- Drinking water during exercise will produce cramps.

Pregame meal. The ideal pregame meal is a light one, approximately 300 kcalories, eaten 2 to 4 hours before the event. It should be high in complex carbohydrates, relatively low in protein, with little fat or fiber.[3] This schedule for the meal gives the body time to digest, absorb, and transform it into stored

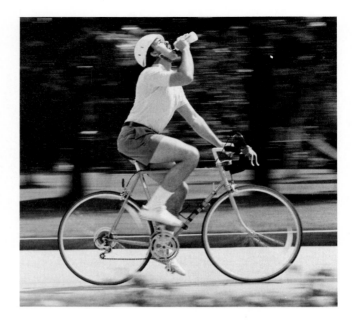

❖ **FIG. 16-1**
Frequent small drinks of cold water during extended exercise prevents dehydration.

❖ TABLE 16-2	*Sample pregame meal* *Approximately 300 kcal, high complex carbohydrate,* *low protein, fat, and fiber*
	1 cup spaghetti, tomato sauce
	1 slice French bread
	1 cup apple juice

glycogen. Good food choices include pasta, bread, bagels, muffins, and cereal with nonfat milk. (See Tables 16-2 and 16-3.)

Hydration. Dehydration can be a serious problem for athletes. Its extent depends on (1) intensity and duration of the exercise, (2) the surrounding temperature, (3) level of fitness, and (4) the pregame or preexercise state of hydration. The thirst mechanism cannot keep up with the exercise. To prevent dehydration, therefore, athletes are advised to drink water frequently, more than they think they need (Fig. 16-1). Cold water absorbs more quickly. They should drink small cups of it every 15 minutes during long athletic events. A number of "sports drinks" with added sugar, electrolytes, and flavorings have been marketed recently (Box 16-2), but questions have been raised about their use or misuse. Adding electrolytes and sugar to the water delays its emptying from the stomach. Except for endurance events, plain cold water is usually the rehydration fluid of choice. Electrolytes will be replaced with the athlete's next meal.

Ergogenic aids. Athletes, of course, always want to win. Since ancient times

❖

BOX 16-2
Sorting Out the Sports Drink Story

The current story of the so-called sports drinks developed from the belief that water alone does not meet hydration needs during exercise. We know now that the ideal fluid to prevent dehydration depends on how demanding the exercise is and how long it lasts.

For regular nonendurance exercise, physically fit athletes do perfectly well on plain water. However, what long-term endurance athletes do need, especially in hot weather, is both water and fuel—carbohydrate. Without carbohydrate replacement, a long-distance marathon runner, for example, would soon run out of muscle glycogen and slow down. Also, in such a demanding run, when the body can sweat as much as 6% of its weight, it cannot keep cool enough and the overall system overheats, leading to heatstroke and collapse. But simply adding sugar to water causes the water to be held in the stomach longer, where it does the body tissues no good for immediate needs.

The first group of sports drinks began with a solution called Gatorade, named by its developers for their university's football team. They reasoned that if they analyzed their players' sweat they could replace lost minerals and water, then add some flavoring, coloring, and sugars to make it more acceptable, and it would do a better job than plain water. Although it was highly profitable for the university and for the manufacturer, subsequent studies showed that regular nonendurance athletes did not need it. Plain water served their needs very well and they obtained their minerals in their diet.

A second category of sports drinks has been developed to meet the dual water-and-energy needs of athletes in longer-lasting endurance events. More dilute 10% sugar solutions, using glucose or glucose polymers (short chains of about five glucose molecules) that are not sweet, are being used. In the more dilute solutions, both energy-sustaining sugars leave the stomach rapidly and provide a continuing fuel and water source for the endurance athlete.

Other products entering the sports drink market have been Gatorade clones that claim to add no sugar yet supply ample amounts of fructose and glucose in their fruit juice base. Fructose does not leave the stomach rapidly and is absorbed from the intestine more slowly than glucose, often causing bloating or diarrhea. Still others add to their fruit juice base multiple vitamins yielding 137% of the RDA in a single 10-ounce bottle, but contain no minerals. All of these vitamins won't help performance at all, and on a hot day a sweating athlete could easily down a megadose in four or five bottles.

It is important to sort out the claims of sports drinks. They are not for everyone. In the long run, special drinks meet needs of the athlete in endurance evants. But for nonendurance activities most persons don't need them. After all, water is the best solution for regular needs—and costs far less.

References

Costill D: Carbohydrates for exercise: dietary demands for optimal performance, Int J Sports Med 9:1, 1988.

Kris-Etherton PM: Nutrition and athletic performance, Nutr Today 25(5):35, 1990.

they have been seeking and experimenting with some "magic" substance or treatment to gain the competitive edge. Today these substances sought by modern athletes are known as *ergogenic* (work-producing) aids. Most are worthless fads, but one current practice—the use of **steroids**—is of great concern because it is dangerous and in athletics, illegal. Public attention was recently focused on this practice when the gold medal winner for the 100-

❖ TABLE 16-3   *Modified depletion-taper precompetition program for glycogen loading*

Day	Exercise	Diet
1	90-minute period at 70%-75% Vo₂ max	Mixed diet 50% carbohydrate (350 g)
2-3	Gradual tapering of time and intensity	Diet above continued
4-5	Tapering of exercise time and intensity continues	Mixed diet 70% carbohydrate (550 g)
6	Complete rest	Diet above continued
7	Day of completion	High-carbohydrate preevent diet

Adapted from Wright ED: Carbohydrate nutrition and exercise, Clin Nutr 7(1):18, 1988.

meter dash in the 1988 Olympic games was disqualified for use of steroids. It has since become common knowledge that this practice is widespread among athletes and body builders, sometimes starting as early as high school or even junior high school. These steroids are synthetic sex hormones that have two actions: (1) *anabolic* (tissue growth), and (2) *androgenic* (masculinization). Athletes often take these drugs in megadoses 10 to 30 times their normal body hormonal output to increase muscle size, strength, and performance. The physiologic side effects, however, can be devastating, varying from premature bone growth closure, thus stunting normal skeletal development, and liver injury, to accelerated heart disease, high blood pressure, sterility, and many other physical effects.[5] Psychologic effects vary from increasing aggressiveness, drug dependence, and mood swings to depression, decreased sex drive, and violent rage. Many serious athletes face a hard choice of not using these dangerous drugs and facing a large field of opponents who are using and reaping the competitive edge—or of using the drugs and risking the side effects and potential official discovery and disqualification.[6]

PLANNING A PERSONAL EXERCISE PROGRAM
Health benefits
Exercise benefits overall health in general. The sense of fitness it brings helps one to "feel good." But in addition to this general sense of well-being, exercise, especially when mixed with aerobic forms, has special benefits for persons with certain health problems.

Coronary heart disease. Several benefits of exercise exist for those persons with coronary heart disease (see Chapter 19). Exercise helps to:
1. Increase heart size and strength (Remember: the heart is a muscle, and exercise strengthens it as it would any muscle.)
2. Increase stroke volume (That is, the heart puts out more blood with each beat, so it does not have to beat as rapidly to circulate the same amount of blood.)
3. Raise blood levels of high-density lipoproteins (HDLs), helping to control cholesterol levels
4. Improve general work of the circulatory system by increasing the blood's oxygen-carrying capacity and volume

Diabetes. Exercise helps control diabetes, especially noninsulin-dependent diabetes mellitus (NIDDM) in obese adults. It improves the action of the person's naturally produced insulin by increasing the number of "insulin receptor" sites, areas where insulin may be carried into cells. In managing insulin-dependent diabetes mellitus (IDDM), the type of exercise and when it is done must be balanced with food and insulin to prevent reactions caused by drops in blood sugar.

Weight management. Exercise is extremely beneficial in weight management because it (1) helps regulate appetite, (2) increases basal metabolic rate, and (3) reduces the genetic fat deposit set-point level (p. 223). Exercise also helps reduce stress-related eating. It helps "work off" the hormonal effects produced by stress in the body.

Bone disease. Exercise increases calcium deposit in bone. Thus it increases bone density and reduces the risk of osteoporosis.

Mental health. Exercise stimulates the production of brain opiates, substances called *endorphins*. These natural substances decrease pain (this is how aspirin works, by stimulating production of endorphins), and improve the mood, including an exhilarating kind of "high."

Personal needs

Health status and personal gains. In planning a personal exercise program, it is important to check first on individual health status, present level of fitness, personal needs, and resources required in equipment or cost. The exercise you choose should be something you enjoy and that has some aerobic value. Also, start slowly and build gradually to avoid discouragement and injury. Moderation and regularity are the chief guides.

Aerobic benefits. To build aerobic capacity, the level of exercise must raise the pulse to within 70% of the individual's maximum heart rate. You can estimate your own *cardiac rate* by subtracting your age from 220. This gives

❖ **TABLE 16-4**   *Target zone heart rate according to age to achieve aerobic physical effect of exercise*

Age	Maximal attainable heart rate (pulse: 220 minus age)	Target zone	
		70% maximal rate	85% maximal rate
20	200	140	170
25	195	136	166
30	190	133	161
35	185	129	157
40	180	126	153
45	175	122	149
50	170	119	144
55	165	115	140
60	160	112	136
65	155	108	132
70	150	105	127
75	145	101	124

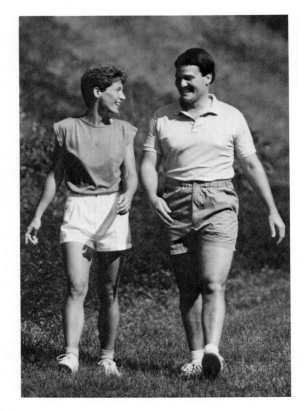

❖ **FIG. 16-2**
Aerobic walking is an enjoyable exercise that can fit into almost anyone's life-style.

❖ **TABLE 16-5**   *Aerobic exercises for physical fitness (maintained at*
aerobic level for at least 30 minutes)

Type of exercise	Aerobic forms
Ballplaying	Handball
	Raquetball
	Squash
Bicycling	Stationary
	Touring
Dancing	Aerobic routines
	Ballet
	Disco
Jumping rope	Brisk pace
Running/jogging	Brisk pace
Skating	Ice skating
	Roller skating
Skiing	Cross country
Swimming	Steady pace
Walking	Brisk pace

your maximum heart rate. About 70% of this figure is your *target zone rate*, the level to which you want to raise your pulse during exercise (Table 16-4). For aerobic benefits, this rate should be maintained 20 minutes and practiced about three times a week. Check your resting pulse before starting the exercise period, then again during and immediately afterward.

Types of physical activity

General exercise. It's best to have a variety of exercises in your plan. Many do not reach aerobic levels but are enjoyable and should be included. Whatever you do, if it isn't fun, you'll soon stop, which benefits no one.

Aerobic exercise. Simple walking can be developed into an aerobic exercise (Fig. 16-2). Start slowly and gradually increase your pace and distance. It is convenient and requires no equipment except good walking shoes. It is also satisfying to many people for whom other forms may not be appropriate. Examples of aerobic forms of exercise are shown in Table 16-5.

Exercise preparation and care. Whatever your exercise choice, preparation and continuing care are important. Before beginning, stretch your muscles to prevent stress or injury. Afterward take time to cool down. Don't go beyond tolerance limits. Listen to your own body. When you are tired, rest. When you hurt, stop. When you want more challenge, increase your exercise level—but only then. Remember, it's *your* exercise plan.

SUMMARY

Many fine muscle fibers and cells, triggered by nerve endings, work smoothly together to make all our physical activity possible. Our primary fuel for energy to run this system is carbohydrate, mainly in the form of complex carbohydrate foods, or starches. The constant body fuels resulting from carbohydrate metabolism are circulating blood sugar and stored glycogen in muscles and liver. Stored body fat supplies additional fuel as fatty acids. Protein, however, provides only insignificant energy for exercise. Vitamins and minerals cannot be burned for energy but are important co-enzyme partners for the process of energy production.

Exercise does increase the need for kilocalories and water. Cold water in small, frequent amounts is the best way to avoid dehydration. Electrolytes lost in sweat are replaced in the next meal. The optimal diet for the athlete is 60% of the kilocalories from carbohydrate (mainly complex starches), 25% from fat, and 15% from protein. The pregame meal should be small, mainly complex carbohydrates (starches), with little fat, protein, or fiber.

General and aerobic exercise have many benefits, which increase with practice. Excellent aerobic exercises include sustained fast walking, swimming, jogging, running, and aerobic dancing or workouts.

❖ REVIEW QUESTIONS

1. Compare and discuss the three energy nutrients in terms of their relative roles as fuel for exercise.
2. Outline the nutrition and physical fitness principles you would discuss with a client who is an athlete. Plan a diet for this person that would meet nutrient and energy needs.

3. Why is fluid balance vital during exercise periods? How is water and electrolyte balance achieved?
4. Decribe the health benefits of exercise for a person with heart disease and for an overweight person with noninsulin-dependent diabetes mellitus (NIDDM).
5. Describe several factors a person should consider in planning a personal exercise program. Define the term *aerobic exercise*. List its benefits.

❖ SELF-TEST QUESTIONS

True-false
For each item you answer "false," write the correct statement.
1. Water containing electrolytes and sugar is the best way to replace these substances lost during exercise.
2. Drinking water immediately before and during an athletic event causes cramps.
3. Cold water is absorbed more quickly from the stomach.
4. Athletes need protein for extra energy.
5. Vitamins and minerals are burned for energy in workouts and training sessions.
6. Protein and fat do not contribute to glycogen stores.
7. Sweating is the main mechanism for dissipating body heat.
8. Aerobic exercise is of limited benefit in control of heart disease and diabetes.
9. Walking can be an excellent form of aerobic exercise.

Multiple choice
1. Which of the following general activities is most likely to provide aerobic exercise?
   a. Golf
   b. Swimming
   c. Tennis
   d. Baseball
2. To develop aerobic capacity, the exercise should:
   a. Raise the pulse to 50% of the maximum heart rate
   b. Be maintained for alternating 10-minute periods
   c. Be practiced consistently every day
   d. Be practiced several times a week at appropriate pulse rate for sustained periods of time
3. Characteristics of a healthful exercise program should include:
   a. Enjoyable activities
   b. Moderation
   c. Regularity
   d. All of these
4. Exercise is beneficial in weight management because it:
   (1) Helps regulate appetite
   (2) Decreases BMR
   (3) Reduces stress-related eating
   (4) Increases the set-point for fat deposit
       a. 1 and 3   c. 1 and 4
       b. 2 and 4   d. 2 and 3
5. Which of these meals would be the best choice as an athlete's pregame meal?
   a. Large grilled steak, fried potatoes, ice cream
   b. Fried fish, vegetable salad with cream dressing, fresh fruit
   c. Spaghetti with tomato sauce, French bread, fruit
   d. Hamburger, french fries, cola

❖ SUGGESTIONS FOR FURTHER STUDY

Analysis of athletes' diets

Interview two athletes in your school or community, one male and one female. Ask them about food habits and attitudes, their own or ones they have observed in teammates. Ask about use of supplements, pregame meals, nutrition advice from coaches, and any other food- or nutrition-related practices.

Analyze your findings in terms of total energy value of diet (kilocalories) and relative percentages of total kilocalories supplied by protein, fat, and carbohydrate. Compare the two athletes' diets, nutrition practices, and beliefs. Present your findings in your class discussion. Follow up your initial interview with any dietary counseling indicated, if it is appropriate.

Discussion group for athletes

Plan with a school or community organization athletic director to hold an informal discussion group with team members to present nutrition information for persons involved in team sports. Discuss their questions about food and nutrition practices and beliefs. Provide a display or appropriate handouts of sound nutrition information, resources, or reference lists for sources of helpful materials.

Survey of Fitness Centers

Visit a variety of fitness centers in your community. Gather information and reference materials about each center's program: services offered, costs, staff resources, diet recommendations, or sale of any nutrition products in relation to their program. Compare and evaluate these programs in a follow-up class discussion.

References

1. Barr SI and Costill DL: Water—can the endurance athlete get too much of a good thing? J Am Diet Assoc 89(11):1629, 1989.
2. Hagan RD: Benefits of aerobic conditioning and diet for overweight adults, Sports Med 5:144, 1988.
3. Clark N: Nancy Clark's sports nutrition guidebook: eating to fuel your active lifestyle, Champaign, Ill, 1990, Leisure Press.
4. Aronsen VA: Vitamins and minerals as ergogenic aids, Physician and Sports Med 14:209, 1988.
5. Hallagen JB and others: Anabolic-androgenic steroid use by athletes, N Engl J Med 321:1042, 1989.
6. Lamb DR and Wardlaw GM: Sports nutrition, Nutri-News, Jan 1991, p 10, Mosby—Year Book.

Further reading

Keith RE and others: Dietary status of trained female cyclists, J Am Diet Assoc 89(11):1620, 1989.

Williams MH: Nutritional ergogenic aids and athletic performance, Nutr Today 24(1):7, 1989.

These two articles indicate that proper nutrition is currently regarded as one of the most important factors in athletic performance success.

17

❖

Nutritional care

KEY CONCEPTS

Valid health care is based on individual needs.

Comprehensive health care is best provided by a team of various health professionals and support staff persons.

A personalized health care plan, based on identified individual needs and goals, guides actions to promote healing and health.

*P*ersons face acute illness or chronic disease and its treatment in a variety of settings: hospital, extended care facility, clinic, or home. In all instances nutritional support is fundamental. Frequently it is the primary therapy. Sensitive care is always based on the individual's personal needs. To meet individual nutritional needs, a broad knowledge of nutritional state, requirements, and ways of meeting these identified needs is essential. The clinical nutritionist (registered dietitian), along with the physician, carries the major responsibility for this nutritional care. Each health team member must help with this care, however, if it is to be person-centered care that meets individual needs.

In this chapter we focus on the comprehensive care of the patient's nutritional needs and explore the basic care process involved. Whatever the need and wherever the place of care, the health care team, including the patient and family, work together to support the healing process and promote health.

THE THERAPEUTIC PROCESS
Setting and focus of care

Health care setting. The modern hospital has become a marvel of medical technology, but these medical advances have also brought increasing confusion to many patients. Their illness places them in the midst of a complex system of care. Various persons come and go, and it is understandable when the course does not always run smoothly. Patients need personal advocates. Primary health care providers such as the nurse and the dietitian can provide such essential support and personalized care.

Health care team. In the area of nutritional care, the clinical nutritionist (registered dietitian) carries the major responsibility. Working closely with the physician, the nutritionist determines individual nutritional therapy needs and plan of care. Throughout this process team support is essential. Nurses especially are in a unique position to provide this important nutritional support, referring patients to the clinical nutritionist when time or skills are lacking.[1] Of all the health care team members, nurses are in the closest continuous contact with patients and their families. A real partnership with patients and their families is essential to valid care.[2] In this developing team relationship, all involved parties need each other's expertise and experience for a successful outcome.

Person-centered care. To be valid, nutritional care must be based on identified individual needs. It must be *person-centered*. Needs must be updated constantly with the patient. Such personalized care demands a great commitment from health workers. Despite all methods, tools, and technologies described here and elsewhere, remember this basic fact: *the most healing tool you will ever use is yourself*. This is a simple yet profound truth, because it is the *human* encounter to which we bring ourselves and our skills.

Phases of the care process

Collecting information. To provide person-centered care, we need to collect as much information about the patient's situation as possible. We must know the nutritional status, food habits, and living situation, as well as the patient's needs, desires, and goals. The patient (Fig. 17-1) and the family are primary

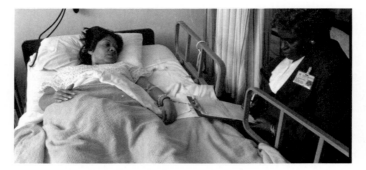

❖   FIG. 17-1

Interviewing patient to plan personal care.

sources of this information. Other sources include the patient's medical chart, oral or written communication with hospital staff, and related research.

Identifying problems. A careful study of all the information you have gathered will reveal basic patient needs. Other needs will develop as the hospitalization continues. You can begin to list these needs to guide care.

Planning care. Appropriate care is planned to meet these identified needs. This written care plan will give attention to personal needs and goals, as well as the identified medical care requirements.

Implementing care. Appropriate and realistic actions then carry out the personal care plan. Nutritional care and teaching, for example, would include an appropriate food plan with examples of food choices, food buying, or food preparation. Such activities might include family members as well.

Evaluating and recording results. Results need to be checked to see if the needs have been met. Then the plan can be revised as needed for continuing care. These actions and results must be carefully recorded in the patient's medical chart.

In the remainder of this chapter, we briefly review each of these five phases of individual health care in terms of nutritional aspects of overall patient care. Nutritional support is an essential component of all health care.

COLLECTING AND ANALYZING NUTRITIONAL INFORMATION
Collection

Body measures. Practice taking body measurements correctly to avoid errors. Also maintain proper equipment and careful technique. Three types of measurements are common in clinical practice.

1. Weight. Weigh hospital patients at consistent times, for example, in the early morning after the bladder is emptied and before breakfast. Weigh clinic patients without shoes in light indoor clothing or examining gown. Ask about the usual body weight and compare it with standard weight-height tables (p. 222).[3] Ask about any recent weight loss: how much over what time period. A rapid weight loss is significant. Also, is the cause known? Similarly, ask about any recent weight gain. Sometimes it is helpful to ask about general weight history over time, peaks and lows at what ages.

2. Height. Use a fixed measuring stick against the wall if possible. Otherwise, use the moveable measuring rod on the platform clinic scales. Have the person stand as straight as possible, without shoes or cap. Note growth of children, as well as diminishing height of older adults.

3. Body composition. The nutritionist usually measures various aspects of body size and composition. These include mid-upper-arm circumference and triceps skinfold, from which mid-upper-arm muscle circumference can be calculated. This provides a good general indication of body leanness and fatness (p. 221). Special calipers measure skinfold thickness (Fig. 17-2).

Medical tests. Many laboratory tests help measure nutritional status and are available to study. Several of these most frequently used are listed here.

1. Plasma protein. Basic measures are hemoglobin, hematocrit, and serum albumin. Additional tests may include serum transferrin or total iron-binding capacity (TIBC), and ferritin. These tests help detect protein and iron deficiencies.

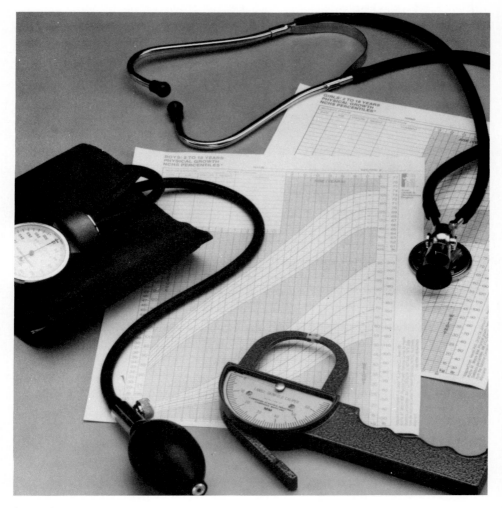

❖ FIG. 17-2

Assessment tools, including skinfold calipers, that measure relative amount of subcutaneous fat tissues at various body sites.

2. *Protein metabolism.* Basic 24-hour urine tests measure products of protein metabolism: urinary creatinine and urea nitrogen. Elevated levels may indicate excess body tissue breakdown.

3. *Immune system integrity.* Basic tests determine the lymphocyte count, the ratio of these special white cells to total white blood cell count. Also, skin testing may be done for sensitivity to common antigens and hence strength of general immunity system.

In general, these medical tests used for nutrition assessment are reliable in persons of any age, but conditions in elderly patients may interfere and need to be considered in evaluating test results. For example, laboratory values are affected by hydration status, presence of chronic diseases, changes in organ function, and by drugs.[4]

❖ **TABLE 17-1** *Clinical signs of nutritional status*

Body area	Signs of good nutrition	Signs of poor nutrition
General appearance	Alert, responsive	Listless, apathetic, cachexic
Weight	Normal for height, age, body build	Overweight or underweight (special concern for underweight)
Posture	Erect, arms and legs straight	Sagging shoulders, sunken chest, humped back
Muscles	Well developed; firm, good tone; some fat under skin	Flaccid, poor tone; undeveloped; tender, "wasted" appearance; cannot walk properly
Nervous control	Good attention span; not irritable or restless; normal reflexes; psychologic stability	Inattentive, irritable, confused; burning and tingling of hands and feet (paresthesia); loss of position and vibratory sense; weakness and tenderness of muscles (may result in ability to walk); decrease or loss of ankle and knee relflexes
Gastrointestinal function	Good appetite and digestion, normal regular elimination, no palpable (perceptible to touch) organs or masses	Anorexia, indigestion, constipation or diarrhea, liver or spleen enlargment
Cardiovascular function	Normal heart rate and rhythm, no murmurs, normal blood pressure for age	Rapid heart rate (greater than 100 beats/minute tachycardia), enlarged heart, abnormal rhythm, elevated blood pressure
General vitality	Endurance, energetic, sleeps well, vigorous	Easily fatigued, no energy, falls asleep easily, looks tired, apathetic
Hair	Shiny, lustrous, firm, not easily plucked, heathy scalp	Stringy, dull, brittle, dry, thin and sparse; depigmented; can be easily plucked
Skin (general)	Smooth, slightly moist, good color	Rough, dry, scaly, pale, pigmented, irritated; bruises; petechiae
Face and neck	Skin color uniform, smooth, pink, healthy appearance, not swollen	Greasy, discolored, scaly, swollen; skin dark over cheeks and under eyes; lumpiness or flakiness of skin around nose and mouth
Lips	Smooth, good color; moist; not chapped or swollen	Dry, scaly, swollen, redness and swelling (cheilosis), or angular lesions at corners of the mouth or fissures or scars (stomatitis)

Mouth, oral membranes	Reddish pink mucous membranes in oral cavity	Swollen, boggy oral mucous membranes
Gums	Good pink color, healthy, red, no swelling or bleeding	Spongy, bleed easily, marginal redness, inflamed, gums receding
Tongue	Good pink color or deep reddish in appearance, not swollen or smooth, surface papillae present, no lesion	Swelling, scarlet and raw, magenta color, beefy (glossitis), hyperemic and hypertrophic papillae, atrophic papillae
Teeth	No cavities, no pain, bright, straight, no crowding, well-shaped jaw, clean, no discoloration	Unfilled caries, absent teeth, worn surfaces, mottled (fluorosis), malpositioned
Eyes	Bright, clear, shiny; no sores at corner of eyelids; membranes moist and healthy pink color, no prominent blood vessels or amount of tissue or sclera; no fatigue circles beneath	Eye membranes pale (pale conjunctivas), redness of membrane (conjunctival injection), dryness, signs of infection; Bitot's spots, redness and fissuring of eyelid corners (angular palpebritis), dryness of eye membrane (conjunctival xerosis), dull appearance of cornea (corneal xerosis), soft cornea (keratomalacia)
Neck (glands)	No enlargement	Thyroid enlarged
Nails	Firm, pink	Spoon shaped (koilonychia), brittle, ridged
Legs, feet	No tenderness, weakness, or swelling, good color	Edema, tender calf, tingling weakness
Skeleton	No malformations	Bowlegs, knock-knees, chest deformity at diaphragm, beaded ribs, prominent scapulas

From Williams SR: Nutritional assessment and guidance in prenatal care. In Worthington-Roberts BS and Williams SR: Nutrition in pregnancy and lactation, ed 4, St Louis, 1989, Mosby–Year Book, Inc.

Observations. Careful observations of the patient's condition in various areas of the body may reveal signs of poor nutrition in comparison to signs of good nutrition. Table 17-1 lists some of these clinical signs of nutritional status. Keep these in mind when providing general patient care.

Diet history. General knowledge of the patient's basic eating habits helps to identify any possible nutritional deficiencies. Box 17-1 shows an example of a general guide for a nutrition history. Sometimes a more specific food intake is obtained using a 24-hour recall, that is, going through the previous day and asking for everything consumed, food items used, and amounts and

---

BOX 17-1

❖ ——————— CLINICAL APPLICATION ——————— ❖

Nutrition History: Activity-Associated General Day's Food Pattern

Name _____ Date _____

Height _____ Weight (lb) _____ (kg) _____ Age _____

Ideal weight _____

Referral
Diagnosis
Diet order
Members of household
Occupation
Recreation, physical activity
Present food intake

	Place	Hour	Frequency, form, and amount checklist
Breakfast			Milk
			Cheese
			Meat
			Fish
			Poultry
Noon meal			Eggs
			Cream
			Butter, margarine
			Other fats
Evening meal			Vegetables, green
			Vegetables, other
			Fruits (citrus)
			Legumes
Extra meals			Potato
			Bread—kind
			Sugar
			Desserts
			Beverages
Summary			Alcohol
			Vitamins
			Candy

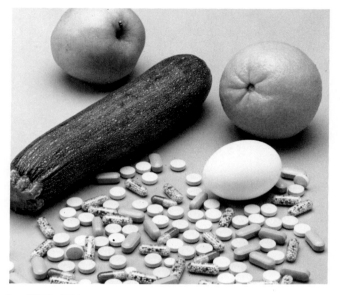

❖ **FIG. 17-3**

Many drugs, foods, and nutrients interact to cause nutritional problems.

methods of preparation. A more extended 3-day food record may give still further information about food habits or problems.

Analysis

Nutritional problems. A study of all the nutrition information collected will help identify nutritional problems. These problems may include nutrient deficiencies, such as evidence of iron deficiency anemia, or underlying disease requiring a special modified diet. Evidence may reveal signs of general malnutrition requiring rebuilding of body tissue and nutrient stores. There may be need for special assistance in eating and swallowing.[5]

Drug-nutrient interactions. Information about all drugs used is essential. This includes over-the-counter self-medications and "street drugs," as well as alcohol use and prescribed drugs. Research each item to determine any possible problems from interactions of all drugs with foods and nutrients (Fig. 17-3). Many such reactions exist and are encountered with multiple drug use, especially encountered in elderly patients with chronic diseases.

Personal needs and goals. Any personal, cultural, and ethnic needs must be considered in helping the patient plan for meeting health needs. Economic needs are paramount for many persons in high-risk populations. Personal goals help establish priorities for immediate as well as long-term care.

PLANNING AND IMPLEMENTING NUTRITIONAL CARE
Basic principles of diet therapy

Normal nutrition base. The primary principle of diet therapy is that it is based on the patient's normal nutritional requirements. This is important for the patient to know. Any therapeutic diet is only a modification of normal

❖ **TABLE 17-2** *Routine hospital diets*

Food	Clear liquid	Full liquid	Soft	Regular
Soup	Clear fat-free broth, bouillon	Same, plus strained or blended cream soups	Same, plus all cream soups	All
Cereal		Cooked refined cereal	Cooked cereal, corn-flakes, rice, noodles, macaroni, sphagetti	
Bread			White bread, crackers, melba toast, zwie-back	All
Protein foods		Milk, cream, milk drinks, yogurt	Same, plus eggs (not fried), mild cheese, cottage and cream cheese, fowl, fish, sweetbreads, tender beef, veal, lamb, liver, bacon, gravy	All
Vegetables			Potatoes: baked, mashed, creamed, steamed, scalloped; tender cooked whole bland vegetables; fresh lettuce, toma-toes	All

Fruit and fruit juices	Fruit juices (as tolerated), flavored fruit drinks	All	Same, plus cooked fruit: peaches, pears, applesauce, peeled apricots, white cherries; ripe peaches, pears, banana, orange and grapefruit sections without membrane	All
Desserts and gelatin	Fruit-flavored gelatin, fruit ices and popsicles	Same, plus sherbet, ice cream puddings, custard, frozen yogurt	Same, plus plain sponge cakes, plain cookies, plain cake, puddings, pie made with allowed foods	
Miscellaneous	Soft drinks (as tolerated), coffee and tea, decaffeinated coffee and tea, cereal beverages such as Postum, sugar, honey, salt, hard candy, Polycoase, residue-free supplements	Same, plus margarine, pepper, all supplements	Same, plus, mild salad dressings	

nutritional needs, and is modified only as the individual's specific condition requires.

Disease modifications. Nutritional components of the normal diet may be modified in three basic ways:

1. *Nutrients.* One or more of the basic nutrients such as protein, carbohydrate, fat, mineral, or vitamin may be modified in amount or form.

2. *Energy.* The total energy value of the diet, expressed in kilocalories (kcal), may be increased or decreased.

3. *Texture.* The texture or seasoning of the diet may be modified, as in liquid or low-residue diets.

Personal adaptation. Successful nutritional therapy can occur only when the diet is *personalized*, that is, adapted to meet individual needs. This can only be done by planning *with the patient or family.* Four areas need to be explored together.

1. *Personal needs.* What personal desires, concerns, goals, or life situation needs must be met?

2. *Disease.* How does the patient's disease or condition affect the body and its normal metabolic functions?

3. *Nutritional therapy.* How and why does the diet need to be changed to meet the needs created by the patient's particular disease or condition?

4. *Food plan.* How do these necessary nutritional modifications affect daily food choices?

Routine house diets. A schedule of routine "house" diets, based on some type of cycle menus, is usually followed in most hospitals. The basic modification is in texture, ranging from clear liquid (no milk), through full liquid (including milk) and soft, to a full regular diet. Table 17-2 summarizes details of currently liberalized routine hospital diets.

Mode of feeding

The method of feeding used in the nutritional care plan depends on the patient's condition. The clinical nutritionist and the nurse work together to manage the diet by using oral, tube, peripheral vein, or total parenteral feeding.

Oral diet. As long as possible, regular oral feedings are preferred. If needed, nutrient supplements may be added. According to the patient's condition, the nurse may need to assist the patient in eating. This can be a special opportunity for nutrition counseling and support.

Tube feeding. When a patient cannot eat but the gastrointestinal tract can be used, tube feeding provides nutritional support. Various commercial formulas are available and usually preferred over locally mixed ones. A blended formula may be calculated and prepared, but greater risk of contamination in preparation and storage exists.

Peripheral vein feeding. If the patient cannot take in food or formula through the gastrointestinal tract, intravenous (IV) feeding is required. Various solutions of dextrose, amino acids, vitamins, minerals, and lipids can be fed through peripheral veins. The nutrient and kilocalorie intake is limited in this method of feeding, however, so it is used only when the nutritional need is not extensive or long term. It is helpful for the patient to understand that this is still a method of "feeding."

Total parenteral nutrition (TPN). When the patient's nutritional need is great, as in massive injury or debilitating disease, and may be required for longer time, feeding through a larger central vein is needed. Total parenteral nutrition (TPN) is a special surgical procedure. It requires special nutrient solutions administered by a team of specialists: physicians, nutritionists, pharmacists, and nurses. Throughout this procedure the patient will need special care and support, including instruction for continued TPN use at home as needed.

EVALUATION OF NUTRITIONAL CARE
General considerations

When the nutritional plan of care is carried out, it is evaluated in terms of the nutritional diagnosis and treatment objectives. This evaluation continues through the period of care and terminates at the point of discharge or the end of the care period. Various questions are important, as listed in the following sections.

Nutritional goals. What is the effect of the diet or feeding method on the illness or the patient's situation? Is there need for any change in the nutrients, kilocalories, meal-snack pattern, or the feeding method?

Accuracy of care plan actions. Must any of the nutritional care plan components be changed? Is it necessary to change the type of food or feeding equipment, environment for meals, counseling procedures, or types of learning activities for nutrition education?

Ability to follow diet. Does any hindrance or disability prevent the patient from following the treatment plan? What is the impact of the diet on the patient, family, or staff? Was all the necessary nutrition information gathered correctly? Do the patient and family understand all the self-care instructions provided? Are needed community resources available or convenient for use? Has any needed food-assistance program been sufficient for the patient's care?

Role of the nurse and nutritionist

The nurse and the nutritionist form an important team for providing nutrition care. The clinical nutritionist determines nutritional needs, plans and manages nutritional therapy, and evaluates and records results. Throughout this entire process, the nurse helps develop, support, and carry out the plan of care. Successful care depends on close nutritionist-nurse teamwork. At varying times, depending on need, the nurse may serve as an essential coordinator, advocate, interpreter, teacher, or counselor.

Coordinator and advocate. Nurses work more closely with patients than any other practitioner. They are best able to coordinate any of the patient's special services and treatments. They can consult and refer as needed. Sometimes hospital-induced malnutrition exists because meals are frequently in conflict with procedures, a situation the nurse can help resolve. For example, an audit in one hospital revealed that in 1 week 5% of the patient trays were not served at all, 24% were held back for patients undergoing medical procedures at mealtime, and 15% were accepted but uneaten because of poor patient appetite.[6] All too often, this situation still occurs today.

Interpreter. The nurse can help reduce the patient's anxiety by careful, brief, easily understood explanations concerning various treatments and plans of care. This includes basic reinforcement of special diet needs, resulting food choices from menus, and illustrations of needs from foods on the tray. With disinterested or unpopular patients, these activities may be difficult, but efforts to understand such patient behavior are important.[7]

Teacher or counselor. Basic health teaching and counseling are essential roles in nursing. Many opportunities exist during daily care for planned conversations about sound nutrition principles, which will reinforce the clinical nutritionist's work with the patient. Clearly, learning about the patient's nutritional needs must begin with hospital admission or initial contact, must carry through the entire period of care, and must continue in the home environment, supported by community resources as needed.

SUMMARY

The basis for effective nutritional care begins with the patient's nutritional needs and must involve the patient and the family. Such person-centered care requires close teamwork among all health team members providing primary care. Careful assessment of factors influencing nutritional status requires a broad foundation of pertinent information: physiologic, psychosocial, medical, and personal. The patient's medical record is a basic means of communication among health care team members.

Nutritional therapy is based on personal and physical needs of the patient. Successful therapy requires a close working relationship among nutrition, medical, and nursing staff in the health care facility. The nurse has a unique position to reinforce nutritional principles of the diet with the patient and family.

❖ REVIEW QUESTIONS

1. Identify and discuss the possible effects of various psychosocial factors on the outcome of nutritional therapy.
2. List and describe commonly used measures for determining nutritional status, including (a) body measures, (b) medical tests, (c) clinical observations, and (d) food habits.
3. Describe the roles of the clinical nutritionist and the nurse in nutritional care.

❖ SELF-TEST QUESTIONS

True-false

For each item answered "false," write the correct statement.

1. Nutritional care is based on individual patient needs.
2. A patient's housing situation has little relation to his illness or his continuing care.
3. History taking is an important skill in planning nutritional care.
4. A patient's social history has little value in planning his diet.
5. Once a diet treatment plan has been established, it should be followed continuously without change.
6. Normal nutrition needs are the basis for diet therapy.
7. The patient's personal goals do not relate to his diet therapy and instruction.
8. A diet modified in energy value may be indicated for an obese patient.
9. Ill patients with little appetite are stimulated to eat by larger food portions.
10. Involvement of the patient's family in his diet therapy and teaching usually creates problems and is best avoided.

Multiple choice

1. Which of the following physical details help to determine a patient's nutritional needs?
   (1) Age and sex
   (2) Disabilities
   (3) Skin condition
   (4) Symptoms of illness
       a. 2 and 4   c. 1 and 3
       b. 1 and 4   d. All of these

2. A nutrition history should include which of the following items of nutritional information?
   (1) General food habits
   (2) Food-buying practices
   (3) Cooking methods
   (4) Food likes and dislikes
       a. 1 and 3   c. All of these
       b. 1 and 4   d. 2 and 4

3. Knowledge of which of the following items is necessary for carrying out valid diet therapy for a hospitalized patient?
   (1) The specific diet and its relation to the patient's disease
   (2) Foods affected by the diet modification
   (3) Mode of the hospital's food service and need of the patient for any eating aids
   (4) The patient's response to the diet
       a. 1 and 2   c. 2 and 4
       b. All of these   d. 2 and 3

4. A special diet may be based on a specific nutrient modification. For example, a 30 g protein diet would include increased amounts of which of the following foods?
       a. Meat and fish
       b. Eggs and poultry
       c. Cheese and milk
       d. Fruits and vegetables

5. Which of the following actions would be helpful to a disabled patient who needs assistance in eating?
   (1) Learning the extent of his disability and encouraging him to do as much of the feeding as he can for himself
   (2) Feeding the patient completely, regardless of the problem, since it saves him time and energy
   (3) Hurrying the feeding to get in as much food as possible before his appetite wanes
   (4) Sitting comfortably by the patient's bed and offering him mouthfuls of food, with ample time to chew, swallow, and rest as needed
       a. 2 and 3   c. 1 and 3
       b. 1 and 4   d. 2 and 4

❖ SUGGESTIONS FOR FURTHER STUDY

Group project: Role of the registered dietitian in patient-client care

Form small groups of two or three students and assign visits to a number of different-sized hospitals available in the community. If possible, include a large medical center, a smaller community hospital, a nursing home, and a community health center. At each of these facilities arrange to interview various dietitians about their roles in patient care. If possible, include the following types of dietitians in your interviews:

1. Clinic dietitian in outpatient setting
2. Administrative dietitian or dietary department director
3. Clinical or patient care dietitian in hospital
4. Consulting dietitian to nursing homes
5. Consulting nutritionist in private practice
6. Public health nutritionist in public health department
7. Nutritionist in community health center or health agency

Include the following questions in your interviews:

1. What system of food service is being used?
2. What is the dietitian's relation to other patient care personnel such as physicians, nurses, social workers, and others?
3. What types of activities does the dietitian conduct with patients and staff?
4. What relationship does dietitian have with the hospital administrator or medical chief-of-staff?

Observe tray service in the hospital. Note the form of tray service used, the types of diets being served, and the nature of the foods being used in each.

Feeding disabled patients or children

Arrange with any available health care facility in the community to assist in the feeding of a disabled patient or small child. Select a variety of community settings such as nursing homes and hospitals.

Observe the patient's reaction and attitudes expressed toward the food. What degree of feeding assistance did the patient require? What plan of feeding assistance did you find worked best? If a rehabilitation center is available, visit the center and observe the variety of self-feeding devices being used by the patients. If you are visiting a pediatric ward, compare the reactions of the children to the food being served.

In a follow-up class discussion, compare the findings of various students in different settings. What recommendations can you make from your experience?

References

1. US Preventive Services Task Force: Nutritional counseling, Am Fam Physician 40:125, Aug 1989.
2. Gilbert J: Partnership—a new paradigm for health care, Hospitals 64:72, June 5, 1990.
3. Weigley ES: Average? Ideal? Desirable? A brief overview of height-weight tables in the United States. J Am Diet Assoc 84(4):417, 1984.
4. Chernoff R: Physiologic aging and nutritional status, Nutr Clin Prac 5:8, Feb 1990.
5. Dilorio C and Price ME: Swallowing—an assessment guide, Am J Nurs 90:42, July 1990.
6. Kared FA, Becker DS, and Finkelstein G: Unreceived meals source of malnourishment, Hospitals 56:47, 1982.
7. Kus RJ: Nurses and unpopular patients, Am J Nurs 90:62, June 1990.

Further reading

Dwyer JT and others: Changes in relative weight among institutionalized elderly adults, J Gerontol 42:246, May 1987.

Matthews LE: Using anthropometric parameters to evaluate nutritional status, J Nutr Elderly 5:67, Winter 1985/1986.

Tramposch TS and Blue LS: A nutrition screening and assessment system for use with the elderly in extended care, J Am Diet Assoc 87(9):1207.

These three articles discuss special assessment needs of elderly persons in long-term-care facilities, using adapted methods and standard reference norms, especially for nonambulatory residents.

18

❖

Gastrointestinal problems

K E Y   C O N C E P T S

Diseases of the gastrointestinal tract and its accessory organs interrupt the body's normal digestion-absorption-metabolism cycle.

Allergic conditions produce sensitivity to certain food components.

Underlying genetic diseases cause specific metabolic defects that block the body's ability to handle specific food nutrients.

*W*hen we eat, we usually take for granted our intricate body system for handling food. We just don't think about it. When something goes wrong with the system, however, it affects our whole being.

When we consider the gastrointestinal tract and its handling of the food we eat, we know that we are looking at much more than the physical system. We are looking at the whole person. The overall system is a sensitive mirror, both directly and indirectly, of the individual human condition. Stressed adults with ulcers avoid upsetting foods. Young children with certain food allergies or genetic disorders learn early to say, "I can't eat that because it will make me sick."

In this chapter we look at this sensitive system that handles our food and its nutrients to provide energy and maintain body tissues. We not only must base our nutritional therapy on the functioning of this finely integrated network, but also must focus on the person whose life it affects.

THE UPPER GASTROINTESTINAL TRACT
Problems of the mouth and esophagus

Dental problems. Although the incidence of dental caries has declined somewhat in the past few years, tooth decay still plagues children. Some of the decline results from increased use of fluoridated public water supplies and fluoridated toothpastes, as well as better dental hygiene. The use of refined sugars, however, mainly as corn sweeteners in processed foods, continues to increase as new products are developed.[1] In elderly persons, loss of teeth or ill-fitting dentures may cause problems with chewing and thus digestion of food. Sometimes a *mechanical soft diet* is helpful. In this diet all foods are soft-cooked, meats are ground and mixed with sauces or gravies, thus requiring less chewing and facilitating eating.

Surgical procedures. A fractured jaw or other mouth or neck surgery poses obvious eating problems. Healing nutrients must be supplied, usually in the form of high-protein, high-caloric liquids. Table 18-1 provides an example of a simple "milkshake." Other commercial formulas are also available. As healing progresses, soft foods requiring little chewing effort can be added, building to a full diet according to individual tolerance.

Hiatal hernia. Normally the lower end of the esophagus enters the chest cavity through an opening in the diaphragm membrane called the *hiatus*. A hiatal hernia occurs when a portion of the upper stomach protrudes up through this opening also, as shown in Fig. 18-1. This is not an uncommon problem, especially in obese adults. In such persons weight reduction is essential. They should eat small amounts of food at a time, avoid lying down after meals, and sleep with the head of the bed elevated to prevent reflux of acid stomach contents. Frequent use of antacids helps control the symptoms of "heartburn," caused by tissue irritation of the lower esophagus and upper herniated area of the stomach by the acid-enzyme-food mixture. From 85% to 90% of persons with this esophagitis and gastritis respond to weight reduction and conservative measures. Large hiatal hernias or smaller sliding hernias may require surgical repair. Also, avoiding tight clothing helps to relieve discomfort.

Peptic ulcer disease

Incidence. Throughout the world peptic ulcer disease affects about 10% of the population. It can occur at any age, but is seen mostly in middle adulthood,

❖ **TABLE 18-1**   *High-protein, high caloric formula*

Ingredients	Amount	Approximate food value	
Milk	1 cup	Protein	40 g
Egg substitute (Egg Beaters)	¼ cup	Fat	30 g
Skim milk powder or	6 to 8 tbsp	Carbohydrate	70 g
Casec	2 tbsp	Kcalories	710
Sugar	2 tbsp		
Ice cream	2.5 cm (1 in) slice or 1 scoop		
Cocoa or other flavoring	2 tbsp		
Vanilla	Few drops, as desired		

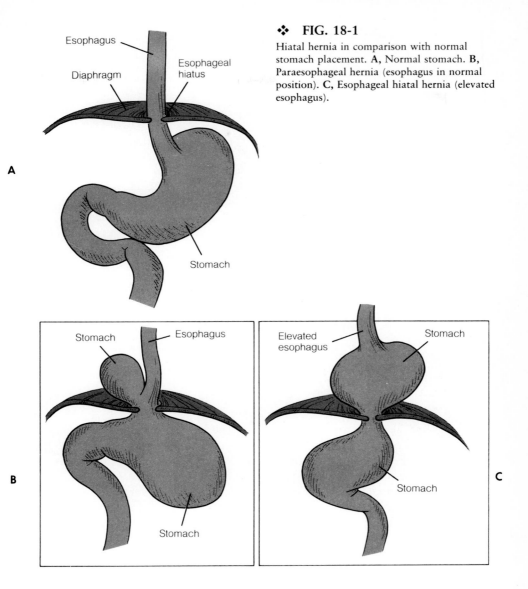

❖ FIG. 18-1

Hiatal hernia in comparison with normal stomach placement. **A,** Normal stomach. **B,** Paraesophageal hernia (esophagus in normal position). **C,** Esophageal hiatal hernia (elevated esophagus).

Esophagus

Esophageal hiatus

Diaphragm

A

Stomach

Stomach

Esophagus

B

Stomach

Elevated esophagus

Stomach

Stomach

C

between ages 45 and 55. Gastric and duodenal ulcers, along with the complication of perforation, occur more often in men. Other diseases and injuries such as burns may cause so-called stress ulcers.

Causes. The exact cause of peptic ulcer is unknown. Some evidence suggests a genetic factor, since relatives of peptic ulcer patients have about three times as many ulcers as members of the general population. Both physical and psychologic factors, however, clearly are involved.

1. Physical factors. The general term *peptic ulcer* refers to an eroded mucosal lesion in the central portion of the gastrointestinal (GI) tract. It can occur in the lower esophagus, stomach, or first portion of the duodenum, the *duodenal bulb.* Most ulcers occur in the duodenal bulb, because the gastric contents

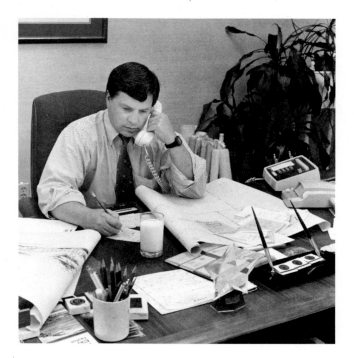

❖ **FIG. 18-2**

Stress may contribute to peptic ulcer disease in predisposed inidividuals.

emptying here are most concentrated. The lesion results from an imbalance between two factors: (1) amount of gastric acid and pepsin (a powerful gastric enzyme for digestion of protein) secretions, and (2) degree of tissue resistance to these secretions.

2. Psychologic factors. The influence of psychologic factors in development of peptic ulcer varies. No distinct personality type is free from the disease. Stress during the young and middle adult years, however, when personal and career strivings are at a peak, may contribute to its development in predisposed individuals (Fig. 18-2). The stress of emergency trauma and injury, as well as long-term rehabilitation processes, often brings on stress ulcers.

Clinical symptoms. General symptoms include increased gastric muscle tone and painful contractions when the stomach is empty. In duodenal ulcers the amount and concentration of hydrochloric acid secretions are increased; in gastric ulcers the secretions may be normal. Low plasma protein levels, anemia, and weight loss reveal nutritional deficiencies. Hemorrhage may be a first signal. Diagnosis is confirmed by x-ray tests and visualization by gastroscopy.

General management. The primary goal of medical management is twofold: to support tissue healing and to provide psychologic rest. Three factors provide the basis of this care.

1. Drug therapy. Antacids buffer excess acid present in the stomach. Other drugs block acid secretion. Sedatives may be used to aid rest.

General directions

- Respect individual responses or tolerances to specific foods experienced at any given time, remembering that the same food may evoke different responses at different times depending on the stress factor.
- Eat smaller meals more often, eat slowly, and savor your food in a calm environment as much as possible.
- Try to avoid caffeine beverages such as coffee, cola, and tea; also avoid alcohol.
- Cut down on or quit smoking cigarettes, not only to help the ulcer but also to help food taste better.
- Avoid excessive pepper on food or concentrated meat broths and extractives.
- Avoid frequent use of aspirin or other drugs that may damage the stomach lining.

Foods	Recommended foods	Controlled foods
Bread, cereals (at least 4 servings daily)	Any whole-grain or enriched bread, cereals, crackers, pasta	None
Vegetables (at least 2 servings daily)	Any vegetable, raw or cooked; vegetable juices	None
Potatoes, other starches	White potatoes, sweet potatoes, or yams; enriched rice, brown rice; corn, barley, millet, bulgur; pasta	Fried forms
Fruits (at least 2 servings daily)	Any fruit, raw or cooked; fruit juices	None
Milk, milk products (2 servings daily as desired)	Any form of milk or milk drink; yogurt; cheeses	None
Meats or substitutes (2 servings daily)	Poultry, fish and shellfish lean meats; eggs, cheeses; legumes—dried beans and peas, lentils, soybeans; smooth peanut butter	Fried forms or too highly seasoned or fatty foods
Soups, stews	Mildly seasoned, less concentrated meat stock base; any cream soups	More highly seasoned or concentrated base
Desserts	Any desserts tolerated	Items containing nuts or coconut; fried pastries
Beverages	Decaffeinated coffee, cocoa, fruit drinks, mineral waters, noncola soft drinks; less strong tea with milk	Regular coffee, strong tea, colas, alcohol
Fats (use in moderation)	Margarine; butter, cream; vegetable oils; mild salad dressings, mayonnaise, oil and vinegar with herbs	Highly seasoned dressings
Sauces, gravies	Mildly flavored, less strong meat bases	Strongly seasoned, especially with pepper, hot peppers, and sauces
Miscellaneous	Salt in moderation (iodized); flavorings; herbs, spices; mustard, catsup, vinegar in moderation, as tolerated	Strongly flavored condiments; popcorn; nuts, coconut as tolerated

2. Rest. Healing requires both physical and mental rest. In addition to or instead of needed sedative therapy, stress-reduction relaxation techniques help provide needed rest.

3. Diet. Nutritional therapy for peptic ulcer has changed considerably. Its basic goal is to support healing and prevent further tissue damage.

Dietary management. In the past a highly restrictive "bland" diet was used in the care of patients with peptic ulcer disease. In some places it may still be used but should be discarded. A bland diet has long since proved to be ineffective and lacking in adequate nutritional support for the healing process. Such a restrictive diet is unnecessary today when newer and better drugs are available to control acid secretions and assist healing. Thus current diet therapy is based on a liberal individual approach, guided by individual responses to any food. This approach recognizes variances in need and provides much more personal, psychologic, physiologic, and nutritional support. Table 18-2 provides a general food guide for this more effective personal approach.

THE LOWER GASTROINTESTINAL TRACT
General functional disorders

Irritable bowel syndrome. This general stress-related disorder of the intestine may occur at any age but develops more frequently in women. Irritation of the mucous membrane is caused by irregular eating and bowel habits and by excessive use of laxatives, enemas, and a variety of other medications. Symptoms vary between spastic constipation and "nervous" diarrhea. General dietary measures are designed to provide optimal nutrition and regular bowel motility. The person should eat additional amounts of fiber foods, such as whole grains, beans, vegetables, and fruits. During alternate periods of diarrhea or excessive flatulence, the fiber content may need to be decreased somewhat. Personal support will help reduce stress factors.

Constipation. This general complaint, real or imagined, is common. In fact, Americans spend a quarter of a billion dollars each year for laxatives to treat their so-called regularity problem. However, intestinal elimination is highly individual; a daily bowel movement is not necessary for good health. This common short-term problem usually results from various sources of nervous tension and worry, changes in routines, constant laxative use, low-fiber diets, or lack of exercise. Improved diet, exercise, and bowel habits usually remedy the situation. Any laxative habit should be avoided. The diet should include increased fiber and adequate fluid intake, based first on an assessment of current fiber and fluid intake, as well as any diuretic drug use. Bowel obstruction from excess bran cereal, a large bowl daily (about 20 g), in a man receiving diuretic therapy for hypertension has been reported.[2]

A recommended daily allowance for dietary fiber has not been established. This is due in part to the wide variance in types of fiber and a lack of a standard acceptable method of fiber analysis.[3] Estimates of intake for U.S. adults range from 2.5 to 5.0 g/day to 11 to 23 g/day, depending on the fiber analysis procedure used.[4] Adequate intake of dietary fiber can be obtained from choosing several servings daily from a variety of fiber-rich foods—whole-grain breads and cereals, legumes (beans and peas), vegetables, fruits, and nuts. A reasonable goal is 10 to 15 g fiber/1000 kcal or a total daily intake of about

❖ **TABLE 18-3** *Dietary fiber and kilocalorie values for selected foods*

Foods	Serving	Dietary fiber (g)	Kcalories
Breads and cereals			
All Bran	⅓ cup	8.5	70
Bran (100%)	½ cup	8.4	75
Bran Buds	⅓ cup	7.9	75
Corn Bran	⅔ cup	5.4	100
Bran Chex	⅔ cup	4.6	90
Cracklin' Oat Bran	⅓ cup	4.3	110
Bran Flakes	¾ cup	4.0	90
Air-popped popcorn	1 cup	2.5	25
Oatmeal	1 cup	2.2	144
Grapenuts	¼ cup	1.4	100
Whole-wheat bread	1 slice	1.4	60
Legumes, cooked			
Kidney beans	½ cup	7.3	110
Lima beans	½ cup	4.5	130
Vegetables, cooked			
Green peas	½ cup	3.6	55
Corn	½ cup	2.9	70
Parsnip	½ cup	2.7	50
Potato, with skin	1 medium	2.5	95
Brussel sprouts	½ cup	2.3	30
Carrots	½ cup	2.3	25
Broccoli	½ cup	2.2	20
Beans, green	½ cup	1.6	15
Tomato, chopped	½ cup	1.5	17
Cabbage, red & white	½ cup	1.4	15
Kale	½ cup	1.4	20
Cauliflower	½ cup	1.1	15
Lettuce (fresh)	1 cup	0.8	7
Fruits			
Apple	1 medium	3.5	80
Raisins	¼ cup	3.1	110
Prunes, dried	3	3.0	60
Strawberries	1 cup	3.0	45
Orange	1 medium	2.6	60
Banana	1 medium	2.4	105
Blueberries	½ cup	2.0	40
Dates, dried	3	1.9	70
Peach	1 medium	1.9	35
Apricot, fresh	3 medium	1.8	50
Grapefruit	½ cup	1.6	40
Apricot, dried	5 halves	1.4	40
Cherries	10	1.2	50
Pineapple	½ cup	1.1	40

Adapted from Lanza E and Butrum RR: A critical review of food fiber analysis and data, J Am Diet Assoc 86:732, 1986.

20 to 30 g.[5] A sample list of food sources is given in Table 18-3. Use of purified fiber or fiber supplements is not generally recommended.

   Diarrhea. Functional diarrhea usually results from general dietary excesses. The fermentation of sugars involved, or excess fiber, can stimulate intestinal muscle function. In some cases it may result from intolerance to specific foods or nutrients. Diarrhea in infants is a more serious problem, especially if it is prolonged, leading rapidly to dehydration and nutrient losses, and is associated with infection.

Organic diseases

   Diverticulosis. This intestinal disease is characterized by the formation of many small pouches, or pockets, along the mucosal lining, usually in the colon. These little pouches are called *diverticula*. Most often they occur in older persons and develop at points of weakened muscles in the bowel wall. When these pockets become infected, a condition called *diverticulitis*, pain develops in the affected area. Sometimes perforation occurs and surgery is indicated. After an episode of diverticulitis, a brief period of a liquid then a low-residue diet may be used. Over time, however, a generally moderate-fiber diet, 10 to 15 g/1000 kcal, is beneficial. Along with sufficient fluid intake to maintain adequate hydration, there should be liberal use of fruits and vegetables, legumes (beans and peas), and whole-grain breads and cereals. Studies have indicated that coarse rather than fine types of fiber are more effective in controlling symptoms.[6] Residue in the colon reduces the painful muscle contractions that are characteristic of the disease.

   Malabsorption syndrome: celiac disease (sprue). Poor absorption of nutrients is caused by damage to the mucosal villi on the absorbing surface of the small intestine. In celiac disease (sprue), the damaging agent is a fraction of the protein *gluten*, which is toxic to sensitive individuals. When gluten, found mainly in wheat, damages the absorbing tissue, the area is then greatly impaired for absorption of all nutrients, especially fat. Diarrhea follows and general malnutrition develops. A general gluten-free diet restricts food sources of the main grain source, wheat, and secondary sources in rye, oats, buckwheat, and barley (Table 18-4).

   Inflammatory bowel disease. The term *inflammatory bowel disease* is used currently to apply to both *ulcerative colitis* and *Crohn's disease*. Their related condition, *short-bowel syndrome*, results from repeated surgical removal of sections of the small intestine as the disease progresses. All of these conditions can have severe, often devastating nutritional results as more and more of the absorbing surface area becomes involved. Restoring positive nutrition is a basic requirement for tissue healing and health. Elemental formulas of amino acids, glucose, fat, minerals, and vitamins are more easily absorbed and support initial healing in response to antibacterial and anti-inflammatory medications. Gradually the diet is advanced to restore optimal nutrient intake. The principles of the continuing diet management include the following requirements: (1) high-protein, about 100 g a day, omitting milk at first since it causes difficulty in many patients; (2) high-energy, about 2500 to 3000 kcal; (3) increased minerals and vitamins, usually with supplements; and (4) low-residue, to avoid irritation until healing is well established. A low residue diet (Table 18-5) is

❖ TABLE 18-4   *Gluten-free diet for adult celiac disease (sprue)*

Characteristics

- All forms of wheat, rye, oat, buckwheat, and barley are omitted, except gluten-free wheat starch.
- All other foods are permitted freely, unless specified otherwise by the physician.
- The diet should be high in protein, calories, vitamins, and minerals.

Foods	Allowed	Not allowed
Milk (2 glasses or more)	As desired	
Cheese	Any, as desired	
Eggs (1 or 2 daily)	As desired	
Meat, fish, fowl (1 or 2 servings)	Any plain meat	Breaded, creamed, or with thickened gravy; no bread dressings
Soups	All clear and vegetable soups; cream soups thickened with cream, cornstarch, or potato flour only	No wheat flour-thickened soup; no canned soup except clear broth
Vegetables (2 servings of green or yellow daily, at least)	As desired, except creamed	No cream sauce or breading
Fruits (at least 2 or 3 daily, including 1 citrus)	As desired	
Bread	Only that made from rice, corn, or soybean flour, or gluten-free wheat starch	All bread, rolls, crackers, cake, and cookies made from wheat and rye, Ry-Krisp, muffins, biscuits, waffles, pancake flour, and other prepared mixes, rusks, zwieback, pretzels; any product containing oatmeal, barley, or buckwheat; no breaded food or food crumbs
Cereals	Cornflakes, cornmeal, hominy, rice, Rice Krispies, puffed rice, precooked rice cereals	No wheat or rye cereals, wheat germ, barley, buckwheat, kasha
Pastas		No macaroni, spaghetti, noodles, dumplings
Desserts	Jell-O, fruit Jell-O, ice or sherbet, homemade ice cream, custard, junket, rice pudding, cornstarch pudding (homemade)	Cakes, cookies, pastry; commercial ice cream and ice cream cones; prepared mixes, puddings; homemade puddings thickened with wheat flour

CAUTION: *Read labels on all packaged and prepared foods.*

❖ **TABLE 18-5** *Low-residue diet*

Foods	Allowed	Not allowed
Beverages	Only 2 glasses of milk, if allowed, boiled or evaporated; fruit juices, coffee, tea, carbonated beverages	Alcohol
Eggs	Prepared in any manner, except fried	Fried eggs
Cheese	Cottage, cream, mild American, Tillamook (used in small amounts)	Highly flavored cheeses
Meat or poultry	Roasted, baked, or broiled tender beef, bacon, ham, lamb, liver, veal, fish, chicken, or turkey	Tough meats, pork; no fried or highly spices meats
Soup	Bouillon, broth, strained cream soups from the foods allowed	Any others
Fats	Butter, margarine, oils, 30 ml (1 oz) cream daily	None
Vegetables	Canned or cooked strained vegetables, such as asparagus, beets, carrots, peas, pumpkin, squash, spinach, young string beans, tomato juice	Raw or whole cooked vegetables
Fruits	Strained fruit juices, cooked or canned apples, apricots, Royal Anne cherries, peaches, pears; diet fruit puree; ripe banana and avocado; all without skins or seeds	All other raw fruits, other cooked fruits
Bread and crackers	Refined bread, toast, rolls, crackers	Pancakes, waffles, whole-grain bread or rolls
Cereals	Cooked cereal such as Cream of Wheat, Malt-O-Meal, strained oatmeal, cornmeal, cornflakes, puffed rice, Rice Krispies, puffed wheat	Whole-grain cereals; other prepared cereals
Potatoes or substitute	Potatoes, white rice, macaroni, noodles, spaghetti	Fried potato, potato chips, brown rice
Desserts	Gelatin desserts, tapioca, angel food or sponge cake, plain custards, water ice or ice cream without fruit or nuts, rennet or simple puddings	Rich pastries, pies, anything with nuts or dried fruits
Sweets	Sugar, jelly, honey, syrups, gumdrops, hard candy, plain creams, milk chocolate	Other candy; jam, marmalade
Miscellaneous	Cream sauce, plain gravy, salt	Nuts, olives, popcorn, rich gravies, pepper, spices, vinegar

followed by a regular diet with high-protein feedings as soon as tolerated. Only heavy roughage need be avoided.

FOOD ALLERGIES AND INTOLERANCES
Food allergies

The problem of allergy. Several conditions may cause certain food allergies or intolerances. The underlying problem relates to the body's immune system or originates genetically. The word *allergy* comes from two Greek words and means "altered reactivity," referring to the abnormal reactions of the immune system to a number of substances in our environment. A particular allergic condition results from a disorder of the immune system; it is immunity "gone wrong."

Common food allergens. Sensitivity to protein is a common basis for food allergy. The three most common food allergens are milk, egg, and wheat. Thus the early foods of infants and children are frequent offenders in sensitive individuals. Substitute milk products, usually with a soy base, are used. In an allergic child's diet, solid foods are usually added slowly to the original formula, with common offenders excluded in early feedings. In some cases, a process of *food elimination* is used to identify offending foods. A core of less-often offending foods is used at first, then other single foods are gradually added to test the response. If a given food causes the allergic reaction to return, the food is then identified as an allergen and eliminated from use. It may be retested later to see if it still has the same effect. Referral to a clinical nutritionist is helpful to provide family education and counseling. Guidance is needed for substitution of foods or special food products and modified recipes to maintain nutritional needs for growth. Children tend to become less allergic as they grow older, but family education concerning label-reading of all food products and cooking guides is essential from the beginning.

Genetic disease and food intolerances

The genetic defect. Certain food intolerances stem from underlying genetic disease. In each genetic disease the specific cell enzyme (all enzymes are proteins) controlling the cell's metabolism of a specific nutrient is missing, so the normal handling of that particular nutrient is blocked at that point. Three examples are phenylketonuria, galactosemia, and lactose intolerance.

Phenylketonuria. This disorder (PKU) results from the missing enzyme that breaks down the essential amino acid *phenylalanine* to tyrosine, another amino acid. If left untreated, this condition causes profound mental retardation and central nervous system damage, with irritability, hyperactivity, convulsive seizures, and bizarre behavior. Today, with mandatory newborn screening programs in all areas of the United States, these babies are identified and treatment is started immediately. Then they grow normally and have healthy lives (Fig. 18-3). The treatment is a special low-phenylalanine diet, using special formulas and low-protein food products. Much family counseling is needed by the metabolic team at each care center.

Galactosemia. This genetic disease affects carbohydrate metabolism. The missing cell enzyme is one that converts *galactose* to glucose. Since galactose comes from the breakdown of *lactose* (milk sugar), all sources of lactose in

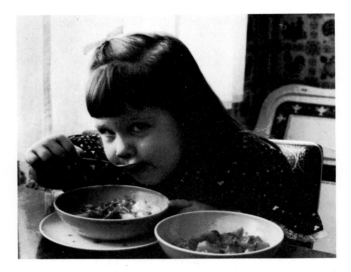

❖ FIG. 18-3

This perfectly developed 2-year-old has phenylketonuria (PKU). Screened and diagnosed at birth, she has eaten a carefully controlled low-phenylalanine diet and is growing normally.

the infant's diet must be eliminated. When not treated this condition causes brain damage and also liver damage. Present newborn screening programs identify these babies as well, so treatment can begin immediately to avoid this damage. The child then grows normally. Treatment is a galactose-free diet, with special formulas and lactose-free food guides.

Lactose intolerance. A deficiency of any one of the disaccharidases (lactase, sucrase, or maltase) in the intestine may produce a wide range of GI problems and abdominal pain because the specific sugar involved cannot be digested (p. 15). Lactose intolerance is the most common. Insufficient lactase is present to break down the milk sugar lactose; thus the lactose accumulates in the intestine causing abdominal cramping and diarrhea. Milk and all products containing lactose are carefully avoided. Milk treated with lactase or soy milk products are substitutes.

PROBLEMS OF THE GASTROINTESTINAL ACCESSORY ORGANS

Three major accessory organs lie beside the gastrointestinal tract. These organs, the liver, gallbladder, and pancreas, produce important digestive agents that enter the intestine and aid in the handling of food substances (Fig. 18-4). Diseases of these organs easily affect normal GI function and cause problems with the handling of specific types of food.

Liver disease

Hepatitis. Acute hepatitis is an inflammatory condition caused by viruses, alcohol, drugs, or toxins. The viral agent of the infection is transmitted by the oral-fecal route, a common one in many epidemic diseases. The carrier is usually contaminated food or water. In other cases the virus may be transmitted by transfusions of infected blood, or by contaminated syringes or needles.

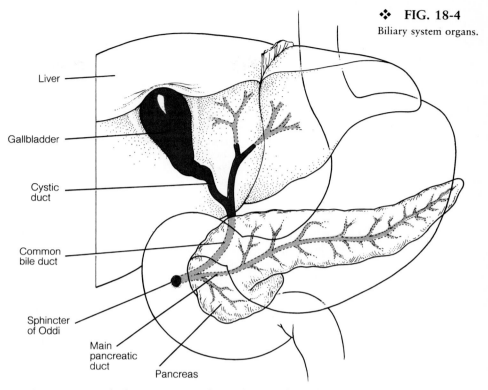

❖ **FIG. 18-4**
Biliary system organs.

Liver

Gallbladder

Cystic
duct

Common
bile duct

Sphincter
of Oddi

Main
pancreatic
duct

Pancreas

Symptoms include anorexia and jaundice, with underlying malnutrition. Treatment centers on bed rest and nutritional therapy to support healing of the involved liver tissue. The following requirements govern the principles of the diet therapy and relate to the liver's function in metabolizing each nutrient.

1. High protein. Protein is essential for building new liver cells and tissues. It also combines with fats and removes them, preventing the damage of fatty infiltration in liver tissue. The diet should supply from 75 to 100 g of high quality protein daily.

2. High carbohydrate. Available glucose restores protective glycogen reserves in the liver. It also helps meet the energy demands of the disease process, as well as preventing the breakdown of protein for energy, thus ensuring its use for vital tissue building needed for healing. The diet should supply from 300 to 400 g of carbohydrate daily.

3. Moderate fat. Some fat helps season food to encourage eating despite the poor appetite. A moderate amount of easily used fat, from milk products as well as vegetable oil, is beneficial. The diet should incorporate about 100 to 150 g of such fat daily.

4. High energy. From 2500 to 3000 kcalories are needed daily to meet energy demands. This increased amount is necessary to support the healing process, to make up losses from fever and general debilitation, and to renew strength for recuperating from the disease.

5. Meals and feedings. At first liquid feedings may be necessary, such as milkshakes high in protein and kilocalories (see Table 18-1) or special formula

BOX 18-1

❖ ——————————— CLINICAL APPLICATION ——————————— ❖

Case Study: Bill's Bout With Infectious Hepatitis

Bill is a college student who spent part of his summer vacation in Mexico. Shortly after he returned home, he began to feel ill. He had little energy, no appetite, and severe headaches. Nothing he ate seemed to agree with him. He felt nauseated, began to have diarrhea, and soon develop a fever. He began to show evidence of jaundice.

Bill was hospitalized for diagnosis and treatment. His tests indicated impaired liver function. His liver and spleen were enlarged and tender. The physician's diagnosis was infectious hepatitis. Bill's hospital diet was high in proteins, carbohydrates, and kcalories and moderately low in fats. However, Bill had difficulty eating. He had no appetite, and food seemed to nauseate him even more.

Questions for Analysis

1. What are the normal functions of the liver in relation to the metabolism of carbohydrates, proteins, and fats? What other nutrient functions does the liver have?
2. What is the relationship of the normal liver functions to the effects, or clinical symptoms, that Bill experienced during his illness?
3. Why does vigorous nutritional therapy in liver disease such as hepatitis present a problem in planning a diet?
4. Outline a day's food plan for Bill. Calculate the amount of kcalories and protein to ensure that he is getting the amount he needs.
5. What vitamins and minerals would be significant aspects of Bill's nutritional therapy? Why?

products for frequent use. As the patient's appetite and food tolerance improve, a full diet as already described is needed, observing likes and dislikes and planning ways to encourage an optimal food intake. Nutrition is the basic therapy.

Cirrhosis. Liver disease may advance to the chronic state of cirrhosis (Fig. 18-5). The most common problem is fatty cirrhosis associated with malnutrition and alcoholism. The relentless malnutrition leads to multiple nutritional deficiences as drinking alcohol increasingly substitutes for eating meals. Alcohol and its metabolic products can also cause direct damage to liver cells. The accompanying fatty infiltration kills liver cells and only nonfunctioning fibrous scar tissue remains. Eventually, low plasma protein levels fall, causing *ascites*, or abdominal fluid accumulation. Scar tissue impairs blood circulation, resulting in elevated venous blood pressure and esophageal *varices*. Often the rupture of these enlarged veins with massive hemorrhage is the cause of death. When alcoholism is the underlying problem, treatment is difficult. Nutritional therapy focuses on as much healing support as possible.

1. Protein according to tolerance. In the absence of impending hepatic coma, the diet should supply about 80 to 100 g of protein a day to correct

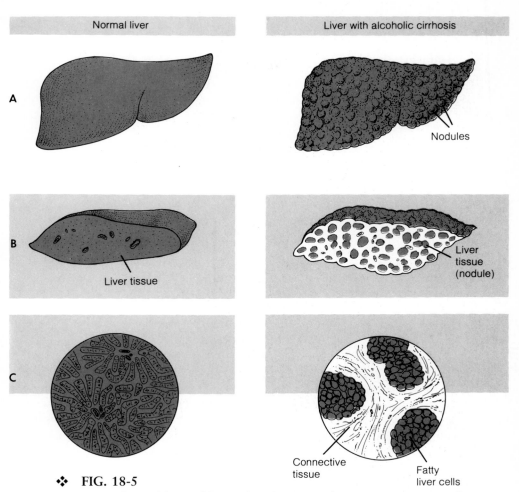

❖ **FIG. 18-5**

Comparison of normal liver and liver with cirrhotic tissue changes. **A,** Anterior view of organ, **B,** cross section, **C,** tissue structure.

the severe malnutrition, heal liver tissue, and restore plasma proteins. If signs of coma begin, the protein must be reduced to individual tolerance.

2. *Low sodium.* Sodium is restricted to about 500 to 1000 mg a day (p. 301) to help reduce the fluid retention (ascites).

3. *Soft texture.* If esophageal varices develop, soft foods help prevent the danger of rupture and hemorrhage.

4. *Optimal general nutrition.* The remaining diet principles outlined for hepatitis are continued for cirrhosis for the same reasons. Kilocalories, carbohydrates, and vitamins, especially B-complex vitamins including thiamin and folate, are important. Moderate fat is used. Alcohol is forbidden. Box 18-2 summarizes this diet for cirrhosis.

Hepatic coma. One of the main functions of the liver is to remove ammonia, and hence nitrogen (see Fig. 4-2, p. 38), from the blood by converting it to urea for urinary excretion. When cirrhosis continues and fibrous scar tissue

❖

BOX 18-2

High-Protein, High-Carbohydrate, Moderate-Fat Daily Diet

1 L (1 qt) of milk
¼ cup egg substitute (Egg Beaters)
224 g (8 oz) lean meat, fish, poultry
4 servings vegetables:
  2 servings potato or substitute
  1 serving green leafy or yellow vegetable
  1 to 2 servings of other vegetables, including 1 raw
3 to 4 servings fruit (include juices often):
  1 to 2 citrus fruits (or other good source of ascorbic acid)
  2 servings other fruit
6 to 8 servings bread and cereal (whole grain or enriched):
  1 serving cereal
  5 to 6 slices bread, crackers
2 to 4 tbsp butter or fortified margarine
Additional jam, jelly, honey, and other carbohydrate foods as patient desires and is
  able to eat them
Sweetened fruit juices to increase both carbohydrate and fluid

---

replaces more and more normal liver tissue, the blood can no longer circulate normally through the liver. Other vessels develop around this scar tissue, bypassing the liver. The blood, carrying its ammonia load, cannot reach the liver for its normal removal of the ammonia and nitrogen. Instead it must follow the bypass and proceed to the brain, producing ammonia intoxication and coma. The resulting *hepatic encephalopathy* brings apathy, confusion, inappropriate behavior, and drowsiness, progressing to coma. Treatment focuses on removal of sources of excess ammonia. Since this is a nitrogen compound and its main source is protein, the main dietary goal is to reduce the protein intake. Table 18-6 provides a guide for reducing the diet's protein to 15 g a day, with additional increases according to individual tolerance.

Gallbladder disease

Function. The basic function of the gallbladder is to concentrate and store bile. Then it releases the concentrated bile into the small intestine when fat is present there. In the intestine the bile emulsifies the fat, preparing it for initial digestion, then carries the fat into the cells of the intestinal wall for its continued metabolism (p. 126).

Cholecystitis and cholelithiasis. Inflammation of the gallbladder, *cholecystitis*, usually results from a low-grade chronic infection. Cholesterol in bile, which is not soluble in water, normally is kept in solution. But when continued infection alters the solubility of bile ingredients, cholesterol separates out and forms gallstones. This condition is called *cholelithiasis*. When infection, stones, or both are present, contraction of the gallbladder causes pain when fat enters the intestion. Thus fatty foods are usually avoided. The treatment is surgical removal of the gallbladder, a *cholecystectomy*. If the patient is obese, some weight loss before surgery may be indicated. Diet therapy in any case will

❖ **TABLE 18-6**   *Low-protein diets: 15 g, 30 g, 40 g, and 50 g protein*

General directions

- The following diets are used when dietary protein is to be restricted.
- The patterns limit foods containing a large percentage of protein, such as milk, eggs, cheese, meat, fish, fowl, and legumes.
- Meat extractives, soups, broth, bouillon, gravies, and gelatin desserts should also be avoided.

Basic meal patterns (contain approximately 15 g of protein)

Breakfast	Lunch	Dinner
½ cup fruit or fruit juice	1 small potato	1 small potato
½ cup cereal	½ cup vegetable	½ cup vegetable
1 slice toast	Salad (vegetable or fruit)	Salad (vegetable or fruit)
Butter	1 slice bread	1 slice bread
Jelly	Butter	Butter
Sugar	1 serving fruit	1 serving fruit
2 tbsp cream	Sugar	Sugar
Coffee	Coffee or tea	Coffee or tea

For 30 g protein

Add: 1 cup milk
   28 g (1 oz) meat, 1 egg, or equivalent

Examples of meat portions

28 g (1 oz) meat = 1 thin slice roast, 4 ×
            5 cm
           (1½ × 2 in)
           1 rounded tbsp cottage cheese
           1 slice American cheese

For 40 g protein

Add: 1 cup milk
   70 g (2½ oz) meat, or 1 egg and 42 g
   (1½ oz) meat

70 g (2½ oz) meat = Ground beef patty
           (5 from
             448 g [1 lb])
           1 slice roast

For 50 g protein

Add: 1 cup milk
   112 g (4 oz) meat, or 2 eggs and 56 g (2
   oz) meat

112 g (4 oz) meat = 2 lamb chops
           1 average steak

center on control of fat. Table 18-7 outlines a general low-fat diet guide, but the degree of its application will depend on individual need.

Pancreatic disease

Pancreatitis. Acute inflammation of the pancreas, *pancreatitis*, is caused by the digestion of the organ tissue by the very enzymes it produces, principally trypsin (p. 126). Obstruction of the common duct through which the inactive enzymes normally enter the intestine causes the enzymes and bile to back up into the pancreas. This mixing of digestive materials activates the powerful enzymes within the gland. In this active form they begin to "digest" the pancreatic tissue itself, causing severe pain. Mild or moderate episodes may subside

❖ **TABLE 18-7** *Low-fat and fat-free diets*

Low-fat diet

General description
- This diet contains foods that are low in fat.
- Foods are prepared without the addition of fat.
- Fatty meats, gravies, oils, cream, lard, and desserts containing eggs, butter, cream, nuts, and avocados are avoided.
- Foods should be used in amounts specified and only as tolerated.
- The sample pattern contains approximately 85 g protein, 50 g fat, 220 g carbohydrates, and 1670 kcalories.

Foods	Allowed	Not allowed
Beverages	Skim milk, coffee, tea, carbonated beverages, fruit juices	Whole milk, cream, evaporated and condensed milk
Bread and cereals	All kinds	Rich rolls or breads, waffles, pancakes
Desserts	Jell-O, sherbet, water ices, fruit whips made without cream, angel food cake, rice and tapioca puddings made with skim milk	Pastries, pies, rich cakes, and cookies, ice cream
Fruits	All fruits, as tolerated	Avocado
Eggs	3 allowed per week, cooked any way except fried	Fried eggs
Fats	3 tsp butter or margarine daily	Salad and cooking oils, mayonnaise
Meats	Lean meat such as beef, veal, lamb, liver, lean fish and fowl, baked, broiled, or roasted without added fat	Fried meats, bacon, ham, pork, goose, duck, fatty fish, fish canned in oil, cold cuts
Cheese	Dry or fat-free cottage cheese	All other cheese
Potato or substitute	Potatoes, rice, macaroni, noodles, spaghetti, all prepared without added fat	Fried potatoes, potato chips
Soups	Bouillon or broth, without fat; soups made with skimmed milk	Cream soups
Sweets	Jam, jelly, sugar candies without nuts or chocolate	Chocolate, nuts, peanut butter
Vegetables	All kinds as tolerated	The following should be omitted if they cause distress: broccoli, cauliflower, corn, cucumber, green pepper, radishes, turnips, onions, dried peas, and beans
Miscellaneous	Salt in moderation	Pepper, spices, highly spices food, olives, pickles, cream sauces, gravies

Suggested menu pattern

Breakfast	Lunch and dinner
Fruit	Meat, broiled or baked
Cereal	Potato
Toast, jelly	Vegetable
1 tsp butter or margarine	Salad with fat-free dressing
Egg 3 times per week	Bread, jelly
Skim milk, 1 cup	1 tsp butter or margarine
Coffee, sugar	Fruit or dessert, as allowed
	Skim milk, 1 cup coffee, sugar

Fat-free diet

General description

The following additional restrictions are made to the low-fat diet to make it relatively fat-free.
1. Meat, eggs, and butter or margarine are omitted.
2. A substitute for meat at the noon and evening meal is 84 g (3 oz) of fat-free cottage cheese.

completely, but the condition has a tendency to recur. Initial care includes measures for acute disease involving shock: intravenous feeding (p. 353), replacement of fluid and electrolytes, blood transfusion, antibiotics, pain medications, and gastric suction. As healing progresses, oral feedings are resumed. A light diet is used to reduce stimulation of pancreatic secretions. Alcohol and excess coffee should also be avoided to decrease pancreatic stimulation.

Cystic fibrosis of the pancreas. Cystic fibrosis is a generalized genetic disease of children. It involves the exocrine glands, especially the pancreas. Thus it affects many tissues and organs of the body. In past years its prognosis was poor; few children survived past 10 years of age. Now we have better knowledge of the disease, improved diagnostic tests, clinical treatment, and antibiotic therapy. As a result, prognosis has improved.

1. Clinical symptoms. Symptoms include (1) diminished digestion of food due to absence of the usual pancreatic enzymes, (2) respiratory problems and chronic pulmonary disease due to malfunction of the mucus glands with accumulation of thick secretions, (3) abnormal secretions of the sweat glands containing large amounts of electrolytes, and (4) possible cirrhosis of the liver from biliary obstruction, increased by malnutrition or infection.

2. Treatment. Three factors guide treatment: (1) control of respiratory infections, (2) relief from the effect of the thick bronchial secretions that make breathing difficult, and (3) maintenance of sound nutrition. Only about half of the food the child eats is broken down and absorbed, so a large appetite and an increased food intake replace these losses.

3. Nutritional therapy. The basic diet objective is to make up for the constant loss of nutrient material in the frequent large stools. Large amounts of protein and carbohydrate are needed, usually supplied in simple forms, but

BOX 18-3

❖ ——————— **CLINICAL APPLICATION** ——————— ❖

Case Study: Paul's Adaptation to Cystic Fibrosis

Paul is a 12-year-old boy with cystic fibrosis of the pancreas. He is hospitalized with pneumonia and has difficulty breathing. He is a thin child with little muscle development. He tires easily, although he has a large appetite. His stools are large and frequent and contain undigested food material.

Questions for Analysis

1. What is cystic fibrosis? Account for the clinical effects of the disease as evidenced by Paul's appearance and symptoms.
2. What are the basic goals of treatment in cystic fibrosis? Why is vigorous nutritional therapy a main part of treatment?
3. Outline a day's food plan for Paul. Check the amount of protein and kcalories by calculating total food values in your food plan to ensure the extra amount he needs.
4. Why does Paul require therapeutic doses of multivitamins, including the B complex? Why does he need to have these in water-soluble form?

❖ **TABLE 18-8**   *Principles of dietary management for children with cystic fibrosis*

Principle	Reason
High calorie	Energy demands of growth and compensation for fecal losses; large appetite usually ensures acceptance of increased amounts of food
High protein	Usually tolerated in large amounts; excess above normal growth needs required to compensate for losses
Moderate carbohydrate	Starch less well tolerated; simple sugars easily assimilated
Low to moderate fat, as tolerated	Fat poorly absorbed, but tolerance varies widely
Generous salt	Food generously salted to replace sweat loss; salt supplements in hot weather
Vitamins	Double doses of multivitamins in water-soluble form (vitamin E supplements sometimes used because low blood levels of the vitamin have been observed); vitamin K supplements with prolonged antibiotic therapy
Pancreatic enzymes	Large amounts given by mouth with each meal (may be mixed with cereal or applesauce for infants) to compensate for pancreatic deficiency—powdered pancreas extract containing steapsin, trypsin, and amylopsin (Pancreatin, or other pancreatic extracts such as Cotazyme or Viokase)

limited tolerance for fats exists. Diet guides, such as the one outlined in Table 18-8, are similar to those used for celiac disease, except that gluten is not involved and more emphasis is placed on quantity of food. Food forms vary according to the age of the child. Nutrient supplements are used according to need. (See Box 18-3.)

SUMMARY

Nutritional management of gastrointestinal disease is based on the degree of interference in the normal ingestion-digestion-absorption-metabolism that the disease causes. Problems in the upper GI tract relate to conditions that hinder chewing or transporting the food mass down the esophagus into the stomach. A hiatal hernia at the entry of the esophagus into the chest cavity interferes with passage of the food into the stomach, causing acid tissue irritation and discomfort after eating.

Peptic ulcer disease, a common GI problem, is an acidic erosion of the mucosal lining of the stomach or the duodenal bulb, which is where the concentrated acidic food mass enters the duodenum, the first section of the small intestine. The ulcerated tissue brings nutritional problems such as anemia and weight loss. Medical management consists of drug therapy and rest. Diet therapy is liberal and individual, with a goal of correcting malnutrition and supporting healing.

Problems of the lower GI tract include common functional disorders such as constipation and diarrhea, for which symptomatic and personalized treatment are indicated. Diseases involving tissue changes, such as diverticulitis and malabsorption problems (celiac disease, inflammatory bowel disease) are more difficult to resolve. Nutritional therapy requires modification of the diet's protein and energy content and food texture, increased vitamins and minerals, and replacement of fluids and electrolytes. Continuous adjustment of the diet is made according to individual need.

Other food intolerances may be caused by allergies or underlying genetic disease. Specific genetic disease results from specific missing cell enzymes that control cell metabolism of specific nutrients. The special diet in each case limits or eliminates the particular nutrient involved.

Diseases of the GI accessory organs also contribute to nutrition problems. Common liver disorders include hepatitis, caused by a viral infection, and cirrhosis, caused by progressive liver disease that damages tissue by such toxins as excessive alcohol. Uncontrolled cirrhosis leads to hepatic coma and eventual liver failure and death. Nutrient and energy levels of the necessary diet therapy vary with the progression of the disease process. Gallbladder disease, infection and stones, involves some limit to fat tolerance, which is modified according to individual need. Pancreatic disease includes pancreatitis, a serious condition requiring immediate measures to counter the shock symptoms, followed by restorative nutritional support. Cystic fibrosis of the pancreas is a genetic disease with generalized effects involving respiration and malnutrition.

❖ REVIEW QUESTIONS

1. What general nutritional guidance would you give to a person with a hiatal hernia? What would be the basic goal for your suggestions?
2. In current practice what are the basic principles of diet planning for patients with peptic ulcer disease? How do these principles differ from former traditional therapy?
3. Describe the causes, clinical signs, and treatment of each of the following diseases: diverticulitis, celiac disease, and inflammatory bowel disease.
4. What is the rationale for treatment in the progressive course of liver disease—hepatitis, cirrhosis, and hepatic coma?

❖ SELF-TEST QUESTIONS

True-false
For each item you answer "false," write the correct statement.
1. A high-fiber diet is indicated for a person with dental problems.
2. Lying down after eating helps a person with hiatal hernia to relieve discomfort.
3. The fundamental cause of peptic ulcer is unknown.
4. Peptic ulcer pain is reduced when the stomach is empty and can rest.
5. A low-residue diet is advocated for treatment of diverticulosis.
6. All food sources of wheat must be eliminated on the gluten-free diet for treatment of celiac disease.
7. PKU is a genetic disease requiring dietary control of the essential amino acid phenylalanine.
8. Soy products are often used for children allergic to milk.
9. The nutritional objective in cystic fibrosis is to compensate for the large nutrient losses.

Multiple choice
1. In a gluten-free diet for celiac disease, which of the following foods would be eliminated?
   a. Eggs
   b. Milk
   c. Rice
   d. Saltine crackers
2. The symptoms of anemia in malabsorption diseases are caused by poor absorption of which of the following nutrients?
   a. Vitamin K
   b. Iron and folic acid
   c. Calcium and phosphorus
   d. Fats
3. Lactose intolerance in certain population groups is caused by a genetic deficiency of which of the following enzymes?
   a. Sucrase
   b. Pepsin
   c. Lactase
   d. Maltase
4. Treatment for hepatic coma includes:
   a. Increased protein to aid healing of liver cells
   b. Decreased protein to reduce blood ammonia levels
   c. Decreased kilocalories to reduce the metabolic load
   d. Increased fluid intake to stimulate output

References

1. Campbell VS: Dietitian's forum: Are children consuming too much sugar? Food Management 25:58, May 1990.
2. Miller DL, Miller PF, and Dekker JJ: Small-bowel obstruction from bran cereal, JAMA 263:813, Feb 9, 1990.
3. Slavin JL: Dietary fiber—mechanisms or magic on disease prevention? Nutr Today 25(6):6, 1990.
4. Council on Scientific Affairs, American Medical Association: Dietary fiber and health, JAMA 262:542, July 28, 1989.
5. Kritchevsky D: Dietary fiber, Ann Rev Nutr 8:301, 1988.
6. Smith AN, Drummond E, and Eastwood MA: The effect of coarse and fine Canadian Red Spring Wheat and French Soft Wheat bran on colonic motility in patients with diverticular disease, Am J Clin Nutr 34(11):2460, 1981.

Further reading

Slavin JL: Dietary fiber—mechanisms or magic on disease prevention? Nutr Today 25(6):6, 1990.

This timely article helps us to understand why it is difficult to make any definite statements about dietary fiber allowances. The more we learn about this nondigestible material in our diet, the more we see that all fiber is not created equal. The author describes this variety of forms and components and explains why an accepted method for fiber and fiber component analysis awaits much more research. She provides a reasoned basis for the recommendation to American consumers: use only a gradual increase in dietary fiber from a variety of food sources.

Coronary heart disease and hypertension

KEY CONCEPTS

Heart disease results from several risk factors, mostly preventable ones associated with our life-style, that contribute to its development.

The "silent" genetic risk factor without symptoms, essential hypertension, can be identified and controlled.

Most cardiovascular risk factors are associated with nutrition and can be reduced by changing food and life-style habits.

*C*ardiovascular disease accounts for more than half of the deaths each year in the United States, approximately 550,000. It is our leading health problem. This same situation exists in most other developed Western societies. Every day thousands of persons suffer heart attacks and strokes, with more than a million others continuing to suffer from various forms of rheumatic and congestive heart disease.

During the past decade our cardiovascular death rate has declined somewhat, mostly because of improved emergency care for heart attacks, but it remains our number-one "killer disease." In this chapter, we look at the primary underlying disease process, atherosclerosis, and the various risk factors involved, especially hypertension. Then we explore ways we can use nutritional approaches to reduce these risk factors and help prevent disease.

CORONARY HEART DISEASE
The basic problem of atherosclerosis

The disease process. The major cardiovascular disease and the underlying pathologic process in coronary heart disease is **atherosclerosis**. Although much has been learned about the disease, recent studies have strengthened the association of key risk factors including diet to the progressive development of the atherosclerotic process.[1] This process is characterized by fatty fibrous plaques that begin in childhood to develop fatty streaks, largely composed of cholesterol, on the inside lining of major blood vessels. When tissue is examined, crystals of cholesterol can be seen with the unaided eye in the softened cheesy debris characteristic of advanced disease. This fatty debris suggested its name to early investigators, from the Greek words *athera* meaning "gruel," and *sclerosis*, "hardening." This fatty fibrous process gradually thickens over time, narrowing the interior part of the blood vessel, and often forming blood clots from its irritation of the vessel tissue. Eventually the thickening of the vessel or a blood clot may cut off blood flow, as shown in Fig. 19-1.

Cells deprived of their normal blood supply will die. The local area of dying or dead tissue is called an *infarct*. If the affected blood vessel is a major artery supplying vital blood nutrients and oxygen to the heart muscle, the *myocardium*, the result is called an acute **myocardial infarction (MI)** or a *heart attack*. If the affected vessel is a major artery supplying the brain, the result is called a **cerebrovascular accident (CVA)** or a *stroke*. The major arteries and their many branches serving the heart are called *coronary* arteries because they lie across the brow of the heart muscle and resemble a crown. Thus the overall disease process is called **coronary heart disease**. A common symptom of its presence is **angina pectoris**, chest pain, usually radiating down the arm and caused by excitement or effort.

Relation to fat metabolism. The major research studies to date have found elevated blood **lipids** associated with coronary heart disease and related heart attacks.[1] *Lipid* is the class name for all fats and fat-related compounds. Lipid substances involved in the disease process are described in Chapter 3 and can be reviewed in more detail there. Here we emphasize three of these substances.

1. Triglycerides. The chemical name for fat, which describes its basic structure, is *triglyceride* (p. 25). All simple fats, whether in our bodies or in our foods, are triglycerides. The blood test for total triglycerides measures this level circulating in our blood. The major research studies of heart disease have also shown a definite association between amount and types of dietary fat and elevated blood lipid level.[1,2]

2. Cholesterol. The fat-related compound now clearly associated with atherosclerosis and heart disease is *cholesterol*. About 60 million American adults have high blood cholesterol levels requiring medical advice and intervention using diet as the primary treatment.[3,4] A reduction in dietary cholesterol has been shown to lower total blood cholesterol levels and reduce the risk of heart disease in predisposed individuals. Cholesterol is produced *only* in animal tissue; thus it can *never* be found in plant foods.

3. Lipoproteins. Because fat is not soluble in water, it is carried in the bloodstream in little packages wrapped with protein, which are called *lipoproteins*. These compounds are produced in the *intestinal wall* after a meal

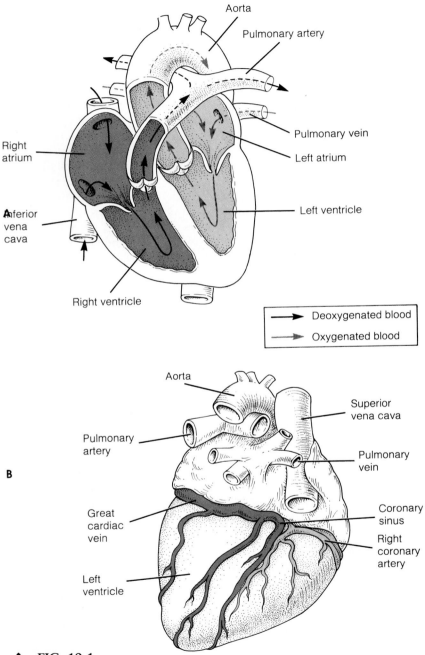

> ━━━▶ Deoxygenated blood
> ┈┈┈▶ Oxygenated blood

❖   **FIG. 19-1**

A and **B,** The normal human heart. **A,** Anterior view showing cardiac circulation. **B,** Posterior external view showing coronary arteries. **C,** Atherosclerotic plaque in artery.

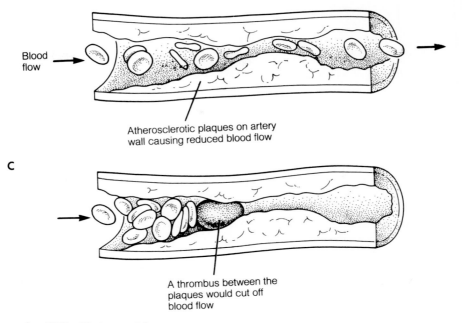

Atherosclerotic plaques on artery
wall causing reduced blood flow

C

A thrombus between the
plaques would cut off
blood flow

❖ **FIG. 19-1, cont'd**

containing fat, and in the *liver* as part of the regular ongoing process of fat
metabolism. They carry fat and cholesterol to tissues for cell metabolism use
and back to the liver for breakdown and excretion as needed. They are grouped
and named according to their fat and cholesterol content and thus their density.
Those with the highest lipid content have the lowest density. Three of these
types of lipoproteins, formed in the liver, are significant in relation to heart
disease risk:

- **Very-low-density lipoproteins (VLDL)** carry a relatively large load of fat
  to cells but also include about 15% cholesterol.
- **Low-density lipoproteins (LDL)** carry, in addition to other lipids, about
  two thirds or more of the total plasma cholesterol to body tissues. They
  are formed in the liver and serum from catabolism of VLDL. Because
  they constantly send cholesterol to tissues, they have been called the "bad
  cholesterol" sources. In our blood lipid tests the total LDL certainly represents the major "cholesterol of concern."
- **High-density lipoproteins (HDL)** carry less total fat and more carrier
  protein and transport cholesterol from the tissues to the liver for catabolism and elimination from the body. Thus, in comparison with LDL
  cholesterol, HDL cholesterol is called the "good cholesterol," and higher
  serum levels are considered protective against cardiovascular disease. The
  normal HDL range is 30 to 80 mg/dl. Thus a value below 30 implies
  significant risk, and a value of 75 or greater contributes definite protection
  and decreased risk.

Risk factors. We have learned several important facts from the major studies of heart disease. First, the underlying disease process of atherosclerosis is

BOX 19-1

❖ —————————— CLINICAL APPLICATION —————————— ❖

Case Study: The Patient With a Myocardial Infarction (Heart Attack)

Charles Carter is a successful young businessman. He works long hours and carries the major responsibility of his struggling small business. At his last physical checkup, the physician cautioned him about his pace. Already he was showing some mild hypertension. His blood cholesterol was elevated and he was overweight. In his desk job he got little exercise and found himself smoking more and eating irregularly because of the stress of his increasing financial pressures.

One day while commuting in the heavy freeway traffic, Mr. Carter felt a pain in his chest and became increasingly apprehensive. When he arrived home, the pain persisted and increased. He broke out into a cold sweat and felt nauseated. When he became more ill after trying to eat dinner, his wife called their physician and Mr. Carter was admitted to the hospital.

After emergency care and tests, the physician placed Mr. Carter in the coronary care unit at the hospital. His test results showed elevated total cholesterol, triglycerides, lipoproteins—especially LDL, but low HDL. The electrocardiogram revealed an infarction of the posterior myocardium wall.

At first, when Mr. Carter was able to take oral nourishment, he had only a liquid diet. As his condition stabilized, his diet was increased to an 800-kcalorie soft diet, low in cholesterol and fat. By the end of the first week, it was increased again to a 1200-kcalorie full diet, low cholesterol, with only 25% of the total kcalories from fat and a P/S ratio of 1/1.

Mr. Carter gradually improved over the next few weeks and was able to go home. The physician, nurse, and clinical dietitian discussed with Mr. Carter and his wife the need for care at home during a period of convalescence. They explained that he had an underlying lipid disorder and was to continue his weight loss and follow a prudent diet.

Questions for Analysis

1. Identify factors in Mr. Carter's personal and medical history that place him at high risk for coronary heart disease. Give reasons why each factor contributes to heart disease.
2. Identify as many of the laboratory tests the physician ordered as you can. Relate these tests to Mr. Carter's condition.
3. Why did Mr. Carter receive only a liquid diet at first? What is the reason for each modification in his first diet of solid food?
4. What occurs in the underlying disease process that causes a heart attack? What relation do fat and cholesterol have to this underlying process?
5. Outline a day's menu for Mr. Carter on his 1200-kcalorie prudent diet.
6. What needs might Mr. Carter have when he goes home? How would you help him prepare to go home? Name some community resources you might use in helping him understand his illness and plan his continuing self-care.

caused by multiple risk factors, as shown in Table 19-1. Second, elevated serum cholesterol is one of the *major* risk factors for the disease process, along with hypertension, which is worsened by obesity, and smoking. Third, dietary fat *can* affect serum cholesterol. The National Institutes of Health Consensus Group for lowering blood cholesterol has defined serum cholesterol values for

❖ **TABLE 19-1**   *Multiple risk factors in cardiovascular disease*

Personal characteristics (no control)	Learned behaviors (intervene and change)	Background conditions (screen-treat)
Sex	Stress/coping	Hypertension
Age	Smoking cigarettes	Diabetes mellitus
Family history	Sedentary life	Hyperlipidemia (especially
	Obesity	hypercholesterolemia)
	Food habits	
	Excess fat	
	Excess sugar	
	Excess salt	

❖ **TABLE 19-2**   *Serum cholesterol levels identifying persons at moderate and high risk who require treatment (diet therapy and weight control; drug therapy only after careful maximal diet therapy)*

Age (years)	Moderate risk	High risk
	Greater than:	Greater than:
2-19	170 mg/dl	185 mg/dl
20-29	200 mg/dl	220 mg/dl
30-39	220 mg/dl	240 mg/dl
40 and older	240 mg/dl	260 mg/dl

From National Institutes of Health: Nutr Today 20(1):13, 1985.

persons at risk (Table 19-2) and emphasized the importance of educating the public about this preventable risk factor.[3,4]

Fat-controlled diets. Since control of dietary fat and cholesterol has been shown to be important in reducing risks for heart disease, the dietary guidelines for healthy Americans (p. 9), issued by the U.S. Departments of Agriculture and of Health and Human Services, as well as national health agencies for heart disease, cancer, and diabetes, recommend dietary decreases in these two nutrients. Two primary factors in a fat-controlled diet are: (1) *Reducing the total amount of fat*: no more than 30% of the total energy (kcalories) intake should come from fat. (2) *Reducing the use of animal fat*: no more than approximately a third of the total fat kcalories should come from saturated animal fat, with the remainder from unsaturated plant fat.

Also, the dietary cholesterol should be reduced to about 300 mg/day.

The prudent diet. This reduced amount of fat and cholesterol, together with the greater use of unsaturated plant fats than saturated animal fats, is included in the general goals of the prudent diet recommended by the American Heart Association and other health agencies, as shown in Table 19-3. Step wise revisions for the prudent diet, shown in Table 19-4, provide further guidelines for lowering elevated blood lipid levels.[5] A simplified low-fat diet with emphasis on polyunsaturated and monounsaturated food fats, mostly from vegetable oil and its products, is the basic guideline. When the risk factor

❖ **TABLE 19-3**   *The prudent diet as compared with the usual American diet*

	Prudent diet	Usual American diet
Total kcalories	Sufficient to maintain ideal body weight	Often excessive for need
Cholesterol	300 mg	600-800 mg
Total fats (% of kcalories)	30%-35%	40%-45%
Saturated	10% or less	15%-20%
Monounsaturated	15%	15%-20%
Polyunsaturated	10%	5%-6%
P/S ratio (polyunsaturated/saturated fat in the diet)	1-1.5/1	0.3/1
Carbohydrate (% of kcalories)	50%-55%	40%-45%
Starch (complex CHO)	30%-35%	20%-25%
Simple sugars	10%	15%-20%
Proteins (% of total kcalories)	12%-20%	12%-15%
Sodium	130 mEq (3 g)	200-250 mEq (4.5-6.0 g)

❖ **TABLE 19-4**   *American Heart Association revised prudent diet guidelines for lowering elevated blood lipid levels*

	Step 1 % total kcalories	Step 2 % total kcalories
Total fat	<30	<30
Saturated	<10	<7
Monounsaturated	10-15	10-15
Polyunsaturated	10	10
Carbohydrate	50-60	50-60
Protein	15-20	15-20
Cholesterol	<300 mg/day	<200 mg/day

of obesity is present, the energy value of the diet (kcalories) is also reduced accordingly, and increased exercise is encouraged. A treadmill exercise tolerance test is used to determine individual exercise limit for a person with a history of cardiac disease (Fig 19-2).

Additional dietary factors. Recent interest has centered on dietary fiber and *omega-3 fatty acids* as additional food factors in reducing risks involved in coronary heart disease (Box 19-2). Each of these factors may need consideration along with the primary focus on fat and cholesterol.

The problem of acute cardiovascular disease

When cardiovascular disease progresses to the point of cutting off the blood supply to major coronary arteries, a critical vascular event, a heart attack, or MI occurs. In the initial acute phase of the attack, additional diet modifications are required to allow healing.

Objective: cardiac rest. All care, including diet, is directed toward ensuring cardiac rest so that the damaged heart may be restored to normal functioning.

Principles of diet therapy. The diet is modified in energy value and texture, as well as in fat and sodium.

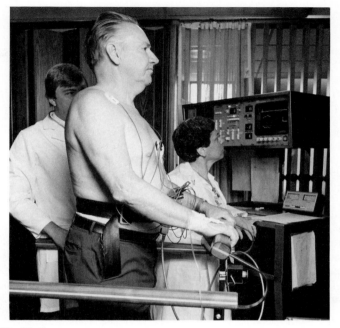

❖ FIG. 19-2

Patient with history of cardiac disease is evaluated for exercise tolerance with treadmill test.

1. *Kcalories.* A brief period of undernutrition during the first day or so after the heart attack reduces the metabolic workload on the damaged heart. The metabolic demands for digestion, absorption, and metabolism of food require a generous cardiac output volume. Thus, to decrease this level of metabolic activity to one that the weakened heart can accommodate, small feedings are spread over the day when an oral diet is started. The patient will progress to eating more as healing occurs. During the initial recovery period, the diet may be limited to about 1200 to 1500 kcalories to continue cardiac rest from metabolic workloads. Afterward, if the patient is overweight, this kcalorie level may continue to help the patient begin very gradual excess weight loss.

2. *Texture.* Early feedings generally include foods relatively soft in texture or easily digested to avoid excess effort in eating. For a time, the patient may need to be fed to reduce the physical effort of eating further and to help ensure sufficient intake if appetite is poor and the patient is weak. Smaller meals served more frequently may give needed nourishment without undue strain or pressure. Temperature extremes in foods, both solids and liquids, should be avoided.

3. *Fat.* The general "prudent" diet will control the amount and types of fat as well as cholesterol (see Tables 19-3 and 19-4).

4. *Sodium.* General attention to a reduced sodium content in the foods selected is also emphasized. Usually a mild sodium restriction to about 2 to 3 g/day is sufficient. This can be achieved by using salt only lightly in cooking, by adding none when eating, and by avoiding salty processed foods.

❖

BOX 19-2
Omega-3 fatty acids and dietary fiber in coronary heart disease therapy

The primary focus of nutritional therapy for coronary heart disease (CHD) centers on control of lipid factors, including cholesterol and saturated fats. Two additional food factors, however, play a different role. In varying ways they also help to protect us from CHD development.

Omega-3 fatty acids

Studies indicate that the omega-3 fatty acids, *eicosapentaenoic acid (EPA)* and *docosahexaenoic acid (DHA)* may have protective functions in their capacity to hinder blood clots from forming. Scientific interest was first sparked by earlier observations among Greenland Eskimos, who eat a diet rich in fish oils but have a low incidence of heart disease. The scientists found that these fish oils contain high levels of long-chain polyunsaturated fatty acids, which they named *omega-3* fatty acids from the nature of their chemical structure. Continuing study supports the potential nutritional and clinical importance of these fatty acids. They are found mostly in seafood and marine oils from fatty fish, such as cod, salmon, mackerel, and menhaden.

On the basis of research results to date, these omega-3 fatty acids can:
- Change the pattern of plasma fatty acids to alter platelet activity and reduce the clumping together of these disk-shaped blood factors to cause blood clotting, thus lowering the risk of coronary thrombosis
- Increase anti-inflammatory effects
- Decrease synthesis of very-low-density lipoproteins

Dietary fiber

Studies indicate that water-soluble types of dietary fiber have significant cholesterol-lowering effect. Soluble fiber includes gums, pectin, certain hemicelluloses, and storage polysaccharides. Foods rich in soluble fiber include oat bran and dried beans, with additional amounts in barley and fruits. Oat bran, for example, contains a primary water-soluble gum, beta-glucan, which is a lipid-lowering agent. Soluble fiber can:
- Delay gastric emptying
- Increase intestinal transit time
- Slow glucose absorption
- Be fermented in the colon into short-chain fatty acids that may inhibit liver cholesterol synthesis and help clear LDL-cholesterol

It would seem, then, that factors in foods such as oats, dried beans, and fatty fish would provide valuable lipid-lowering additions to our diets.

References

Anderson JW and Gustafson NJ: Dietary fiber and heart disease: current management concepts and recommendations, Top Clin Nutr 3(2):21, 1988.

Simopoulos AP: Omega-3 fatty acids in growth and development: dietary implications, Nutr Today 23(3):12, 1988.

BOX 19-3
Restrictions For a Mild Low-Sodium Diet (2 to 3 g Sodium)

Do not use
1. Salt at the table (use salt lightly in cooking)
2. Salt-preserved foods such as salted or smoked meat (bacon and bacon fat, bologna, dried or chipped beef, corned beef, frankfurters, ham, kosher meats, luncheon meats, salt pork, sausage, smoked tongue), salted or smoked fish (anchovies, caviar, salted and dried cod, herring, sardines) sauerkraut, olives
3. Highly salted foods such as crackers, pretzels, potato chips, corn chips, salted nuts, salted popcorn
4. Spices and condiments such as bouillon cubes,* catsup,* chili sauce,* celery salt, garlic sauce, onion salt, monosodium glutamate, meat sauces, meat tenderizers,* pickles, prepared mustard, relishes, Worcestershire sauce, soy sauce
5. Cheese,* peanut butter*

* Dietetic low-sodium kind may be used.

The problem of chronic heart disease

In chronic heart disease a condition of **congestive heart failure** may develop over time. The progressively weakened heart muscle is unable to maintain an adequate cardiac output to sustain normal blood circulation. The resulting fluid imbalances cause *edema*, especially **pulmonary edema**, to develop. This condition brings added problems in breathing and places more stress on the laboring heart.

Objective: control of cardiac edema. The basic objective of diet therapy in this condition is control of the fluid imbalance resulting in cardiac edema.

Principles of diet therapy. Because of the role of sodium in tissue fluid balance (p. 109), the diet used to treat cardiac edema restricts the sodium intake. The main source of dietary sodium is common table salt, sodium chloride. The taste for salt is an acquired one. Some persons salt food heavily by habit without even tasting it first and habituate their taste to high salt levels. Others acquire a taste for less salt by the habit of using smaller amounts. In the American diet, therefore, common daily adult intakes of sodium range widely, according to habit, from about 3 to 4 g to as high as 10 to 12 g with heavy use. Besides salt used in cooking or added at the table, a large amount is used in food processing. Remaining sources of sodium include that found as a naturally occurring mineral in certain foods. The American Heart Association has outlined three main levels of sodium restriction, which can be achieved by progressively deleting these main dietary sodium sources.

1. Mild sodium restriction (2 to 3 g). Salt may be used *lightly* in cooking, assuming the use of fresh foods, but *no added salt* is allowed. In addition, no salty processed foods are used, such as pickles, olives, bacon, ham, corn chips, or potato chips. Box 19-3 provides a general deletion list for mild sodium restriction. Some processed foods with less salt added are beginning to appear on our food market shelves.

2. Moderate sodium restriction (1000 mg). There is no salt used in cooking, no added salt, and no salty foods. Beginning at this level some control of foods

❖

BOX 19-4

Restrictions For a Moderate Low-Sodium Diet
(1000 mg Sodium)

Do not use

1. Salt in cooking or at the table
2. Salt-preserved foods such as salted or smoked meat (bacon and bacon fat, bologna, dried or chipped beef, brains, corned beef, frankfurters, ham, kosher meats, luncheon meats, salt pork, sausage, smoked tongue, kidneys), salted or smoked fish (anchovies, caviar, salted and dried cod, herring, sardines, frozen fish fillets, canned salmon,* tuna*), sauerkraut, olives
3. Highly salted foods such as crackers, pretzels, potato chips, corn chips, salted nuts, salted popcorn
4. Spices and condiments such as bouillon cubes,* catsup,* chili sauce,* celery salt, garlic salt, onion salt, monosodium glutamate, meat sauces, meat tenderizers,* pickles, prepared mustard, relishes, Worcestershire sauce, soy sauce
5. Cheese,* peanut butter*
6. Buttermilk (unsalted buttermilk may be used) instead of skimmed milk
7. Canned vegetables,* canned vegetable juices*
8. Frozen peas, frozen lima beans, frozen mixed vegetables, any frozen vegetables to which salt has been added
9. More than 1 serving of any of these vegetables in 1 day: artichokes, beet greens, beets, carrots, celery, dandelion greens, kale, mustard greens, spinach, Swiss chard, turnips (white)
10. Regular bread, rolls,* crackers*
11. Dry cereals,* except puffed rice, puffed wheat, and shredded wheat
12. Quick-cooking Cream of Wheat
13. Shellfish: clams, crab, lobster, shrimp (oysters may be used)
14. Salted butter, salted margaine, commercial French dressings,* mayonnaise,* other salad dressings*
15. Regular baking powder,* baking soda, or anything containing them; self-rising flour
16. Prepared mixes: pudding,* gelatin,* cake, biscuit
17. Commercial candies

* Dietetic low-sodium kinds may be used.

with natural sodium is started. Vegetables higher in natural sodium are limited. Fresh foods are used, rather than those processed with salt. Salt-free baked products are generally used. Meat and milk, foods higher in natural sodium, are used in only moderate portions. Box 19-4 provides a general deletion list for moderate sodium restriction.

   3. Strict sodium restriction (500 mg). In additions to the mild and moderate deletions, the natural sodium food sources of meat, milk, and eggs are used in smaller portions. Milk is limited to 2 cups in any form, meat to 5 ounces, and eggs to one. Higher-sodium vegetables are deleted. Box 19-5 provides a general deletion list for strict sodium restriction.

❖

BOX 19-5
Restrictions For a Strict Low-Sodium Diet (500 mg Sodium)

Do not use

1. Salt in cooking or at the table
2. Salt-preserved foods such as salted or smoked meat (bacon and bacon fat, bologna, dried or chipped beef, brains, corned beef, frankfurters, ham, kosher meats, luncheon meats, salt pork, sausage, smoked tongue, kidneys), salted or smoked fish (anchovies, caviar, salted and dried cod, herring, sardines, frozen fish fillets, canned salmon,* tuna*), sauerkraut, olives
3. Highly salted foods such as crackers, pretzels, potato chips, corn chips, salted nuts, salted popcorn
4. Spices and condiments such as bouillon cubes,* catsup,* chili sauce,* celery salt, garlic salt, onion salt, monosodium glutamate, meat sauces, meat tenderizers,* pickles, prepared mustard, relishes, Worcestershire sauce, soy sauce
5. Cheese,* peanut butter*
6. Buttermilk (unsalted buttermilk may be used) instead of skimmed milk
7. More than 2 cups skimmed milk a day, including that used on cereal
8. Any commercial foods made of milk (ice cream, ice milk, milk shakes)
9. Canned vegetables,* canned vegetables juices*
10. Frozen peas, frozen lima beans, frozen mixed vegetables, any frozen vegetables to which salt has been added
11. These vegetables: artichokes, beet greens, beets, carrots, celery, dandelion greens, kale, mustard greens, spinach, Swiss chard, turnips (white)
12. Regular bread,* rolls,* crackers
13. Dry cereals,* except puffed rice, puffed wheat, and shredded wheat
14. Quick-cooking cream of wheat
15. Shellfish: clams, crab, lobster, shrimp (oysters may be used)
16. Salted butter, salted margaine, commercial French dressings,* mayonnaise,* other salad dressings*
17. Regular baking powder,* baking soda, or anything containing them; self-rising flour
18. Prepared mixes: pudding,* gelatin,* cake, biscuit
19. Commercial candies

* Dietetic low-sodium kinds may be used.

ESSENTIAL HYPERTENSION
The problem of hypertension

Incidence and nature. Hypertension, or high blood pressure, is a health problem in the lives of some 60 million Americans. About 30% of American adults have high blood pressure, with the numbers increasing with age. The incidence ranges from a low of 2% for white women aged 18 through 24, to 83% for black women aged 65 through 74.[6] Actually, when speaking of the chronic disease of elevated blood pressure, the term *hypertension* is more correct than *high blood pressure*, because the blood pressure may occasionally be elevated temporarily in situations such as overexertion or stress. In general, the disease hypertension means **essential hypertension**; 90% of cases fall in this category, and we don't really know what causes it.

Hypertension has been called the "silent" disease because no signs indicate its presence, but it can have serious effects if not detected, treated, and controlled. It is usually an inherited disorder; children of hypertensive parents may develop the condition at early ages, often in their adolescent years. Hypertension occurs more frequently in blacks than in whites.[7] Obesity makes the condition worse because it forces the heart to work harder, thus maintaining higher blood pressure, to circulate blood through all the excess tissue. Smoking also increases blood pressure because the nicotine constricts the small blood vessels. Other risk factors include lack of exercise, chronic stress, certain drugs such as birth control pills, and for some sensitive persons, caffeine.

Types of hypertensive blood pressure levels. Common blood pressure measurements indicate the pressure of the blood surge in the arteries of the upper arm with each heart beat. The power of each surge is measured in units called *millimeters of mercury*, abbreviated *mm Hg*. Two forces are counted and represented by two numbers. The first number on the top of the fraction measures the force of the blood surge when the heart contracts; it is called the *systolic* pressure. The second number on the bottom measures the pressure remaining in the arteries when the heart relaxes between beats; it is called the *diastolic* pressure. Adult blood pressure is usually considered normal if it is less than 140/90 mm Hg. Current hypertension screening and treatment programs identify persons with hypertension according to degree of severity of these pressures as mild, moderate, or severe. Then specific care is outlined for each type, seeking to limit drugs as much as possible.[7]

1. Mild hypertension. Diastolic pressure is 90 to 104 mm Hg. Initial focus is on nondrug approaches of diet therapy to reduce excess weight and restrict sodium.

2. Moderate hypertension. Diastolic pressure is 105 to 119 mm Hg. In addition to the diet therapy for the mild form, drugs are used according to need, usually including a diuretic agent. Continuous use of some *diuretic drugs*, though not all, causes loss of potassium along with the increased loss of water from the body. Since potassium is necessary for maintaining normal heart muscle action, a depletion could become dangerous. Potassium replacement is necessary. Dietary replacement by increased use of potassium-rich food choices is an important part of therapy. These foods include fruits, especially bananas and orange juice, vegetables, legumes, nuts, whole grains, and meat.

3. Severe hypertension. Diastolic pressure is 120 to 130 mm Hg or greater. In addition to the diet for the moderate form, vigorous drug therapy is necessary. Nutritional support is important for all types of hypertension, along with other nondrug therapies of physical exercise and stress reduction activities.

The principles of nutritional therapy

Weight management. According to individual need, weight management requires losing excess weight and maintaining an appropriate weight for height. A sound approach to managing weight loss is given in Chapter 15 and guidance for increasing physical exercise in Chapter 16. Because the overweight state has been closely associated with hypertension risk factors, a wisely planned personal program of weight reduction and physical activity is a cornerstone of therapy.

Sodium control. In sodium-sensitive persons, additional attention is given to sodium restriction in the diet. Generally the mild 2 g sodium level is sufficient (see Box 19-2). In more severe cases of hypertension, the moderate 1 g sodium level may be indicated (see Box 19-3).

Other minerals. In addition to sodium control, especially for sodium-sensitive persons, other minerals have been discussed in relation to hypertension. Some evidence suggests that increased calcium intake is beneficial for some hypertensive persons. Also, as indicated, increased potassium to replace loss with diuretic use and to supply normal dietary needs is an important part of diet therapy.

The prudent diet. As outlined for general coronary heart disease, the accepted prudent diet in current use for controlling fat and cholesterol is also recommended for persons with any level of hypertension (see Tables 19-3 and 19-4). It is a sound basic diet for general health promotion and risk reduction.

EDUCATION AND PREVENTION
Practical food guides

Food planning and purchasing. The general dietary guidelines for Americans (p. 9) provide a basic outline to guide food habits. The food exchange lists, described in Chapter 20 and listed in the Appendix for reference, give food groups with fat and sodium modifications discussed here. They also provide a guide for control of kcalories to help plan for any needed weight management. An important part of purchasing food is reading labels carefully. All processed food products making any health claims must provide nutrition information on the label (p. 184). A good general guide is to use primarily fresh foods with informed selection of processed foods only as necessary. Refer to Chapter 13 for background material about food supply and health.

Food preparation. Numerous guides for good preparation of primary foods with less use of fat and salt are currently available since the public is more aware of these health needs. Many seasonings such as herbs, spices, lemon, wine, onion, garlic, nonfat milk and yogurt, and fresh fat-free meat broth can help train the taste for less salt and fat. Less meat in leaner and smaller portions can be combined with more complex carbohydrate foods—starches such as potato, pasta, and beans—to make more healthful main dishes. Whole-grain breads and cereals can provide needed fiber and more use of fish can add healthier forms of fat in smaller quantities. A variety of vegetables, steamed and lightly seasoned, and fruits add interest, taste appeal, and nourishment to meals. The American Heart Association Cookbook is an excellent guide to newer, lighter, tasteful, and healthier food preparation.

Special needs. Individual adaptation of diet principles is important in all nutrition teaching and counseling. Special attention needs to be given to personal desires, ethnic diets, individual situations, and food habits as discussed in Chapter 14. No diet can be followed unless it meets personal needs.

Education principles

Start early. Prevention of hypertension and heart disease begins in childhood, especially with children of high-risk families. With close attention to normal growth needs, some preventive measures in family food habits can relate to weight control and avoidance of foods high in salt and fat. For adults with heart disease and hypertension, learning should be an integral part of all therapy. When a heart attack does occur, learning should begin early in convalescence, not at discharge, to give patients and their families clear and practical knowledge of positive needs.

Focus on high-risk groups. Education concerning the risks of heart disease and hypertension should be directed particularly to persons and families with these risks (see Table 19-1). For example, hypertension has been closely associated with certain high-risk groups, including blacks, persons with strong family histories, and obese individuals.

Use a variety of resources. As more is being learned about heart disease and hypertension, the American Heart Association and other health agencies are providing many excellent resources. The American Dietetic Association provides a series of pamphlets that are helpful in client education, several of which apply here: *Weight Expectations, Fiber Facts, Cholesterol Countdown,* and *The Sodium Story* (PO Box 10960, Chicago, IL 60610). Also, as the public and professionals have become more aware of health needs and disease prevention, an increasing number of resources and programs can be found in most communities. These include various weight management programs, registered dietitians in private practice or in health care centers who provide nutrition counseling, and practical food preparation materials found in a number of recent "light cuisine" cooking classes and cookbooks. Bookstores and public libraries, as well as health education libraries in health centers and clinics, provide more materials in health promotion and self-care. Local health care centers, for example, teach persons with hypertension and their families how to take their own blood pressure, so they can assume more control in managing their health needs, and provide resources for such self-care.

SUMMARY

Coronary heart disease is the leading cause of death in the United States. Its underlying blood vessel disease is *atherosclerosis*, which involves the buildup of a fatty substance containing cholesterol on the interior surfaces of blood vessels, interfering with blood flow and damaging the blood vessels. If this fatty buildup becomes severe, it cuts off supplies of oxygen and nutrients to tissue cells, which in turn die. When this occurs in a major coronary artery, the result is a *myocardial infarction*, or heart attack.

The risk for atherosclerosis increases with the amount and type of blood lipids (fats), or *lipoproteins*, available. Elevated *serum cholesterol* is a primary risk factor in development of atherosclerosis.

Current recommendations to help prevent coronary heart disease involve a prudent diet, weight management, and increased exercise. Such a diet limits fats to 25% to 30% of total diet kcalories, limits sodium intake to 2 to 3 g per day, and reduces cholesterol intake. Dietary recommendations for acute cardiovascular disease (heart attack) include measures to ensure cardiac rest, such as caloric restriction, soft foods, and small meals, modified in fat, cholesterol, and sodium. Persons with chronic heart disease involving congestive heart failure benefit from a low-sodium diet to control cardiac edema. Persons with hypertension can improve their condition with weight control, exercise, sodium restriction, and adequate calcium and potassium.

❖ REVIEW QUESTIONS

1. Why are fat and cholesterol primary factors in heart disease? How are they carried in the bloodstream? Which of these "fat packages" carry so-called good cholesterol and which carry bad cholesterol, the cholesterol of concern? How can we influence the relative amounts of these fat and cholesterol carriers in our blood? Describe food changes involved.
2. Identify the risk factors for heart disease. What control do we have over these risk factors?
3. Identify four diet recommendations for the patient after a heart attack. Describe how each of these helps recovery.
4. Discuss the three main levels of sodium restriction, describing general food choices and preparation methods.
5. What does the term *essential hypertension* mean? Why would weight control and sodium restriction contribute to its control? What other nutrient factors may be involved in hypertension?

❖ SELF-TEST QUESTIONS

True-false

For each item you answer "false," write the correct statement.

1. In the disease process underlying heart disease, atherosclerosis, the fatty deposits in blood vessel linings are composed mainly of cholesterol.
2. Hypertension occurs more frequently in white populations than in black ones.
3. The problem of cardiovascular disease could be solved if cholesterol could be removed entirely from the body.
4. Cholesterol is a dietary essential because humans depend entirely on food sources for their supply.
5. Lipoproteins are the major transport form of lipids in the blood.
6. The basic clinical objective in treating acute cardiovascular disease, a heart attack, is cardiac rest.
7. In chronic congestive heart disease the heart may eventually fail because its weakened muscle must work at a faster rate to pump out the body's needed blood supply.
8. The taste for salt is instinctive in humans to ensure a sufficient supply.
9. Sodium is an effective therapy in congestive heart failure and in hypertension.
10. Essential hypertension can be cured by drugs and diet.

Multiple choice

1. A low-cholesterol diet would restrict which of the following foods?
   (1) Fish   (3) Eggs
   (2) Liver   (4) Nonfat milk
      a. 1 and 3   c. 3 and 4
      b. 2 and 3   d. 1 and 4
2. Helpful seasonings to use for a sodium restricted diet include:
   (1) Lemon juice   (4) Seasoned salt
   (2) Soy sauce   (5) Garlic and celery salt
   (3) Herbs and spices   (6) MSG (Accent)
      a. 1 and 3   c. 5 and 6
      b. 2 and 4   d. 1, 3, and 6
3. Which of the following foods may be used freely on any low-sodium diet?
   a. Fruits   c. Meat
   b. Milk   d. Spinach and carrots

❖ SUGGESTIONS FOR FURTHER STUDY

Market survey

Visit your local market, individually or in small groups, and make a detailed survey of food products:

1. **Fat-related foods.** Look at foods containing both saturated fats from animal sources (dairy products, meats, etc.) and unsaturated fats from plant sources (vegetable oils, dairy substitute products, etc.). Read all labels carefully and note nutrition information given. Compare the various products in both amount and kind of fat included. Do you find the two saturated plant oils, palm oil and coconut oil, used in any food products? What health claims are made and how valid do you think they are? Compare fat-modified products.

2. **Sodium (salt) in foods.** Make a similar survey of processed foods and their labels. Note references to salt or any other sodium compounds used. Compare any sodium-modified products you can find.

3. **Sugar and fiber in foods.** Since amounts of both sugar as a source of kcalories, and fiber as a possible intestinal binder of cholesterol, have roles in a basic healthy diet to help reduce heart disease risks, make a survey of processed foods containing sugar and fiber. Read labels carefully and note any nutrition information given and any health claims made.

Evaluate the various products you discovered and make a summary report to present in class. Discuss your findings in comparison with those of other groups in the class.

References

1. Committee on Diet and Health, Food and Nutrition Board, National Research Council: Diet and health—implications for reducing chronic disease risks, Washington, DC, 1989, National Academy Press.
2. Sempos C and others: The prevalence of high blood cholesterol levels among adults in the United States, JAMA 262:45, 1989.
3. National Institutes of Health: Consensus Development Conference Statement: Lowering Blood Cholesterol, Nutr Today 20(1):13, 1985.
4. National Heart, Lung, and Blood Institute: Report of the expert panel on detection, evaluation, and treatment of high blood cholesterol in adults, National Cholesterol Education Program, Washington, DC, 1988, US Department of Health and Human Services.
5. Ginsberg HN and others: Reduction of plasma cholesterol levels in normal men on an American Heart Association Step 1 diet or a step 1 diet with added monounsaturated fat, N Engl J Med 322:574, Mar 1, 1990.
6. US Department of Health and Human Services, Public Health Service: Healthy people 2000—national health promotion and disease prevention objectives, Chapter 15: Heart disease and stroke, Washington, DC, 1990, US Government Printing Office.
7. National Heart, Lung, and Blood Institute: The 1988 report of the joint national committee on detection, evaluation, and treatment of high blood pressure, Washington, DC, 1988, US Department of Health and Human Services.

Further reading

Barnett R: Fat—where it's at, Am Health 8:84, Jan/Feb 1989.

Barton D: Down home at the diner, Am Health 8:104, Jan/Feb 1989.

These two articles from a popular health magazine for consumers provide a great deal of information to indicate that Americans are becoming more concerned about fat in their diets. A recent Gallup poll shows that 85% of Americans questioned said that they are doing something to cut fat intake, and the fat content of many new food products being marketed is lower to meet customer demands. The classic "diner" menu list with fat modification recipes shows that lower-fat food can still "stick to the ribs" and bring comfort.

❖

Diabetes mellitus

KEY CONCEPTS

Diabetes mellitus is a metabolic disorder of energy balance with many contributory causes and forms.

Consistent sound diet is the keystone of all diabetes care and control.

Good self-care skills practiced daily enable the person with diabetes to remain healthy and reduce risks of complications.

A personalized care plan, balancing food intake, exercise, and insulin activity, is essential to successful diabetes management.

One in 20 Americans, nearly 11 million, have diabetes. Of these persons, 15% are insulin dependent and 85% are non-insulin dependent. Diabetes complications have become our fifth-ranking cause of death from disease.

Diabetes mellitus is an ancient disease, claiming the lives of its victims at a young age. But in modern times, greater knowledge of the disease and sound self-care have enabled many persons with diabetes to live long and fruitful lives. For the most part, with professional guidance and support, the person with diabetes can remain healthy and reduce risk of health problems through consistent practice of good self-care skills.

In this chapter we look at diabetes mellitus to learn its nature and understand why daily self-care is essential for good control and health. Then we will see that diabetes education is vital not only for persons with diabetes themselves and their families, but also for all health team members and the public as well.

THE NATURE OF DIABETES
History and definition

Early history and naming. Diabetes mellitus is an ancient disease. Its symptoms were described on the Egyptian Ebers Papyrus, dating about 1500 BC. In the first century the Greek physician Aretaeus wrote of a malady in which the body "ate its own flesh" and gave off large quantities of urine. He gave it the name *diabetes*, from the Greek word meaning "siphon" or "to pass through." Much later, in the 17th century, the word *mellitus*, from the Latin word meaning "honey," was added because of the sweet nature of the urine. This name addition distinguished it from another disorder, *diabetes insipidus*, in which large urine output was observed. However, diabetes insipidus is a much more rare and quite different disease caused by lack of the pituitary antidiuretic hormone (ADH). Today the simple term "diabetes" refers to diabetes mellitus. We will follow this common usage in this chapter for simplicity.

Diabetic dark ages. During the Middle Ages and the dawning of our scientific era, many early scientists and physicians continued to puzzle over the mystery of diabetes, but the cause remained obscure. For physicians and their patients these years could be called the "Diabetic Dark Ages." Patients had short lives and were maintained on semistarvation and high-fat diets.

Discovery of insulin. A first breakthrough came from a clue pointing to the involvement of the pancreas in the disease process. This clue was provided by a young German medical student, Paul Langerhans, who found special clusters of cells scattered about the pancreas forming little "islands" of cells. Although he did not yet understand their function, he could see that these cells were different from the rest of the tissue and must be important. When his suspicions later proved true, these little clusters of cells were named for their young discoverer—the *islands of Langerhans*. Soon after, in 1922, using this important clue, two Canadian scientists, Frederick Banting and his assistant, Charles Best, together with two other research team members, physiologists J.B. Collip and J.J.R. Macleod, extracted the first insulin from animals. It proved to be a hormone that regulates the oxidation of blood sugar and helps to convert it to heat and energy. They called the new hormone *insulin*, from the Latin word *insula*, meaning "island." It did prove to be the effective agent for treating diabetes. The first child treated in January 1922, Leonard Thompson, lived to adulthood but died at age 27, not from his diabetes but from coronary heart disease caused by his "diabetic diet" of the day, which was based on 70% of its total kcalories from fat! It is not surprising that the autopsy showed marked atherosclerosis.[1]

Successful use of diet and insulin. The insulin discovery team was more successful on their third attempt with a young girl diagnosed as having diabetes at age 11.[1] She had initially been put on a "starvation" diet of that time and her weight fell from 75 to 45 pounds (34 to 21 kg) over a 3-year period. Fortunately, however, the medical research team had learned the importance of a better "regular" diet for normal growth and health. Thus, with good diet and the new insulin therapy, this child, Elizabeth Hughes, gained weight and vigor and lived a normal life. She married, had three children, took insulin for

58 years and died at age 73 of heart failure. No diabetes has appeared among her descendants.

Current therapy based on contributory causes

Since those early years of insulin discovery and development, continued research has increased our knowledge about diabetes and helped us develop better means of care. During the last few years we have learned that diabetes is not a single disease. Rather, it is currently recognized as a syndrome of many disorders and degrees, characterized by **hyperglycemia** (elevated blood sugar) and, in many persons, various complications. We have also learned that diabetes has multiple causes centering around insulin activity, heredity, and weight, which help give direction for current individual therapy.

Insulin activity. Diabetes is an underlying metabolic disorder developing from various causes, all involving some deficiency in the action of insulin in controlling the body's overall energy balance. It is now evident that diabetes is a condition with multiple forms, resulting from (1) lack of insulin, as in *insulin-dependent diabetes mellitus (IDDM)*, or from (2) insulin resistance, as in *non-insulin-dependent diabetes mellitus (NIDDM)*.

Heredity. Diabetes, especially in insulin-dependent forms, has usually been defined in terms of heredity. Now there is increasing evidence that considerable *genetic variation* exists in both major forms or classes *IDDM* and *NIDDM*. Environmental factors, especially those contributing to obesity, play a role in bringing out the underlying genetic predisposition for diabetes.

Weight. Diabetes has long been associated with weight. Early clinicians observed that diabetes in overweight persons improved with weight loss, and they described diabetes as "fat diabetes" and "thin diabetes."[2] All of these observations preceded any knowledge about insulin or a relationship between diabetes and the pancreas. Current research has reinforced the association between the overweight state and NIDDM.

Types of diabetes

An international work group of the National Institutes of Health has provided an improved classification for the diabetes syndrome.[2] Two broad classes or types are identified as the basis for continued study of subtypes.

Insulin-dependent diabetes mellitus (IDDM). In its insulin-dependent form, diabetes develops rapidly and tends to be more severe and unstable. IDDM occurs more frequently in children, although it also occurs in young adults. The person is usually underweight. Acidosis often occurs.

Non-insulin-dependent diabetes mellitus (NIDDM). In its non-insulin-dependent form, diabetes develops more slowly and is usually milder and more stable. NIDDM occurs mainly in adults, and the person is usually overweight. Acidosis appears infrequently. Most of these overweight adults improve with weight loss and are maintained on diet therapy alone. Sometimes an oral hypoglycemic medication is also needed for control.

Symptoms of diabetes

Initial signs. Early signs of diabetes include three primary symptoms: (1) increased thirst—*polydipsia*, (2) increased urination—*polyuria*, and (3) increased hunger—*polyphagia*. The weight status may be weight loss with IDDM or obesity with NIDDM.

Laboratory test results. Various laboratory tests show the following results: **glycosuria** (sugar in the urine), **hyperglycemia** (elevated blood sugar), and abnormal glucose tolerance tests.

Other possible symptoms. Additional signs may include blurred vision, skin irritation or infection, and general weakness and loss of strength. In elderly persons with diabetes the skin irritation may appear as perineal itching and the weakness as a general drowsiness.

Progressive results. Continued symptoms may occur as the uncontrolled condition becomes more serious. These may include water and electrolyte imbalance, ketoacidosis, and coma.

THE METABOLIC PATTERN OF DIABETES
Energy balance and normal blood sugar controls

Energy balance. Diabetes has been called a disease of carbohydrate metabolism. We now know that it is a general metabolic disorder involving all three of the energy nutrients—carbohydrate, fat, and protein. It is especially related to the metabolism of the two main fuels, carbohydrate and fat, in the body's overall energy system, as described in Chapter 16.

Normal blood sugar balance. Control of blood sugar within its normal range of 70 to 120 mg/dl is vital to life. Normal controls are "built in" to ensure that we always have sufficient circulating blood sugar, glucose, to meet our constant energy needs, even basal metabolic energy needs during sleep, because glucose is the body's major fuel. Note these balanced sources and uses of blood glucose as illustrated in Fig. 20-1.

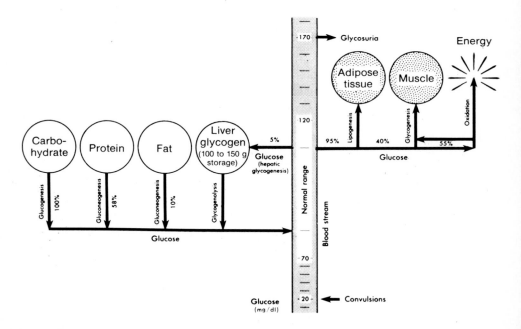

❖ **FIG. 20-1**

Sources of blood glucose (food and stored glycogen) and normal routes of control.

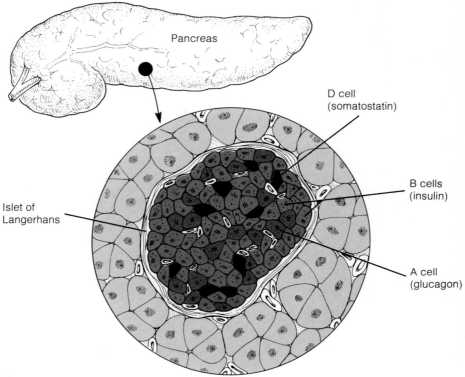

❖ **FIG. 20-2**

Islets of Langerhans, located in the pancreas.

Sources of blood glucose. To ensure a constant supply of the body's main fuel, two sources of blood glucose exist: (1) **diet**—the energy nutrients in our food, dietary carbohydrate, fat, and, as needed, protein; and (2) **glycogen**— the backup source from constant turnover of stored glycogen in liver and muscles.

Uses of blood glucose. To prevent a continued rise of blood glucose above normal range, the body "drains off" glucose as needed by using it in three ways: (1) burns it by cell oxidation for immediate energy needs; (2) changes it to glycogen, which is briefly stored in muscles and liver, then withdrawn to change back into glucose for short-term energy needs; and (3) changes it to fat, which is stored for longer periods as body fat.

Pancreatic hormonal control. The specialized cells of the islets (islands) of Langerhans in the pancreas provide three hormones that work together to regulate blood glucose levels: (1) insulin, (2) glucagon, and (3) somatostatin. This specific arrangement of human islet cells is illustrated in Fig. 20-2.

1. Insulin. Insulin is the major hormone controlling the level of blood glucose. It helps transport circulating glucose into cells by way of specialized insulin receptors; helps change glucose to glycogen and store it in liver and muscles; stimulates change of glucose to fat for storage as body fat; inhibits breakdown of tissue fat and protein; promotes uptake of amino acids by skeletal muscles, increasing tissue protein synthesis; and influences the burning of glucose for constant energy as needed. Insulin is produced in the B cells of the islets, which fill its central zone and make up about 60% of each islet gland.

2. *Glucagon.* Glucagon is a hormone that acts in an opposite manner to insulin to balance the overall blood glucose control. It can rapidly break down stored glycogen and, to a lesser extent, fat. This action raises blood sugar as needed to protect brain and other tissues during sleep hours or fasting. Glucagon is produced in the A cells of the pancreatic islets, which are arranged around the outer rim of each of these glands, making up about 30% of its total cells.

3. *Somatostatin.* Somatostatin is the pancreatic hormone that acts as a "referee" for several other hormones that affect blood glucose levels, synthesizing their various actions. Somatostatin is produced in the D cells of the pancreatic islets, scattered among the A and B cells and making up about 10% of each islet's cells. Because it has more generalized functions in regulating circulating blood sugar, it is also produced in other parts of the body such as the hypothalamus.

Abnormal metabolism in uncontrolled diabetes

When normal insulin activity is lacking, as in uncontrolled diabetes, the normal controls of blood sugar levels do not operate. As a result, abnormal metabolic changes and imbalances occur among the three energy nutrients.

Glucose. Glucose cannot enter cells and be oxidized through its normal cell pathways to produce energy. Thus it builds up in the blood, creating hyperglycemia.

Fat. Fat tissue formation (*lipogenesis*) decreases, and fat tissue breakdown (*lipolysis*) increases. This increased fat breakdown leads to excess formation of **ketones,** intermediate products of fat breakdown, and their accumulation in the body, causing **ketoacidosis.** The appearance of one of these ketones, **acetone,** in the urine indicates the development of ketoacidosis.

Protein. Protein tissues are also broken down in the body's effort to secure energy sources. This causes weight loss and urinary nitrogen loss.

Long-term complications

Poorly controlled diabetes increases risks of long-term diabetic complications. These health problems relate mainly to tissue changes, affecting blood vessels in vital organs.

Retinopathy. These changes involve small hemorrhages from broken arteries in the retina of the eye, with yellow, waxy discharge or retinal detachment. This complication can eventually cause blindness. Retinopathy is not to be confused with the blurry vision that sometimes occurs as one of the first signs of diabetes. Blurry vision is caused by the increased glucose concentration in the fluids of the eye, bringing brief changes in the curved light-refracting surface of the eye.

Nephropathy. These changes involve the nephrons of the kidneys and can lead to renal failure. This extensive intercapillary *glomerulosclerosis* (p. 333) has been named the *Kimmelstiel-Wilson syndrome,* for the German-American pathologist and English physician who first described it.

Neuropathy. These changes involve injury and disease in the peripheral nervous system, especially in the legs and feet, causing prickly sensations, increasing pain, and eventual loss of sensation due to damaged nerves. This loss of nerve reaction can lead to further tissue damage and infection from unfelt foot injuries such as bruises, burns, and deeper **cellulitis.**

Atherosclerosis. Coronary heart disease from underlying atherosclerosis occurs in persons with diabetes about four times as often as in the general population. Peripheral vascular disease occurs about 40 times as often. This large risk factor accounts for the dietary recommendation to reduce dietary fats and cholesterol.

GENERAL MANAGEMENT OF DIABETES
Early detection and monitoring
The guiding principles for treating diabetes are early detection and prevention of complications. Community screening programs and testing of family members help to identify persons with elevated blood sugar levels for follow-up *glucose tolerance test* (fasting and 2-hour tests with a measured glucose dose) and medical diagnosis of results. An additional monitoring aid is the *hemoglobin A1c test.* This provides an effective tool for evaluating long-term management of diabetes and degree of control, since the glucose attaches itself to the particular hemoglobin over the life of the red blood cell. Thus it reflects the level of blood glucose over a long period of time.

Basic goals of care
Overall objectives. The health care team should be guided by three basic objectives in working with the person with diabetes.

1. Maintenance of optimal nutrition. The first objective is to sustain a high level of nutrition for general health promotion, adequate growth and development, and the maintenance of an appropriate lean weight.

2. Avoidance of symptoms. This objective seeks to keep the person relatively free from symptoms of *hyperglycemia* and *glycosuria*, which indicate poor control.

3. Prevention of complications. This third objective recognizes the increased risk a person with diabetes carries for developing the significant tissue changes already described. Consistent control of blood sugar levels helps to reduce these risks.

Importance of good self-care skills. To accomplish these objectives, the person with diabetes must learn and regularly practice good self-care. Daily self-discipline and informed self-care are necessary for sound diabetes management because ultimately all persons with diabetes must treat themselves with the support of a good health care team. Currently, more emphasis is being given to comprehensive diabetes education programs that encourage self-monitoring of blood glucose levels and self-care responsibility.

DIET THERAPY BASED ON THE BALANCE CONCEPT
The Committee on Food and Nutrition of the American Diabetes Association has issued a report updating their nutritional recommendations and principles for individuals with diabetes mellitus.[3] These comprehensive recommendations largely incorporate health promotion principles such as those in the U.S. dietary guidelines for healthy Americans.[4] The core problem in diabetes is energy

balance, the regulation of the body's primary fuel, blood glucose. Based on this concept of balance, the three main principles of nutritional therapy are total energy balance, nutrient balance, and food distribution balance. Personal diet is then expressed in terms of (1) total kcalories required for energy; (2) ratio of these kcalories in relative amounts of the three energy nutrients carbohydrate, fat, and protein; and (3) a food distribution pattern for the day. A fundamental personal principle underlies the whole plan—*the diet for any person with diabetes is always based on the normal nutritional needs of that individual for positive health.*

Total energy balance

Weight management. Since IDDM usually begins in childhood (average age, 11 years), the normal height-weight charts for children provide a standard for adequate growth. In their adult years, maintaining a lean weight continues to be a basic goal. Since NIDDM usually occurs in overweight adults, the major goal is weight reduction and control.

Total kcalories. The total energy value of the diet for a person with diabetes should be expressed as kcalories sufficient to meet individual needs for normal growth and development, physical activity, and maintenance of a desirable lean weight. The RDA standards for children and adults (see inside book covers) can serve as guides for total energy needs, with appropriate reductions in kcalories for overweight adults, as described in Chapter 15.

Nutrient balance

The ratio of carbohydrate, fat, and protein in the diet is based on current recommendations for ideal glucose regulation and lower fat intake to reduce risks of cardiovascular complications (Table 20-1).

Carbohydrate. A more liberal use of carbohydrates, mainly in complex starch forms with fiber, is recommended. About 50% to 60% of the total kcalories of the diet are assigned to carbohydrate.

1. Complex carbohydrate. As indicated most of the dietary carbohydrate kcalories, about 40% of the total kcalories, should come from complex forms, the starches. In most cases these complex carbohydrates break down more slowly than simple sugars and release their available glucose over time, thus producing a smoother blood sugar level.

2. Glycemic index. Some recent study seems to indicate that different carbohydrate foods have different effects on blood sugar levels. This varying effect has been called the glycemic index of the foods. However, not enough is known yet about this effect to determine how it may be used realistically in diet planning.

3. Fiber. Different kinds of dietary fiber in plant foods, such as whole grains, vegetables, and fruits, influence the rate of absorption of the carbohydrate and alter its effect on blood sugar level. An increased fiber content in the diet, about 30 g total or 15 g/1000 kcal for persons on low caloric diets, is recommended as an important factor in regulating blood glucose levels.

4. Simple carbohydrates. The remainder of the carbohydrate kcalories, about 15%, can come from simple carbohydrates, natural sugars as in fruits and milk. Sucrose-sweetened foods should be carefully controlled. These simple

❖ **TABLE 20-1** *Distribution of major nutrients in normal and diabetic diets (as percentages of total calories)*

	Starch and other polysaccharides* (%)	Sugars† and dextrins (%)	Fat (%)	Protein (%)	Alcohol (%)
Typical American diet	25-35	20-30	35-45	12-19	0-10
Traditional diabetic diets	25-30	10-15‡	40-45 ⅔ saturated	16-21	0
Newer diabetic diets: current therapy	30-45	5-15‡	25-35 Less than ½ saturated	12-24	0-6

* A substantial majority of these calories are starch, but complex carbohydrates also include cellulose, hemicellulose, pentosans, and pectin.
† Monosaccharides and disaccharides, mainly sucrose, but also included are fructose, glucose, lactose, and maltose.
‡ Almost exclusively natural sugars, mainly in fruit and milk (lactose).

carbohydrates are readily absorbed and have a more immediate effect on blood sugar level. Honey is a form of simple sugar, mainly fructose, and is *not* a sugar substitute.

5. *Sugar substitute sweeteners.* The most commonly used nonnutritive sweetener has been saccharin, but there is still debate about its continued use. Aspartame, a recently marketed agent also known as Nutrisweet or Equal, is made from two amino acids, phenylalanine and aspartic acid, and is metabolized as such.

Protein. Most Americans eat much more protein than they need. Normal age requirements as outlined in the RDA standards can be a guide. For adults, 0.8 g/kg is recommended for diabetes control. In general, about 15% to 20% of the total kcalories as protein is sufficient to meet growth needs in children and maintain tissue integrity in adults. Lean food forms are recommended to control fat intake.

Fat. No more than 25% to 30% of the diet's total kcalories should come from fat. Fat should always be used in moderation with less use of saturated fats from animal food sources. Also, less cholesterol intake, no more than 300 mg/day, is recommended. This control of fat-related foods helps reduce the high risk diabetes contributes to the development of atherosclerosis and coronary heart disease.

Current diet recommendations of the American Diabetic Association, the American Heart Association, and the American Dietetic Association are compared in Table 20-2.

Food distribution balance

As a general rule, fairly even amounts of food should be eaten at regular intervals throughout the day, adjusted to blood glucose self-monitoring. This basic pattern will help provide a more even blood sugar supply and prevent swings between low and high levels. Snacks between meals may be needed.

Daily activity schedule. Food distribution needs to be planned ahead, especially by persons using insulin, and adjusted according to each day's scheduled activities and blood sugar monitoring to prevent episodes of **hypoglycemia** from insulin reactions. Practical consideration should be given to work demands, social events, and stress periods.

❖ **TABLE 20-2**   *Comparison of AHA and ADA Diet Recommendations**

	AHA Step 1 (% total kcal)	AHA Step 2 (% total kcal)	ADA/ADA (% total kcal)
Total fat	30	30	30
Monounsaturated	10-15	10-15	12-14
Saturated	10	7	10
Polyunsaturated	Up to 10	Up to 10	6-8
Carbohydrate	50-60	50-60	55-60
Protein	15-20	15-20	0.8 g/kg
Cholesterol	300 mg/day	200 mg/day	300 mg/day

* AHA, American Heart Association; ADA, American Diabetes Association and American Dietetic Association.

Exercise. For persons using insulin, it is especially important that any exercise period or additional physical activity be covered in the food distribution plan. For adults with NIDDM, regular exercise is an essential part of a successful weight management program.

Drug therapy. The food distribution pattern will also be influenced by any form of drug therapy—type and amount and dose schedule of insulin or an oral hypoglycemic agent—that is required for control of the diabetes.

Diet management

General planning according to type of diabetes. Since forms of diabetes vary widely, the nature of an individual's own diabetes and its treatment will largely determine the personal diet management required. Table 20-3 provides guidelines for diet strategies needed for each of the two main types of diabetes, IDDM and NIDDM.

Individual needs. Every person with diabetes is unique, having not only a particular form and degree of diabetes but also an individual living situation, background, and food habits. All of these personal needs must be considered, as discussed in Chapters 14 and 17, if appropriate and realistic care is to be planned. The nutrition counselor, usually the clinical dietitian, always seeks to discover these various individual needs in a careful initial nutrition history, including medical and psychosocial needs. This information provides the basis for determining the diet prescription and calculating nutritional requirements. Then a personal diet plan using the balance principles can be outlined.

❖ **TABLE 20-3**   *Dietary strategies for the two main types of diabetes mellitus*

Dietary strategy	IDDM (non-obese)	NIDDM (usually obese)
Decrease energy intake (kcalories)	No	Yes
Increase frequency and number of feedings	Yes	Usually no
Have regular daily intake of kcalories of carbohydrate, protein, and fat	Very important	Not important if average caloric intake remains in low range
Plan consistent daily ratio of protein, carbohydrate, and fat for each feeding	Desirable	Not necessary
Use extra or planned food to treat or prevent hypoglycemia	Very important	Not necessary
Plan regular times for meals and snacks	Very important	Not important
Use extra food for unusual exercise	Yes	Usually not necessary
During illness, use small, frequent feedings of carbohydrate to prevent starvation ketoacidosis	Important	Usually not necessary because of resistance to ketoacidosis

Food exchange system. A basic system widely used for planning personal food patterns to control diabetes and provide optimal nutrition is called the food exchange system. In this system commonly used foods are grouped into *exchange lists* according to approximately equal food values in the portions indicated. Thus a variety of food choices may be made from these lists to fulfill the basic food plan determined by the dietitian, while maintaining the basic diet prescription of total kcalories and balanced ratio of nutrients. These exchange lists are based on current principles and recommendations for wise diabetes control and health promotion.[5] The booklet *Exchange Lists for Meal Planning* is available from both the American Diabetes Association and the American Dietetic Association. Its colorful illustrations and clear content and style provide a helpful tool for patient and client education. These exchange lists are included in Appendix. Table 20-4 illustrates a calculated 2200 kcal diet and resulting food pattern using the exchange system. Box 20-1 gives a sample menu based on this food pattern.

Special concerns. A number of special concerns come up in daily living and become an important part of ongoing diet counseling. Some suggestions for these needs are given here.

1. Special diet food items. Little need exists for special "dietetic" or "diabetic" foods. The diet for a person with diabetes is a regular, well-balanced diet modified in the same areas of fat, cholesterol, sugar, fiber, and salt that are recommended for the general population to promote health and prevent disease. This kind of a healthful diet primarily uses regular fresh foods from all the basic food groups, with limited use of processed foods and more nonfat seasonings. The simple principles of *moderation* and *variety* guide food choices and amounts.

2. Alcohol. Occasional use of alcohol in a diabetic diet can be planned, but caution must be the guide. Occasional use is defined as moderate intake, less than 6% of the total kcalories on a given day, and not more than 2 equivalent portions once or twice a week.[3] An equivalent portion is 1 ounce liquor, 4 ounces of wine, or 12 ounces of beer. The same precautions regarding the use of alcohol that apply to the general public apply to people with diabetes. When a person with IDDM uses a small amount of alcohol, it should *not* be substituted for food exchanges in the diet, but only used in addition, to avoid the possibility of hypoglycemic reactions. Alcohol may be used in cooking as desired, since it vaporizes in the cooking process and contributes only its flavor to the finished product.

3. Physical activity. For any unusual physical activity, the person using insulin needs to make special plans to cover the event.[6] This is especially true of a young person with a "brittle" form of diabetes engaging in strenuous athletic competition or practice (Table 20-5). The energy demands of exercise are discussed in Chapter 16.

4. Illness. When general illness occurs, food and insulin may need to be adjusted accordingly. The texture of the food can be modified to use easily digested and absorbed liquid foods (Table 20-6). This type of liquid substitution can be used for meals not eaten.[7] In general, the person with diabetes who is ill should:

- Maintain intake of food every day, not skipping meals

❖ **TABLE 20-4** Calculation of diabetic diet: Short method using exchange system (2200 kcal)

Food group	Total day's exchanges	Carbohydrate: 275 g (50% kcal)	Protein: 110 g (20% kcal)	Fat: 75 g (30% kcal)	Breakfast	Lunch	Dinner	Snacks PM	Snacks HS
Milk (low-fat)	2	24	16	10	1				1
Vegetable	3	15	6			1	2		
Fruit	3	45			1	1		1	
		84							
Bread	13	195	39		3	3	3	2	2
		279	61						
Meat	7		49	35	1	2	3	1	
			110	45					
Fat (polyunsaturated)	6			30	1	1	2	1	1
				75					

❖

BOX 20-1

Sample Menu Prescription: 2200 kcal

275 g carbohydrate (50% kcal)
110 g protein (20% kcal)
 75 g fat (30% kcal)

Breakfast

1 medium, sliced fresh peach
Shredded Wheat cereal
1 poached egg on whole-grain toast
1 bran muffin
1 tsp margarine
1 cup low-fat milk
Coffee or tea

Lunch

Vegetable soup with wheat crackers
Tuna sandwich on whole-wheat bread
   Filling: Tuna (drained ½ cup)
          Mayonnaise (2 tsp)
          Chopped dill pickle
          Chopped celery
Fresh pear

Afternoon snack

10 crackers with 2 tbsp peanut butter
Orange

Dinner

Pan-broiled pork chop (trimmed well)
1 cup brown rice
½-1 cup green beans
Tossed green salad
  Italian dressing (1-2 tbsp)
½ cup applesauce
1 bran muffin

Evening snack

3 cups popped, plain popcorn
1 oz cheese
1 cup low-fat milk

❖ **TABLE 20-5**   *Meal-planning guide for active people with IDDM*

Moderate activity	Exchange needs	Sample menu
30 minutes	1 bread OR 1 fruit	1 bran muffin OR 1 small orange
1 hour	2 bread + 1 meat OR 2 fruit + 1 milk	Tuna sandwich OR ½ cup fruit salad + 1 cup milk

Strenuous activity	Exchange needs	Sample menus
30 minutes	2 fruit OR 1 bread + 1 fat	1 small banana OR ½ bagel + 1 tsp cream cheese

1 hour	2 bread + 1 meat +
	1 milk OR
	2 bread + 2 meat +
	2 fruit
		Meat and cheese sandwich + 1
		  cup milk OR
		Hamburger + 1 cup orange
		  juice

❖ **TABLE 20-6** *How to modify a diabetic meal plan for sick days*

Usual food intake	Exchange	Carbohydrate (g)
½ chicken breast, roasted	3 meat	0
1 tsp margarine	1 fat	0
½ cup rice	1 bread	15
Tossed green salad, lemon wedge	Free food	0
¾ cup strawberries	1 fruit	10
1 cup skim milk	1 milk	12
		TOTAL 37

Sick day intake*	Exchange	Carbohydrate (g)
2 cups broth	Free food	0
1 cup gelatin	2 fruit	20
1 cup ginger ale (regular)	2 fruit	20
2 cups herbal tea	Free food	0
		TOTAL 40

* OBJECTIVE: To provide required amounts of carbohydrate for times when the person with diabetes has a poor appetite.

- Not omit insulin, but follow an adjusted dosage if needed
- Replace carbohydrate solid foods with equal liquid or soft foods
- Monitor blood sugar level frequently
- Contact physician if the illness lasts more than a day or so

5. *Travel.* When a trip is planned, the diet counselor and the client should confer to decide on food choices according to what will be available to the traveler. In general, preparation activities can include:

- Reviewing meal-planning skills, number and type of exchanges at each meal, basic portion sizes, and tips on eating out
- Learning about foods that will be available, such as ordering a diabetic diet ahead from airlines
- Selecting appropriate snacks to carry and planning time intervals for their use
- Planning for any time zone changes
- Carrying some quick-acting form of carbohydrate at all times and telling companions about signs, symptoms, and treatment of hypoglycemia
- Wearing an ID bracelet or pendant
- Securing physician's cover letter concerning syringes and insulin prescription

6. *Eating out.* In general, the person with diabetes should plan ahead so that accommodations for food eaten at home before and after the meal out can maintain the continuing day's balance. Also, choosing restaurants that have appropriate food available makes menu selection easier.

7. *Stress.* Any form of physiologic or psychosocial stress will affect diabetes control because of hormonal responses that are antagonistic to insulin action. Persons with diabetes, especially those using insulin, should learn useful stress-reduction exercises and activities as part of their self-care skills and practices.

DIABETES EDUCATION PROGRAM
Goal: person-centered self-care

The traditional roles of health care professionals and their patients and clients have been changing in current health care practice. Patients and clients are taking a much more active and informed role in their own health care. This action is especially true in the case of persons with diabetes. By the nature of the disease process and the necessity of daily "survival" skills, the person with diabetes must practice regular, daily self-care (Box 20-2). Thus any effective and successful diabetes education program must focus on personal needs and informed self-care skills. Professional communication must reflect this personal focus and supportive concern.

Content: tools for self-care

Necessary skills. Diabetes educators and the American Diabetes Association

---

BOX 20-2

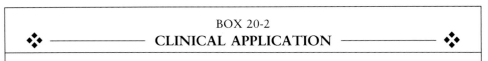

CLINICAL APPLICATION

Case Study: Richard Manages His Diabetes

Richard Smith, age 21, has insulin-dependent diabetes mellitus. He gives himself two injections a day, each a combination of medium-acting insulin and regular short-acting insulin. He gives one injection before breakfast and one before dinner. He usually tests his blood glucose level before each meal and at bedtime. He is a college student, usually active in athletics.

This is final exam week, however, and his schedule is irregular. He is putting in long hours of study and is under considerable stress. One the day before a particularly difficult examination, he is reviewing his study materials at home and forgets to do his blood test or eat lunch. About midafternoon he begins to feel faint and realizes that his blood sugar is low and an insulin reaction is approaching if he does not get a quick source of energy. He looks in the kitchen, and all he can find is orange juice, milk, butter, a loaf of bread, and a jar of peanut butter.

Questions for analysis

1. Which of the foods should Richard eat first, immediately?
2. Why did you make this choice?
   Later, when he is feeling better, he makes a peanut butter and butter sandwich, pours a glass of milk, and eats his snack while he continues studying.
3. What carbohydrate food sources of energy are in his snack?
4. Are these carbohydrate sources in a form the cells can burn for energy? What changes must Richard's body make in these sources to get them into the basic carbohydrate fuel form? What is the complex form of carbohydrate in his snack? Why is this a valuable form of carbohydrate in his diet? What is the basic form of carbohydrate fuel circulating in the blood for use by the cells?
5. What is the relationship of carbohydrate and fat in the final production of energy in the body? If Richard did not take his insulin to provide the necessary control agent for metabolizing the carbohydrate, what would happen to him as the result of improper handling of fat and accumulation of ketones?

have developed guidelines for diabetes education based on learning needs and the necessary skills and content areas required for self-care of diabetes. Persons with diabetes must have essential skills for the best possible control, as well as favorable surrounding factors related to life situations and psychosocial needs. These tools for self-care involve seven basic content areas.

1. *Nature of diabetes.* Persons should have a basic general knowledge of the nature of diabetes and how their form and degree of diabetes relates to this process. This means comparison of the "big" picture in general and their "personal" picture in particular. This would include initial basic survival needs as well as fulfillment of their own fundamental needs, especially support for personal concerns and feelings, in dealing with their diabetes.

2. *Nutrition.* Persons with diabetes should develop a sound food plan based on individual nutritional needs, living and working situations, and food habits. This would include understanding the relation of this food plan to maintaining good diabetes control and promoting positive health.

3. *Insulin.* Persons should understand types and combinations of insulin use or oral medication, their effects and how to regulate them. This would include learning good insulin injection technique, how the insulin used works in the body, and how its action relates to the food plan (Fig. 20-3).

4. *Monitoring glucose levels.* Monitoring of both blood glucose levels and urine sugar, as well as urinary acetone, is important. This includes learning accurate self-testing procedures as well as understanding the meaning of the results and knowing what action to take accordingly in relation to food, insulin, or exercise.

5. *Control of emergencies.* Persons should recognize the early signs of hypoglycemia and its causes and treatment. This would include knowledge of its relation to the balances among insulin, food, and exercise (Fig. 20-4) and how to prevent such episodes, as well as the immediate emergency treatment with some form of quick-acting simple carbohydrate to counteract it, followed by a snack of complex carbohydrate and protein to sustain a normal blood sugar level.

6. *Illness and special needs.* Persons with diabetes should learn how to deal with illness and other special needs, several of which were discussed earlier. These needs include knowledge of how to adjust diet and insulin, as well as planning ahead for events of daily living such as travel, eating out, exercise, or stress.

7. *Personal ID.* Persons with diabetes also should learn how to obtain a personal identification bracelet or pendant through registration with Medic Alert, an international agency located in Turlock, California. This includes understanding why having such identification at all times is important, especially for persons using insulin.

Levels of educational needs. These educational needs can be organized in a diabetes education program on three levels as a learning aid: (1) survival level, (2) home management level, and (3) life-style level.

Resources. A number of useful resources are available from health agencies such as the American Diabetes Association and the American Heart Association, including informational materials and a useful cookbook with nutritional values of recipes. Also, the press is offering more cookbooks for the current consumer market on the newer "light" cooking that reduces fat, sugar,

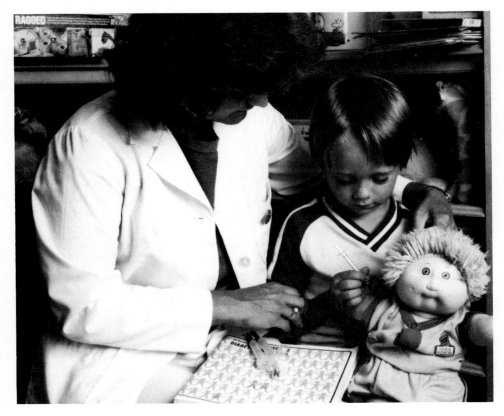

❖ FIG. 20-3

Young child with newly diagnosed insulin-dependent diabetes mellitus (IDDM) learning to inject his own insulin.

and salt and suggests many alternative seasonings and methods of preparation. In addition, resource persons include hospital and clinic dietitians, clinical nutritionists in private practice, public health nutritionists, and local chapters of the American Diabetic Association. Any resources used will need evaluation in terms of individual needs.

Staff education

In the final analysis, the success of the diabetes education program in any health care facility will depend on the sensitivity and training of the staff conducting the program. Continuing education for all professionals and their assistants is essential. Often educational games are useful tools as part of the staff education program, which in turn the staff can use in teaching their patients and clients. The recently developed journal, *The Diabetes Educator*, provides an excellent resource for teaching material. For example, one report describes three educational games: (1) "Tic-Tac-Diabetes," similar to a popular television program, with nine categories of questions, one of which is titled "Thick and Thin" and focuses on questions about meal planning and diet; (2) "What's Wrong with This Picture?" highlights the ADA Exchange Lists; and

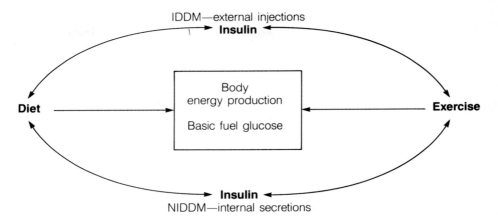

❖ **FIG. 20-4**

Basis of diabetes management: body energy balance. Interacting relations among diet (energy source), insulin (hormone controlling body use of basic fuel glucose), and exercise (physical activity using blood glucose. *IDDM*: Insulin-dependent diabetes mellitus. *NIDDM*: Non-insulin-dependent diabetes mellitus.

(3) "Can You Guess Your Blood Sugar?" helps staff become familiar with the different types of home blood glucose monitors.[8] Another report describes visual aids that demonstrate treatment for hypoglycemia, showing the difference between quick-energy foods needed immediately and the importance of follow-up with longer-acting complex carbohydrates and protein to maintain blood sugar levels.[9] Many such resources can be developed.

SUMMARY

Diabetes mellitus is a syndrome of varying forms and degrees with the common characteristic of hyperglycemia and other symptoms. Its underlying metabolic disorder involves all three of the energy nutrients—carbohydrate, fat, and protein—and influences energy balance. The major controlling hormone involved is insulin from the pancreas; diabetes results from either a lack of insulin or a resistance to its action.

Insulin-dependent diabetes mellitus (IDDM) affects approximately 15% of all persons with diabetes. It occurs primarily in children and is more severe and unstable. Its treatment involves regular meals and snacks balanced with insulin and exercise. Self-monitoring of blood glucose levels indicates needed corrective actions.

Non-insulin-dependent diabetes mellitus (NIDDM) occurs mostly in adults, especially those who are overweight. Acidosis is rare. Its treatment involves weight reduction and maintenance along with regular exercise.

For all forms of diabetes, the keystone of care is sound diet therapy. The basic food plan should be rich in complex carbohydrates and dietary fiber, low in simple sugars, fats (especially saturated fats), and cholesterol; and moderate in protein. Food should be distributed throughout the day in fairly regular amounts and at regular times, and tailored to meet individual needs.

❖ REVIEW QUESTIONS

1. Define diabetes mellitus. Describe the nature of the underlying metabolic disorder. What is the one common characteristic of all forms of diabetes mellitus?
2. Describe the major characteristics of the two main types of diabetes mellitus. Explain how these characteristics influence differences in nutritional therapy. List and describe medications used to control these conditions.
3. Identify and explain symptoms of uncontrolled diabetes mellitus.
4. Describe the possible long-term complications of poorly controlled diabetes mellitus.
5. Describe the principles of a sound diet for a person with diabetes mellitus in terms of the balance concept.

❖ SELF-TEST QUESTIONS

True-false

For each item you answer "false," write the correct statement.

1. The majority of persons with non-insulin-dependent diabetes mellitus (NIDDM) are underweight at the time the disease is discovered.
2. The two nutrients whose metabolism is most closely affected in diabetes are fat and protein.
3. Insulin is a hormone produced by the pituitary gland.
4. Insulin action is influenced by both glucagon and somatostatin.
5. Acetone in the urine of a person with diabetes usually indicates that the diabetes is in poor control.
6. In current practice, persons with diabetes are usually taught to test their own blood glucose daily and regulate their insulin, food, and exercise accordingly.
7. Coronary artery disease occurs in persons with diabetes at about four times the rate in the general population.
8. Diabetic complications occur in a relatively small number of the persons with long-term diabetes.
9. A diabetic diet is a combination of specific foods that should remain constant.
10. Persons with unstable insulin-dependent diabetes mellitus (IDDM) should follow a low-carbohydrate diet for better control.

Multiple choice

1. The caloric value of the diet for a person with diabetes should be:
   a. Increased above normal requirements to meet the increased metabolic demand
   b. Decreased below normal requirements to prevent glucose formation
   c. Sufficient to maintain the person's appropriate lean weight
   d. Contributed mainly by fat to spare the carbohydrate for energy needs
2. In the exchange system of diet control an ounce of cheese equals:
   (1) The same amount of meat
   (2) One cup of milk
   (3) Two tablespoons of peanut butter
   (4) One half cup ice milk

a. 1 and 3	c. 1 and 4
b. 2 and 4	d. 2 and 3
3. The exchange system of diet control is based on principles of:
   (1) Equivalent food values
   (2) Variety of food choices
   (3) Nutritional balance
   (4) Reeducation of eating habits

a. 1 and 3	c. 2 and 3
b. 2 and 4	d. All of these

BASIC PHYSIOLOGY OF THE KIDNEY
Fundamental role of the kidneys

The kidneys perform two major functions. First, they produce urine and in it excrete most of the end products of body metabolism. Second, they control the concentrations of most of the constituents of the body fluids, especially the blood. Tremendous quantities of fluid, about 180 L, are filtered through the kidneys each day. All but 1 to 1.5 L of this fluid is reabsorbed into circulation to maintain necessary body fluids, particularly the circulating blood volume and all its essential components. Thus, as the blood continuously circulates through the kidneys, these marvelous twin organs "launder" the blood repeatedly to monitor and maintain its precious quantity and constituents. Indeed, the composition of the body fluids is determined not so much by what the mouth takes in as by what the kidneys keep. They are the "master chemists" of our internal environment.

Renal nephrons

Basic functional unit. The basic functional unit of the kidney is the **nephron**. The two kidneys together contain about 2,400,000 nephrons, each of which is capable of forming urine by itself. Many of today's advances in treating kidney disease are based on providing maximal support for the nephron's vital functions. Each minute nephron structure is adapted in fine detail to its vital function of maintaining our balanced internal fluid environment necessary for life. At birth each of us has far more nephrons than we actually need. However, we begin to lose them gradually after age 30. Many researchers have related this loss to the excessive protein in our typical Western high-meat diet.[1]

Nephron functions. Each kidney contains about 1 million nephrons. As the body fluid flows through these finely built units, four life-supporting tasks are performed.

1. Filtration. Most of the entering blood's materials are filtered out, except for the larger components of red blood cells and proteins.

2. Reabsorption. As the filtrate continues through the winding tubules, substances the body needs are selectively reabsorbed and returned to the blood.

3. Secretion. Along the tubules, additional hydrogen ions $(H+)$ are secreted as needed to maintain acid-base balance.

4. Excretion. Unneeded waste materials are excreted in the now concentrated urine.

Nephron structures

These unique metabolic tasks that maintain body balance and life are performed by specific nephron structures. These key parts of the nephron include the **glomerulus** and the different tubules, as shown in Fig. 21-1.

Glomerulus. At the head of each nephron, a cup-shaped membrane holds the entering blood capillary and its branching tuft of smaller vessels. Here the blood is filtered across this closely held enveloping basement membrane. This cupped membrane and its tuft or cluster of branching capillaries is called the glomerulus, from the Latin word *glomus* meaning "ball." Only the larger blood proteins and cells remain behind in the circulating blood as it leaves the glomerulus.

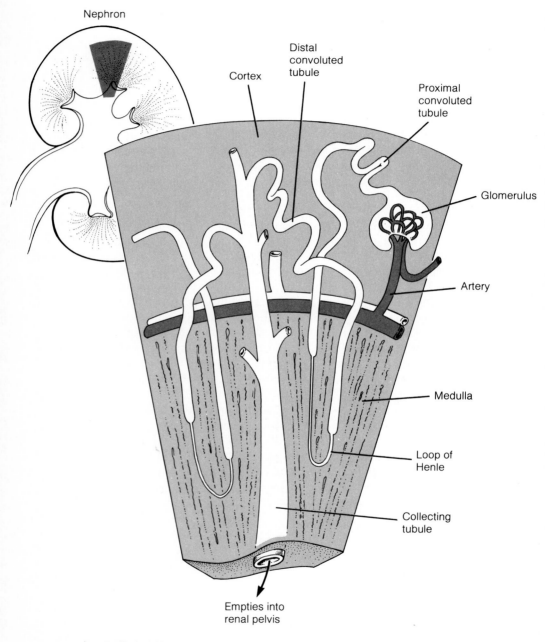

❖ FIG. 21-1

The nephron, functional unit of the kidney.

Tubules. From the cupped head of each nephron a small tubule carries the filtered fluid through its winding pathway and empties into the central area of the kidney. Specific materials are reabsorbed along the way in each of the four parts of these tubules.

1. *Proximal tubule.* Most of the needed nutrients in the fluid are reabsorbed in this first part of the tubule and returned to the blood. Usually all of the glucose and amino acids, as well as about 80% of the water and other substances, are reabsorbed here. Only about 20% of the filtered fluid remains to enter the next section of the tube.

2. *Loop of Henle.* This midsection of the tubule narrows and dips down into the central part of the kidney. Here important exchange of sodium and water takes place to concentrate the surrounding fluid in this central area of the kidney. This concentrated fluid environment maintains the necessary *osmotic pressure* to concentrate the urine as it passes through this central area later on its way out.

3. *Distal tubule.* This latter part of the tubule winds back up into the outer area of the kidney. Here secretion of H+ occurs as needed to provide acid-base balance. Also, sodium is reabsorbed as needed under the influence of the adrenal hormone **aldosterone** (p. 115).

4. *Collecting tubule.* In the final section of the tubule a normal concentrated urine is produced by two important water-reabsorbing actions: (1) influence of the pituitary hormone **antidiuretic hormone** (ADH), also called *vasopressin,* and (2) the osmotic pressure of the more dense surrounding fluid in the central area of the kidney. The volume of the urine now concentrated and ready for excretion is only 0.5% to 1.0% of the original fluid and its materials filtered through the glomerulus at the head of the nephron.

NEPHRON DISEASE PROBLEMS
General causes of kidney disease

Several disease conditions may interfere with this normal functioning of the nephrons and cause kidney disease.

Inflammatory and degenerative disease. The small blood vessels and membranes in the nephrons may become inflamed for a short time, as in acute *glomerulonephritis.* In other cases entire nephrons or nephron sections may be involved, stopping normal function and producing *nephrotic syndrome.* These nephrotic lesions may continue to affect more and more nephrons, leading to progressive *chronic renal failure.* As a result, the impaired metabolism of protein, electrolytes, and water creates nutritional disturbances.

Damage from other diseases. Circulatory disorders such as prolonged poorly controlled hypertension can cause degeneration of the small renal arteries and interfere with normal nephron function. Then increased demand on other nephrons can in turn cause more hypertension and still more damage to nephrons. Uncontrolled insulin-dependent diabetes mellitus (IDDM) can also damage small renal arteries leading to *glomerulosclerosis,* loss of functioning nephrons, and eventual chronic renal failure. Kidney abnormalities present from birth may lead to poor function, infection, or obstruction.

Infection and obstruction. Bacterial urinary tract infection may range from occasional mild discomfort from bladder infection to more involved chronic recurrent disease and obstruction from kidney stones. Obstruction anywhere in the urinary tract blocks drainage and causes further infection and general tissue damage.

Damage from other agents. Various environmental agents such as chemical pesticides, solvents, and similar materials are poisons that can cause kidney damage.[2] Animal venom, certain plants, and drugs may also harm renal tissue.

Nutritional therapy in renal disease

In the treatment of renal disease, nutritional therapy in each case is based on the nature of the disease process and individual responses.

Length of disease. In short-term acute disease, medical therapy with antibiotics usually controls the disease and nutritional therapy is largely optimal nutrition support for healing and normal growth. Long-term chronic disease will involve more specific nutrient modifications.

Degree of impaired renal function. In milder acute disease with only a few nephrons involved, less interference occurs with general renal function as the large number of backup nephrons can meet basic needs. In progressive chronic disease, however, more and more nephrons become involved and renal failure finally results. In these cases, extensive nutritional therapy is required to help maintain renal function as long as possible.

Individual clinical symptoms. In continuing disease, nutrient modifications are designed to meet individual needs according to specific clinical symptoms. This personalized nutritional therapy becomes especially important in advanced renal disease treated with dialysis.

In this chapter we focus primarily on the more serious degenerative process of chronic renal failure and dialysis, which require much special nutritional therapy. Brief reviews of nutrition support for short-term conditions will provide reference for general nutritional care.

Glomerulonephritis

Disease process. This inflammatory process affects the glomeruli, the small blood vessels in the cupped membrane at the head of the nephron. It occurs mostly in young children and usually follows a brief course in its acute form.

Clinical symptoms. Classic symptoms include **hematuria** and **proteinuria**. There may be some **edema** and mild **hypertension**. The patient usually has little appetite, which contributes to feeding problems. If the disease progresses to more renal involvement, signs of **oliguria** or **anuria** may develop.

Nutritional therapy. General care in uncomplicated disease centers mainly on bed rest and antibiotic drug therapy. Pediatricians and nutritionists favor overall optimum nutrition support for growth with adequate protein. Salt is usually not restricted. In most patients with acute short-term disease, especially children with poststreptococcal disease, diet modifications are not crucial. Fluid intake is adjusted to output as a rule.

If the disease process advances, however, more specific nutritional therapy may be indicated according to individual needs.

1. *Protein.* If the **blood urea nitrogen** (**BUN**) is elevated and urine output decreased, dietary protein must be restricted. Usually the diet is modified to a

lowered protein intake of 0.5 g/kg ideal body weight. As long as renal function is adequate enough to maintain a normal BUN level, dietary protein intake may be held at 1 g/kg body weight.

2. *Carbohydrate.* To provide sufficient energy in dietary kcalories, carbohydrates should be given liberally. This intake will also help combat catabolism of tissue protein and prevent starvation **ketosis**.

3. *Sodium.* If low urine output indicates impaired renal function, the sodium may be restricted to 500 to 1000 mg/day (p. 302). As recovery occurs, normal sodium intake of 2 to 3 g/day may be resumed.

4. *Potassium.* If oliguria becomes severe, renal clearance of potassium will be impaired. Thus potassium intake must be monitored carefully according to individual needs.

5. *Water.* Fluid intake is restricted according to urine output. If restriction is not indicated, fluids can be consumed as desired.

Nephrotic syndrome

Disease process. The nephrotic syndrome, or **nephrosis**, results from nephron tissue damage to both glomerulus and tubule. The primary damage is in the major filtering membrane of the glomerulus, allowing large amounts of protein to pass into the tubule. This high protein concentration of the fluid in turn causes further damage to the tubule. Both filtration and reabsorption functions of the nephron are disrupted. This condition may be caused by progressive glomerulonephritis; by other diseases such as diabetes or connective tissue disorders—**collagen disease**; or by other agents such as drugs, heavy metals, or toxic venom from stinging insects such as bees.

Clinical symptoms. Nephrotic syndrome is characterized by a group of symptoms resulting from the nephron tissue damage and impaired function. The large protein loss leads to massive edema and **ascites**, as well as proteinuria. The abdomen becomes distended as the fluid accumulates. The plasma protein level is greatly reduced, especially in the albumin fraction, because of the large loss in the urine. As protein loss continues, tissue proteins are broken down and general malnutrition follows. The severe edema and ascites often masks the extent of the body tissue wasting.

Nutritional therapy. The former standard recommendation for patients with nephrotic syndrome was a high-protein diet, sometimes as high as 3 to 4 g/kg per day. However, current evidence indicates that high-protein diets may accelerate loss of renal function, and that moderately low-protein diets reduce albuminuria and albumin catabolism, with no change in glomerular filtration rate (GFR).[3] Thus physicians and clinical nutritionists are now managing these patients with diets containing less protein.

1. *Protein.* Protein intake should be moderately low, usually 0.6 to 0.8 g/day. An addition of 1.0 g/day of high-biologic protein (p. 42) is given for each gram of urinary protein loss daily. Thus individual total protein will vary according to daily losses.

2. *Kcalories.* Sufficient kcalories must always be provided to free protein for tissue rebuilding. High daily intakes of 50 to 60 kcal/kg may be required. Because appetite is usually poor, food must be as appetizing as possible and in a form most easily tolerated. Much support is needed.

3. Sodium. Dietary sodium may be moderately reduced to approximately 1000 mg/day if needed to help prevent edema.

4. Other minerals and vitamins. There is no need for potassium restriction. Iron and vitamin supplements may be helpful.

CHRONIC RENAL FAILURE
Disease process

Acute renal failure. Acute renal failure may result from some metabolic insult or traumatic injury to normal kidneys. The cause may be severe tissue damage as in extensive burns or crushing injuries. It may also result from infectious disease such as peritonitis, or from various toxic agents. Its effects are sudden and life threatening. Its major sign is oliguria.

Chronic renal failure. On the other hand, chronic renal failure comes from progressive degenerative renal disease and marked impairment of all renal

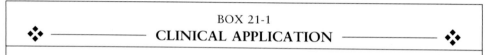

BOX 21-1

❖ ———— CLINICAL APPLICATION ———— ❖

Case Study: The Patient With Chronic Renal Failure

Charles Brown, age 49, is an active man working in a large company. Over a period of time he has begun to tire more easily. He has little appetite and feels generally ill most of the time. Recently he has noticed some ankle swelling and some blood in his urine. Finally, at his wife's insistence, he decided to see his physician.

After a complete workup, the physician's findings included: (1) no prior illness except a case of "flu" with throat infection during Charles' overseas service in the Army; (2) laboratory tests: albumin, red and white cells in the urine; elevated BUN and GFR (glomerular filtration rate); (3) other symptoms: hypertension, edema, headache, occasional vision blurring, and low grade fever. The physician discussed the findings with Charles and his wife, the serious prognosis of advanced renal disease, and together they explored the immediate medical and nutritional needs for treatment. They also discussed the ultimate need for medical management with dialysis. The physician began medications to control Charles' growing symptoms and discomfort.

As time went by, Charles' symptoms increased. He lost more weight, was anemic, and having increased bone and joint pain. Gastrointestinal bleeding and nausea also increased, and he had occasional muscle twitching or spasms. Numerous small mouth ulcers made eating a painful effort. Visits to the clinic nutritionist were made, so Charles and his wife could learn how to manage his present predialysis diet at home.

Questions for Analysis

1. What metabolic imbalances in chronic renal failure do you think accounted for the symptoms Charles was having?
2. What are the objectives of treatment in chronic renal failure?
3. What are the basic principles of Charles' predialysis diet? Describe this type of diet. What foods would be included? Plan a 1-day menu for Charles.
4. What nutrient-related medications and supplements would Charles' physician and clinical nutritionist probably use in his treatment plan? Why?

functions. Few functioning nephrons remain, and gradually these deteriorate. A downhill course inevitably follows. The disease process takes its toll from the "aging Western kidney" made vulnerable by our lifetime of large protein meals.[4] Now, in many Western countries, our adult diet averages about 3000 kcalories and more than 100 g of protein, largely meat, *daily*.

Clinical symptoms

Depending on the nature of the underlying renal disease, the chronic renal changes may involve extensive scarring of renal tissue. This distorts the kidney structure and brings vascular changes from prolonged hypertension. As the nephrons are lost one by one, the remaining ones gradually lose their ability to sustain vital body metabolic balances.

Water balance. Increasingly the kidney cannot reabsorb water and excrete a normal concentrated urine. Dehydration follows and may become critical. At other times when fluid intake exceeds output, water intoxication may occur.

Electrolyte balances. Several imbalances among electrolytes result from decreasing nephron function. The failing kidney cannot appropriately respond to maintain the vital sodium-potassium balance that guards body water (p. 109). A concentration of materials is produced by metabolism of food, such as phosphate, sulfate, and organic acids, which causes metabolic acidosis. The disturbed metabolism of calcium and phosphate from lack of activated vitamin D, a process that occurs in the kidney (p. 68), brings bone pain from a disease called **osteodystrophy.**

Nitrogen retention. Increasing loss of nephron function brings elevated amounts of nitrogenous metabolites such as **urea** and **creatinine**.

Anemia. The damaged kidney cannot accomplish its normal participation in the production of red blood cells. Thus fewer red cells are produced and those that are made survive a shorter time.

Hypertension. When blood flow to renal tissue is increasingly impaired, renal hypertension develops. In turn the hypertension causes cardiovascular damage and further deterioration of the kidneys.

Azotemia. The elevated BUN, serum creatinine, and serum uric acid levels are reflected in the characteristic laboratory finding of azotemia.

General signs and symptoms. Increasing loss of renal function brings progressive weakness, shortness of breath, general lethargy, and fatigue. Thirst, appetite loss, weight loss, diarrhea, and vomiting may occur. Increasing capillary fragility brings skin, nose, oral, and gastrointestinal bleeding. Nervous system involvement brings muscular twitching, burning sensations in the extremities, or convulsions. Irregular cyclic breathing (Cheyne-Stokes respiration) indicates acidosis. There is ulceration of the mouth, a bad taste, and fetid breath. Malnutrition lowers resistance to infection. Bone and joint pain continues.

Nutritional therapy

Basic objectives. Treatment must always be individual. In general, however, basic therapy objectives in care of chronic renal failure are to:
- Reduce protein breakdown
- Avoid dehydration or excess hydration

❖ **TABLE 21-1**   *Protein and nitrogen needs in chronic renal failure*

Creatinine clearance (ml/min)	Nitrogen* (g/day)	Protein (g/day)
40 and above	Unrestricted	Unrestricted
10-40	9.6	60
5-20	6.4	40†
2-10	2.5-3.0 (+ 1.3-2.6)	20 (+ EAA/ana-logues)†
8 and below	Transplantation Dialysis	
5 and below	Dialysis	

*Total protein/6.25.
†EAA. Essential amino acids/alpha-keto-, alpha-hydroxy-analogues of EAA.

- Correct acidosis
- Correct electrolyte imbalances
- Control fluid and electrolyte losses from vomiting and diarrhea
- Maintain optimal nutritional status
- Maintain appetite, general morale, and sense of well-being
- Control complications of hypertension, bone pain, and nervous system involvement
- Retard rate of renal failure, postponing ultimate need for dialysis

Principles of nutritional therapy. Nutrition for chronic renal failure involves variable nutrient adjustments according to individual need.

1. Protein. The critical problem is to provide just enough protein to maintain tissue but avoid a damaging excess. Protein is generally limited to 0.5 to 0.6 g/kg/day, of which at least 0.35 g/kg/day is from high-biologic value protein (p. 42) to ensure an adequate intake of essential amino acids. Some clinicians adjust protein according to *creatinine* clearance, indicating no need to restrict protein intake until this renal function falls below 40 ml/min. Then dietary protein must be decreased as renal function declines (Table 21-1). A very low 20 g protein diet, supplemented with essential amino acids, is used in advanced renal disease to slow progression of renal insufficiency.[5]

2. Amino acid supplements. Mixtures of essential amino acids or amino acid **precursors** provide necessary protein supplementation for low-protein diets. Other supplements consist of nitrogen-free "copies" of essential amino acids called **analogues.**

3. Kilocalories. Carbohydrate and fat must supply sufficient nonprotein kcalories to spare protein for tissue protein synthesis and to supply energy. Approximately 300 to 400 g of carbohydrate is needed daily. Sufficient fat, 75 to 90 g/day, is added to give the patient 2000 to 2500 total kcalories daily.

4. Water. With predialysis patients, fluid intake should be sufficient to maintain adequate urine volume. Usually intake is balanced with output.

5. Sodium. The need for sodium varies. If hypertension and edema are present, sodium intake needs to be restricted. Usually sodium intake ranges from 500 to 2000 mg/day (p. 302).

6. *Potassium.* The damaged kidney cannot clear potassium adequately; thus the dietary intake is kept at about 1500 mg/day.

7. *Phosphate and calcium.* Moderate dietary phosphorus restriction to about 500 to 600 mg/day, along with the protein restriction, is an effective means of delaying progressive renal failure. A calcium supplement is used to correct the hypocalcemia.

8. *Vitamins.* A multivitamin supplement is usually added to the diet of renal patients on protein restriction. A diet of 40 g protein or less does not contribute the full daily need of all the vitamins.

Kidney dialysis

The lives of an estimated 50,000 persons in the United States who develop kidney disease each year have been prolonged by **dialysis** and kidney transplants. A scarcity of organ donors and rejection problems, however, limit transplants. Thus dialysis has become the major treatment for advanced renal disease, especially since coverage of its considerable cost, approximately $1.4 billion each year, by Medicare. Two forms of dialysis are used: hemodialysis and ambulatory peritoneal dialysis.

Hemodialysis. Hemodialysis using an artificial kidney machine (Fig. 21-2) removes toxic substances from the blood and helps restore normal blood levels of the nutrients and their metabolites. To prepare the patient for hemodialysis therapy, a surgical fistula is made by joining an artery and a vein on the forearm just beneath the skin. After this attachment has healed, a needle is inserted through the healed tissue and connected by tubes to the dialysis machine. A patient with chronic renal failure usually requires two to three treatments a week, each treatment lasting 4 to 8 hours. During each treatment the patient's blood makes several round trips through the dialysis solution in the machine, removing excess waste material to maintain normal blood levels of life-sustaining substances that the patient's own kidneys can no longer accomplish. There are two compartments in the machine. One contains blood from the patient carrying all the excess fluids and waste materials, and the other contains the *dialysate*, a solution that may be thought of as a "cleaning fluid." A filter separates the two compartments. As in normal capillary filtration, the blood cells are too large to pass through the pores in the filter. The remaining smaller molecules in the blood, however, pass through the filter and are carried away by the dialysate. If the patient's blood is deficient in certain materials, these may be added to the dialysate.

The diet of a hemodialysis patient plays an important role in maintaining biochemical control. Several basic objectives govern each individual's diet, which is designed to (1) maintain protein and kcalorie balance, (2) prevent dehydration or fluid overload, (3) maintain normal serum potassium and sodium levels, and (4) maintain acceptable phosphate and calcium levels. Control of infection is always an underlying goal. Nutritional therapy in most cases can be planned with more liberal nutrient allowances.

1. *Protein.* For most adult dialysis patients, a standard protein allowance of 1 g/kg lean body weight, carefully calculated for each patient by the dialysis center's clinical dietitians, provides for nutritional needs, maintains positive nitrogen balance, does not produce excessive nitrogenous waste, and replaces the amino acids lost during each dialysis treatment. At least 75% of this daily

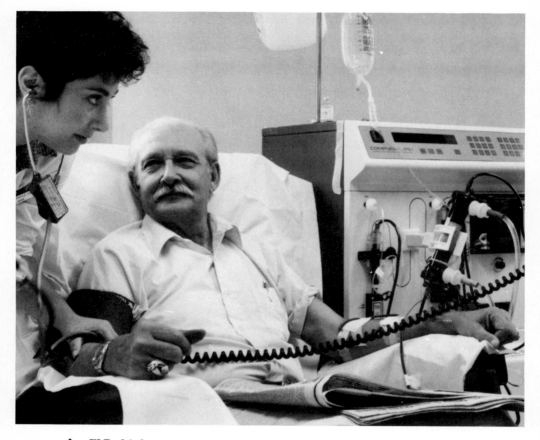

❖ FIG. 21-2

Patient with end-stage chronic renal disease undergoing hemodialysis treatment.

allowance should consist of protein foods of high biologic value, such as eggs, meat, fish, and poultry, but little if any milk. Milk is restricted because it adds more fluid and has a high content of sodium, phosphate, and potassium.

2. *Kilocalories.* A generous amount of carbohydrates with some fat will continue to supply needed kcalories for energy and protein sparing. The usual prescription is for 40 kcal/kg lean body weight. Simple carbohydrate foods should supply most of the carbohydrate, with control of complex carbohydrates such as grains and legumes because they contain incomplete protein and should not take up large amounts of the limited protein allowance.

3. *Water balance.* Fluid is usually limited to 400 to 500 ml/day, plus an amount equal to urine output, if any.

4. *Sodium.* To control body fluid retention and hypertension, sodium is limited to 1000 to 2000 mg/day.

5. *Potassium.* To prevent potassium accumulation, which can cause cardiac problems, potassium intake is restricted to 1500 to 2000 mg/day.

6. *Vitamins.* A supplement of the water-soluble vitamins, B complex and C, is given to replace their loss during the dialysis treatment.

Ambulatory peritoneal dialysis

An alternate form of treatment for some patients is *peritoneal* dialysis. This form has the convenience of home use. In this process, the patient introduces the dialysate solution directly into the peritoneal cavity, four or five times a day, where it can be exchanged for fluids that contain the metabolic waste products. Since the dialysis resulting is continuous within the body between solutions being added and drained, this process is called *continuous ambulatory peritoneal dialysis (CAPD)*. First, the patient is prepared by surgical insertion of a permanent catheter. Then each treatment is done by attaching a disposable bag containing the dialysate solution to the abdominal catheter leading into the peritoneal cavity, waiting 20 to 30 minutes for the solution exchange, then lowering the bag to allow the force of gravity to cause the waste-containing fluid to drain into it. When the bag is empty, it can be folded around the waist or tucked into a pocket, affording the patient mobility. Intermittent use of peritoneal dialysis, self-administered at home, gives the patient more mobility and a sense of being in control. Sometimes an automated device is used to provide several solution exchanges during night sleep hours and one continuous exchange during the day. This technique is called *continuous cyclic peritoneal dialysis (CCPD)*. With peritoneal dialysis and good self-care, a more liberal diet may be used. The patient can:

- Increase protein intake to 1.2 to 1.5 g/kg body weight
- Limit phosphorus to 1200 mg/day by restricting phosphorus-rich foods, such as nuts and legumes, to one serving/week and dairy products, including eggs, to a half-cup portion or one egg or its equivalent each day
- Increase potassium by eating a wide variety of fruits and vegetables each day
- Encourage liberal fluid intake to prevent dehydration
- Avoid sweets and fats to control triglycerides and low-density lipoprotein levels
- Maintain lean body weight by incorporating the kcalories provided by the dialysate solution into the total meal plan

RENAL CALCULI PROBLEMS
Disease process

The basic cause of renal calculi is unknown. However, many factors relating to the nature of the urine itself or to the conditions of the urinary tract environment contribute to their formation. The four major stones formed are calcium, struvite, uric acid, and cystine stones. Fig. 21-3 illustrates the formation of these various stones.

Calcium stones. Approximately 96% of kidney stones are composed of calcium compounds, mainly calcium oxalate or calcium oxalate mixed with calcium phosphate.[6] Excessive urinary calcium may result from several factors: (1) excess intake from large amounts of high-calcium foods or hard water; (2) excess vitamin D, which increases calcium absorption; (3) prolonged immobilization, as in body casting or extended illness or disability, which increases calcium withdrawal from bone; or (4) hyperparathyroidism, which causes excess calcium excretion. In some persons, because of some error in handling

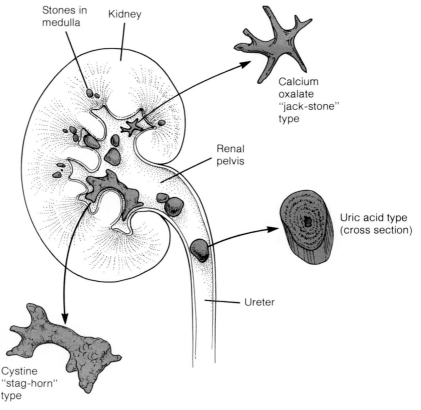

Stones in medulla   Kidney

Calcium oxalate "jack-stone" type

Renal pelvis

Uric acid type (cross section)

Ureter

Cystine "stag-horn" type

❖   **FIG. 21-3**

Renal calculi: stones in kidney, pelvis, and ureter.

oxalates, the oxalate forms compounds with calcium. This formation accounts for about half of all the calcium stones. Oxalates occur naturally in only a few foods (Box 21-2).

Struvite stones. Of the remaining 4% of all kidney stones, struvite stones occur most frequently. These stones are composed of a single compound, magnesium ammonium phosphate ($MgNH_4PO_4$). They are often called *infection stones* since their main cause is urinary tract infection, not an association with any specific nutrient. Thus no specific diet therapy is involved. These are usually large "stag-horn" stones that are removed surgically.

Uric acid stones. Excess excretion of uric acid may be caused by some impairment with the metabolism of **purine**, from which uric acid is formed. This impairment occurs in diseases such as gout. It can also occur in rapid tissue breakdown during wasting disease.

Cystine stones. The most rare kidney stones are cystine stones. They are caused by a genetic metabolic defect in the renal reabsorption of the amino acid cystine. This defect results in an accumulation of cystine in the urine, a condition called **cystinuria**. Since this disorder is of genetic origin, it occurs rarely and only in children with this genetic history.

❖

BOX 21-2
Food Sources of Oxalates

Fruits	*Vegetables*	*Nuts*	*Beverages*	*Other*
Berries, all	Baked beans	Almonds	Chocolate	Grits
Currants	Beans, green	Cashews	Cocoa	Tofu, soy
Concord	and wax	Peanuts	Draft beer	products
grapes	Beets	Peanut	Tea	Wheat germ
Figs	Beet greens	butter		
Fruit cocktail	Celery			
Plums	Chard, Swiss			
Rhubarb	Chives			
Tangerines	Collards			
	Eggplant			
	Endive			
	Kale			
	Leeks			
	Mustard greens			
	Okra			
	Peppers, green			
	Rutabagas			
	Spinach			
	Squash, summer			
	Sweet, potatoes			
	Tomatoes			
	Tomato soup			
	Vegetable soup			

General symptoms and treatment

Clinical symptoms. The main symptom of kidney stones is severe pain. Many other urinary symptoms may result from the presence of the stones. There is usually general weakness and sometimes fever. Laboratory examination of the urine and any stone passed help determine treatment.

Treatment. General treatment may include several considerations.

1. Fluid intake. A large fluid intake is a primary therapy. It helps to produce a more dilute urine and prevent accumulation of materials that form stones.

2. Stone composition. In some cases dietary control of the stone constituents may help reduce the recurrence of such stone formation. This would help to prevent the accumulation of these metabolic substances in the urine available for stone formation.

3. Urinary pH. This factor in relation to diet therapy for renal stones has been given much emphasis in the past, but now is being questioned. Research has indicated that acidification of the urine by traditional acid/alkaline ash diets may have little effect on urinary tract infections or the formation of stones in the urinary tract, because calculation methods for determining urinary pH effect of specific foods have not proved to be valid.[7] It is only in general, not precise, terms that vegetables, fruits, and milk are called "alkaline ash foods" or that meat, cheese, eggs, and whole grains are called "acid ash foods." Thus a desired pH of the urine is better achieved by medical means than traditional acid/alkaline ash diets.

4. Binding agents. Materials that bind potential stone elements in the intestine can prevent their absorption and eliminate them from the body. For example, sodium phytate is used to bind calcium and aluminum gels are used to bind phosphate. Glycine has a similar effect on oxalates.

Nutritional therapy

The nutritional plan of care is mainly related to the nature of the stone. The diet is designed to reduce intake of nutrients leading to formation of the particular type of stone.

❖ **TABLE 21-2** *Low-calcium diet (approximately 400 mg calcium)*

Group	Foods allowed	Foods not allowed
Beverage*	Carbonated beverage, coffee, tea	Chocolate-flavored drinks, milk, milk drinks
Bread	White and light rye bread or crackers	
Cereals	Refined cereals	Oatmeal, whole-grain cereals
Desserts	Cake, cookies, gelatin desserts, pastries, pudding, sherbets, all made without chocolate, milk, or nuts; if egg yolk is used, it must be from one egg allowance	
Fat	Butter, cream (2 tbsp daily) French dressing, margarine, salad oil, shortening	Cream (except in amount allowed), mayonnaise
Fruits	Canned, cooked, or fresh fruits or juice except rhubarb	Dried fruit, rhubarb
Meat, eggs	224 g (8 oz) daily of any meat, fowl, or fish except clams, oysters, or shrimp; not more than one egg daily including those used in cooking	Clams, oysters, shrimp, cheese
Potato or substitute	Potato, hominy, macaroni, noodles, refined rice, spaghetti	Whole-grain rice
Soup	Broth, vegetable soup made from vegetables allowed	Bean or pea soup, cream or milk soup
Sweets	Honey, jam, jelly, sugar	
Vegetables	Any canned, cooked, or fresh vegetables or juice except those listed	Dried beans, broccoli, green cabbage, celery, chard, collards, endive, greens, lettuce, lentils, okra, parsley, parsnips, dried peas, rutabagas
Miscellaneous	Herbs, pickles, popcorn, relishes, salt, spices, vinegar	Chocolate, cocoa, milk gravy, nuts, olives, white sauce

*Depending on calcium content of local water supply. In instances of high calcium content, distilled water may be indicated.

Calcium stones. A low-calcium diet of about 400 mg/day is usually given (Table 21-2). This is about half the average adult intake of 800 mg. This lower level is achieved mainly by removal of milk and dairy products, the main dietary sources of calcium. Other secondary calcium sources are whole grains and leafy vegetables. If the stone is calcium phosphate, the additional sources of phosphorus would be controlled—meats, legumes, and nuts. If it is a calcium oxalate stone, foods high in oxalate (Box 21-2) would be avoided.

As indicated, there is little value in trying to acidify the urine by dietary means in an effort to prevent formation of alkaline stones such as calcium-based ones. Although cranberry juice has been advocated for this purpose, for example, the concentrations and volumes involved in study of its effect are not practical for clinical use. Commercial cranberry juices on the consumer market are far too dilute to be effective, since they contain only about 26% cranberry juice, and a very large amount would be required for any consistent urinary effect. Instead, to achieve a sustained effect on urinary pH, most physicians rely on drugs.

Uric acid stones. Since uric acid is a metabolic product of purines, a low-purine diet is sometimes used, although modern medical treatment achieves more effective control with specific drugs. If dietary control of purines is desired, it can easily be achieved by a vegetarian diet that eliminates most meat, especially organ meats, and concentrated meat extracts and gravies, and that is moderately low in fat.

Cystine stones. Since cystine is derived from the essential amino acid *methionine*, sometimes a low-methionine diet may be used. However, since this diet is essentially a low-protein diet and the rare genetic cystinuria condition occurs mainly in children, the treatment of choice is usually a regular diet to support growth. Medical drug therapy would be used to control infection or produce a more alkaline urine.

SUMMARY

The nephrons are the functional units of the kidneys. Through these unique structures, the kidney maintains life-sustaining blood levels of materials required for life and health. The nephrons accomplish their tremendous task by constantly "laundering" the blood over and over many times each day, returning to the blood what it needs and eliminating the remainder in a concentrated urine. Various diseases that interfere with this vital nephron function can, if damage is extensive, cause serious renal disease.

Chronic renal failure at its end stage is treated by dialysis and kidney transplant. Dialysis patients require close monitoring for protein, water, and electrolyte balance. Renal diseases have predisposing factors. For example, recurrent urinary tract infections may lead to renal calculi, and progressive glomerulonephritis may lead to chronic nephrotic syndrome and renal failure. The Western diet is suspect as a predisposing factor in the development of chronic renal failure. Our modern diet of excess protein may overtax human nephrons, which were not originally designed to handle a steady diet of protein-rich foods.

❖ REVIEW QUESTIONS

1. For each of the following conditions, outline the nutritional components of therapy, explaining the impact of each on kidney function: glomerulonephritis, nephrotic syndrome, and chronic renal failure.
2. List the nutritional factors that must be monitored in persons undergoing renal dialysis.
3. Outline the medical and nutritional therapy for various types of renal stones. Why are acid/alkaline diet modifications no longer valid therapy?

❖ SELF-TEST QUESTIONS

True-false
For each item you answer "false," write the correct statement.
1. The basic functional unit of the kidney is the nephron.
2. There are only a few nephrons in each kidney, so a metabolic stress load can easily cause problems.
3. The operation of the nephrons has little relation to the rest of the body.
4. The task of the glomerulus is filtration.
5. The tasks of the various parts of the nephron tubules are reabsorption, secretion, and excretion.
6. Dietary modifications in acute glomerulonephritis usually involve crucial restrictions of protein and sodium.
7. The primary symptom in nephrotic syndrome is massive albuminuria.
8. The nephrotic syndrome is best treated by a moderately low-protein diet.
9. The multiple symptoms of advanced chronic renal failure result basically from metabolic imbalances in the body's inability to handle protein, electrolytes, and water.
10. Prolonged immobilization, as in full body casts or disability, may lead to withdrawal of bone calcium and the formation of calcium renal stones.

Multiple choice
1. Acute glomerulonephritis is best treated by:
   (1) Reducing protein, since filtration is impaired
   (2) Using normal amount of protein for optimum tissue nutrition and growth
   (3) Restricting sodium to help control edema
   (4) Allowing moderate salt use in uncomplicated cases
      a. 1 and 3   c. 1 and 2
      b. 2 and 4   d. 3 and 4
2. Diet therapy in nephrotic syndrome is designed to:
   (1) Increase protein to replace the massive losses
   (2) Decrease protein moderately to reduce albumin losses
   (3) Increase kcalories to provide energy and spare protein for tissue need
   (4) Decrease kcalories to reduce metabolic workload
   (5) Restrict sodium moderately to help prevent edema
   (6) Restrict sodium only mildly to aid food taste and improve appetite
      a. 2, 3, and 5   c. 1, 4, and 5
      b. 1, 4, and 6   d. 1, 3, and 6

3. The general diet needs in chronic renal failure include:
   (1) Reduced protein intake
   (2) Increased carbohydrate and moderate fat for needed energy
   (3) Careful control of sodium and potassium according to need
   (4) Increased fluids to stimulate kidney function
       a. 1, 2, and 3   c. 1, 3, and 4
       b. 2, 3, and 4   d. 1, 2, and 4

❖ SUGGESTIONS FOR ADDITIONAL STUDY

Individual or group project: kidney dialysis center
Assign students in the class to visit a kidney dialysis center if one is available in your community. Observe the operation of the center. Interview one of the staff nurses and a clinical nutritionist about the dialysis procedure and the dietary management used with the patients. If any teaching materials or diet guides are available, bring copies back to class for use in reporting your visit.

References

1. Brenner BM, Meyer TW, and Hostetter TH: Dietary protein intake and the progressive nature of kidney disease, N Engl J Med 307(11):652, 1982.
2. Abuelo JG: Renal failure caused by chemicals, foods, plants, animal venoms, and misuse of drugs, Arch Intern Med 150:505, March 1990.
3. Coggins CH and Cornell BF: Nutritional management of nephrotic syndrome, in Mitch WE and Klahr S, editors: Nutrition and the kidney, ed 1, Boston, 1988, Little Brown & Co.
4. Piper CM: Very-low-protein diets in chronic renal failure: nutrient content and guidelines for supplementation, J Am Diet Assoc 85(10):1344, 1985.
5. Methany N: Renal stones and urinary pH, Am J Nurs 82:1372, 1982.
6. Dwyer J and others: Acid/alkaline ash diets: time for assessment and change, J Am Diet Assoc 85(7):841, 1985.

Further reading

Curtis JA: The renal patient's guide to good eating: A cookbook for patients by a patient, Springfield, Ill, 1989, Charles C Thomas, Publisher.

    This is an excellent resource filled with ideas for following a renal diet, from the author's own experience as a renal patient herself. It can be recommended to patients.

Van Duyn MA: Acceptability of selected low-protein products for use in diet therapy for chronic renal failure, J Am Diet Assoc 87(7):909, 1987.

    This survey report identifies several acceptable low-protein products that can be used in diets for patients with renal failure to help increase needed kcalories and still maintain the necessary protein restriction.

22

❖

Nutritional care
of surgery patients

K E Y   C O N C E P T S

*Surgical treatment requires added nutritional support
for tissue healing and rapid recovery.*

*Special nutritional problems of gastrointestinal
surgery require diet modifications according to
effect of the surgery on normal food passage.*

*Diet management for surgery patients to ensure optimal nutritional
support involves both oral and venous feeding methods.*

$\mathcal{M}$ alnutrition continues to occur among hospitalized patients, many of whom are surgical patients. Surveys in both American and European hospitals show that almost 50% of the surgical patients have clinical signs of protein-energy malnutrition. This poor state of nutrition hinders healing. Effective nutritional support can reverse this malnutrition, greatly improve prognosis, and speed recovery. The surgical process also places physiologic and psychologic stress on patients, bringing added nutritional demands and risks of clinical problems.

In this chapter we look at these nutritional needs of surgery patients. We see that careful attention to both preoperative and postoperative nutritional support can reduce complications and provide essential resources for healing and health.

NUTRITIONAL NEEDS OF GENERAL SURGERY PATIENTS

A patient undergoing surgery faces great physiologic and psychologic stress on the body. As a result, during this period nutritional demands are greatly increased. Deficiencies can easily develop. If these deficiencies are allowed to develop and are not met, serious malnutrition and clinical problems can occur. It is imperative, therefore, that careful attention be given to the patient's nutritional status in preparation for surgery and to the individual nutritional therapy needs that follow. If these needs are met, there is less risk that complications will develop, and resources will be provided for better wound healing and a more rapid recovery.

Preoperative nutritional care: nutrient reserves

When the surgery is elective, not an emergency, body nutrient stores can be built up to fortify the patient for the demands of the surgery and the immediate period following the period of limited food intake. Particular needs center on protein, energy, vitamins, and minerals.

Protein. Protein deficiencies among surgical patients are far more common than one would assume. Surveys of surgical wards in large city hospitals have revealed obvious protein-energy malnutrition and multiple postsurgical complications. Every patient facing surgery needs to be fortified with adequate body protein in tissue and plasma reserves to counteract blood losses during surgery and to prevent tissue breakdown in the immediate postoperative period.

Energy. Sufficient kcalories must always be provided when increased protein is required for tissue building. The increased kcalories support the added energy demands and spare the protein for its tissue-building work. For example, increased carbohydrate is needed to maintain optimal glycogen stores in the liver as a necessary resource for immediate energy fuel, thus directing protein to its tissue synthesis task. Also, if the patient is underweight, extra kcalories are needed to increase the weight to ideal maintenance level before surgery. If the person is overweight, some weight reduction may be indicated to help reduce surgical risks.

Vitamins and minerals. When increased protein and kcalories are required for any purpose, an appropriate intake of vitamins and minerals involved in protein and energy metabolism must also be supplied. Any deficiency state, such as anemia, should be corrected. Water balance should be ensured, since both electrolytes and fluids are necessary to prevent dehydration.

Immediate preoperative period. Usual preparation for surgery calls for nothing to be taken orally for at least 8 hours before the surgery. This is necessary to ensure that the stomach holds no retained food at surgery. Food in the stomach may cause complications resulting from vomiting or aspiration of food particles during anesthesia or recovery from anesthesia. In addition, any food present in the stomach may interfere with the surgical procedure itself or increase the risk of postoperative gastric retention and expansion. Especially before gastrointestinal surgery, a nonresidue diet (p. 362) may be followed for several days to clear the operative site of any food residue. Commercial low-residue, chemically defined formulas, or **elemental formulas**, such as Vivonex, can provide a complete diet in liquid form. Such formulas can be made more palatable for oral use with flavorings provided. Otherwise they may be fed by tube.

Emergency surgery. If the surgery is an emergency, no time is available for building up ideal nutritional reserves. This makes it more important for persons to maintain a good nutritional status through a healthy diet as a regular habit. In this way, optimum nutrient reserves will be available to supply needs at any time of stress.

Postoperative nutritional care: nutrient needs for healing

Nutritional support is necessary to aid recovery from surgery. In surgical disease, as well as in related surgical procedures, nutrient losses are greatly increased. At the same time food intake is greatly diminished or even absent for a period. To supply this additional nutritional support, several nutrients require particular attention.

Protein. Optimal protein intake in the postoperative recovery period is of primary concern for all patients. Protein is needed to replace losses during surgery and to supply the increased demands of the healing process. During the period immediately after surgery the body tissues usually undergo considerable **catabolism**. This means that the process of tissue breakdown and loss exceeds the process of tissue buildup (p. 37). During this time a negative nitrogen balance of as much as 20 g/day may occur. This negative balance represents an actual loss of tissue protein of more than 0.5 kg (1 pound)/day. In addition to these protein losses from tissue breakdown caused by metabolic imbalances, other losses of protein from the body also occur. These include plasma protein loss through hemorrhage, wound bleeding, and various body fluid losses or **exudates**. In addition, increased loss may occur from extensive tissue destruction, inflammation, infection, and trauma. If any degree of prior malnutrition or chronic infection existed, the patient's protein deficiency could easily become severe and cause serious complications. Several reasons exist for this increased protein demand.

1. Building tissue. The process of wound healing requires building a great deal of new body tissue. This can only be done when a sufficient amount of the essential amino acids from protein intake or body stores can be brought to the tissue by the circulating blood (p. 36). The nine essential amino acids cannot be made by the body and must be present for tissue building. These necessary amino acids must come from diet protein, or from intravenous feeding (p. 353) if the patient is unable to eat normally for an extended period. Usually these tissue protein deficiencies can be met by oral feedings. Thus it is important that a patient be helped to eat as soon as possible after surgery. Sometimes dietary protein intake must be increased to 100 to 150 g/day to restore lost protein and build new tissues at the wound site.

2. Controlling shock. A sufficient supply of plasma protein, mainly albumin, is necessary to protect the blood volume (p. 110). If the plasma protein level drops, insufficient pressure exists to keep tissue fluid circulating between the capillaries and the cells. If this situation occurs, water leaves the blood capillaries and cannot be drawn back into circulation. Shock symptoms result from a shrinking blood volume and the body's effort to restore it.

3. Controlling edema. When the serum protein level is low, **edema** develops as a result of this loss of the osmotic pressure required to maintain the normal movement of fluid between the capillaries and the surrounding tissue. This condition of edema is characterized by puffiness or swelling of the tissue from the excess fluid being held there rather than being returned to circulation. Generalized edema may affect heart and lung action. Local edema at the wound site also interferes with closure of the wound and hinders the normal healing process.

4. Healing bone. Any bone surgery, as in orthopedic problems, involves extensive bone healing. Protein, as well as mineral matter, is essential in the bone tissue for proper bone formation. Protein provides a matrix for the laying down of calcium and phosphorus to form proper bone **callus** and hardening. Thus protein anchors the minerals to build strong bone tissue.

5. Resisting infection. The major components of the body's immune system, which provide its defense against infection, are protein tissues. These defense agents include special white cells called *lymphocytes* (p. 370), as well as antibodies and various other blood cells, hormones, and enzymes. The tissue strength is a major defense barrier against infection at all times.

6. Transporting lipids. Fat is also an important component of tissue structure. It forms the center of cell walls and participates in many other necessary metabolic activities. Protein is required to carry fat in the bloodstream to all tissues (p. 293) for maintaining tissue structures and activities. Also, protein is necessary to carry fat to the liver for necessary work in fat metabolism. Protein present in the liver combines with fat and removes it, thus avoiding the danger of fatty infiltration that would lead to liver disease.

From this list of important protein functions in recovery from surgery, protein deficiency at this time obviously can lead to many clinical problems. These problems include poor wound healing, rupture of the suture lines (**dehiscence**), delayed healing of fractures, depressed heart and lung action, anemia, failure of gastrointestinal **stomas** (p. 361) to function, reduced resistance to infection, liver damage, extensive weight loss, and increased mortality risk.

Water. Water balance after surgery is a constant concern. Sufficient fluid intake is necessary to prevent dehydration, especially in elderly persons whose thirst mechanism may be depressed and cannot be depended on to ensure adequate fluid intake. In patients who have complications or who are seriously ill and have extensive drainage, as much as 7 L (almost 7½ quarts) of fluid daily may be required. In addition, during the postoperative period large water losses may occur from vomiting, hemorrhage, fever, or excessive urination. A comparison of daily water volume needs of surgical patients is given in Table 22-1. The usual intravenous fluids after surgery will supply some initial needs. However, oral intake should begin as soon as possible and be maintained in sufficient quantity.

Energy. As always when increased protein is demanded for tissue building, a sufficient amount of nonprotein kcalories must be supplied for energy to spare protein for its vital tissue-building function. The fuel nutrients, carbohydrate and fat, must therefore be in sufficient supply in the total diet. Since

❖ **TABLE 22-1** *Daily water requirements of the surgical patient*

Type of case and fluid needs	Average fluid required (ml)
Uncomplicated cases	
For vaporizations	1000-1500
For urine	1000-1500
TOTAL	2000-3000
Complicated cases (sepsis, elevation of temperature, humid weather, renal damage)	
For vaporization	2000-2500
For urine	1000-1500
TOTAL	3000-4000
Seriously ill patients with drainage	
For vaporization	2000
For urine	1000
For replacement of body fluid losses	
1000 ml bile drainage	1000
3000 ml Wangensteen drainage	3000
TOTAL	7000

Modified from Zintel HA: Nutrition in the care of the surgical patient. In Wohl M and Goodhart R editors: Modern nutrition in health and disease, ed 3, Philadelphia, 1964, Lea & Febiger.

excess fat presents general health problems, carbohydrate becomes the major source of needed fuel. The total kcalories in the postsurgery diet must be increased to 2500 to 3000 kcal/day before protein can be used entirely for tissue building and not be converted in part to fuel. In situations of acute metabolic stress, as in extensive surgery or burns, kcalorie needs may increase to as much as 4000 to 5000 kcal/day. Carbohydrate not only spares protein for tissue building, but also helps avoid liver damage by maintaining glycogen reserves in the liver tissue. Excessive fuel storage as body fat should be avoided, however, since fatty tissue heals poorly and is more susceptible to infection.

Vitamins. Several vitamins require particular attention in wound healing. Vitamin C is necessary for building strong tissue. It deposits a cementlike substance between the cells, thus strengthening the tissue formed. Vitamin C helps to build connective tissue, new capillary walls, and general tissue ground substance. If extensive tissue building is required, as much as 1 g vitamin C/ day may be needed. Also, as kcalories and protein are increased, the B vitamins, especially thiamin, riboflavin, and niacin, that have important coenzyme roles in protein and energy metabolism must be increased. Other B-complex vitamins, folic acid, B_{12}, pyridoxine, and pantothenic acid, also play important roles in building hemoglobin, and thus must be adequate to meet the demands of an increased blood supply and general metabolic stress. Vitamin K, essential for blood clotting, is usually present in sufficient amount through its synthesis by intestinal bacteria.

Minerals. Attention to any mineral deficiencies, that is, continued adequate amounts in the diet, is essential. When tissue is broken down, as after surgery, cell potassium and phosphorus are lost. Also, electrolyte imbalances of sodium and chloride result from fluid losses. Iron deficiency anemia may develop from blood loss or faulty iron absorption. Another mineral important in wound healing is zinc. An adequate amount of protein usually meets this need, since most dietary zinc is found in protein foods of animal origin. Sometimes in extensive surgery and poor zinc stores, zinc supplements may be used.

GENERAL DIETARY MANAGEMENT

Initial intravenous fluid and electrolytes. Remember that routine postoperative intravenous (IV) fluids are used to supply hydration needs and electrolytes, not to sustain energy and nutrients. Ordinary postsurgical IVs are not designed to supply full nutrient needs or compete with oral feedings. For example, a 5% dextrose solution (D5W) with normal saline (0.9% NaCl solution) contains only 5 g dextrose/dl, about 20 kcalories, or 200 kcal/L, when the total energy need is about 10 times that amount. A rapid return to regular eating should be encouraged and maintained.

Methods of feeding. Only two basic types of methods for dietary management are available: (1) **enteral**—taking in nourishment through the regular gastrointestinal route as long as it can be used, either by regular oral feedings or by tube feedings; or (2) **parenteral**—taking in nourishment through veins, either smaller peripheral veins or a larger central vein. This chapter and Chapter 23 describe these alternate feeding methods.

Oral (enteral) feedings. Most general surgical patients can and should progress to oral feedings as soon as possible. Oral feedings allow for greater additions of needed nutrients and help to stimulate normal action of the gastrointestinal tract. Food can usually be taken orally as soon as regular bowel sounds return. When oral feedings do begin, the patient usually progresses from clear to full liquids and then to a soft or regular diet. Examples of these progressive "routine house diets" used in hospitals are given in Table 17-2 (p. 262). Individual tolerance and needs will always be the guide, but encouragement and help should be supplied in general care of postsurgery patients to enable them to eat as soon as possible.

Parenteral feeding. In cases of major surgery or complications, especially involving the gastrointestinal tract, or when the patient is unable to obtain sufficient nourishment orally, parenteral feeding may be necessary. It provides crucial nutritional support from solutions containing larger amounts of glucose, amino acids, electrolytes, minerals, and vitamins. Fat in the form of lipid emulsions is also used to supply needed kcalories and the essential fatty acid, linoleic acid. For smaller nutrient loads over a brief period of time, peripheral vein feeding may be used. However, for larger nutrient demands over a longer period of time, complete feeding by a larger central vein, **total parenteral nutrition (TPN)**, is required (p. 381). The placement of this larger catheter in a central vein, usually the subclavian vein leading into the heart by way of the superior vena cava, is illustrated in Fig. 22-1. More concentrated nutrient solutions can be fed through this larger vein. A basic TPN solution may contain 2.75% crystalline amino acids and 25% dextrose with added electrolytes, vitamins, and trace elements. The physician and the clinical dietitian determine the needed formula based on individual nutrition assessment, and the pharmacist carefully mixes the solutions according to the prescription. Then the administration of the solution is an important nursing responsibility (Box 22-1). Long-term home use of TPN has been a life-saving measure for many persons but is expensive.[1]

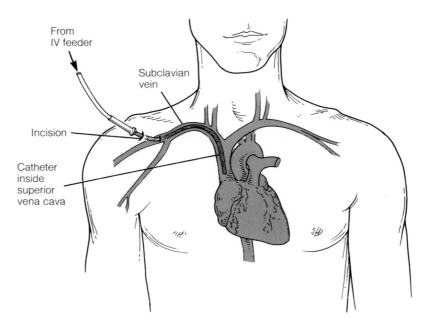

❖ FIG. 22-1

Catheter placement for total parenteral nutrition (TPN) made for feeding via subclavian vein to superior vena cava.

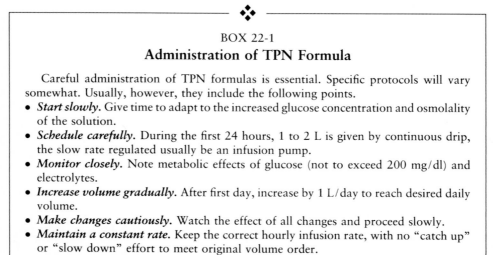

❖

BOX 22-1

Administration of TPN Formula

Careful administration of TPN formulas is essential. Specific protocols will vary somewhat. Usually, however, they include the following points.

- *Start slowly.* Give time to adapt to the increased glucose concentration and osmolality of the solution.
- *Schedule carefully.* During the first 24 hours, 1 to 2 L is given by continuous drip, the slow rate regulated usually be an infusion pump.
- *Monitor closely.* Note metabolic effects of glucose (not to exceed 200 mg/dl) and electrolytes.
- *Increase volume gradually.* After first day, increase by 1 L/day to reach desired daily volume.
- *Make changes cautiously.* Watch the effect of all changes and proceed slowly.
- *Maintain a constant rate.* Keep the correct hourly infusion rate, with no "catch up" or "slow down" effort to meet original volume order.
- *Discontinue slowly.* Take patient off of TPN feeding gradually, reducing rate and daily volume about 1 L/day.

SPECIAL NUTRITIONAL NEEDS AFTER GASTROINTESTINAL SURGERY

Since the gastrointestinal system is uniquely designed to handle food, a surgical procedure on any part of this system requires special dietary attention or modification.

Mouth, throat, and neck surgery

Surgery involving the mouth, throat, or neck requires modification in the mode of eating. Usually the patient cannot chew or swallow normally, and accommodations must be made in each case according to individual limitations.

Oral liquid feedings. Concentrated liquid feedings should be planned to ensure adequate nutrition in less volume of food. An enriched commercial formula such as Ensure can be used several times a day, or a formula can be prepared in a blender using enriching foods to secure the needed base of protein, kcalories, vitamins, and minerals. Nonfat dry milk or a commercial protein supplement such as Casec can be added for further enrichment. An example of such a high-protein, high-caloric formula is given in Table 18-1. This type of concentrated formula can be used for frequent feedings to supply needed nourishment.

Tube feedings. In cases of radical neck or facial surgery, or when the patient is comatose or severely debilitated, tube feedings may be indicated. Current developments in small-bore feeding tubes have made this method of feeding easier. For long-term need, improved equipment and standardized commercial formulas have made continued home tube feeding possible for many patients. Usually a nasogastric tube is used (p. 379). However, if there is obstruction in the esophagus, the tube is inserted into an opening in the abdominal wall, which the surgeon makes at surgery. This procedure is called a **gastrostomy.** In general the tube-feeding formula will be prescribed by the physician and clinical nutritionist according to the patient's nutritional need and tolerance. In any form of tube feeding, it is important to regulate the amount of formula and the rate at which it is given. Usually 2 L are sufficient for a 24-hour period. Feedings should not exceed 240 to 360 ml (8 to 12 ounces) in each 3- to 4-hour interval. A problem encountered in as many as 60% of ill patients receiving liquid formula diets, especially those on tube feedings, is diarrhea. Studies have shown that formulas supplemented with the soluble fiber pectin in a 1% solution (1 ml pectin/100 ml formula) improved bowel function and reduced the incidence of diarrhea.[2] Two general types of formula may be used.

1. Commercial formulas. A wide variety of commercial formulas are available. Their composition is designed to meet particular needs. These products may be made from *intact nutrients* for use with an intact system able to digest and absorb them. Others may be made from "predigested" *elemental nutrients,* which are readily absorbed with only minimal residue. Still others may be formulas for special problems, or single-nutrient products of protein, carbohydrate, and fat, which may be mixed together as calculated by the clinical nutritionist to meet the patient's specific needs. Commercial formulas have the advantage of being standard in composition and immediately available for use. They are also sterile and may be stored. However, the expense involved in long-term use may be a disadvantage for some families.

❖ TABLE 22-2   *Sample tube-feeding formula (2500 ml, 3000 kcalories)*

Ingredients	Amount	Protein	Fat	Carbohydrate
Homogenized milk	1 L	32	40	48
Eggs	3	21	16	
Apple juice	400 ml			55
Vegetable oil	30 ml		30	
Strained baby food (112 g|4 oz|jars)				
Beef liver	4 jars	56	12	14
Beets	2 jars	3		20
Peaches	2 jars	1	1	59
Sustagen	1½ cups (225 g)	52	7	150
(Water as needed to total 2500 ml)				
TOTALS		165	106	346
TOTAL CALORIES			2998	

2. Blended food mixtures. Alternative formulas may be calculated using regular foods mixed in a blender. Some patients, especially elderly persons, may feel needed comfort from the use of their own well known "regular foods," and such a formula is certainly less expensive for long-term home use. However, if the food mixture is unduly diluted to go through the tube, its nutrient density may not compare with that of a commercial formula. Also, with home-prepared formula, the risk of contamination is greater, so strict rules for cleanliness of all equipment, surface areas, and hands, as well as adequate refrigeration, must be followed. Any prolonged exposure to room temperature in the feeding process must be controlled to avoid possible bacterial contamination in formulas. Foods that will liquify in a high-speed blender may be used, and a protein supplement such as Sustagen may be added. The measured amount for a single feeding would need to be at room temperature before giving to the patient. An example of such a formula is shown in Table 22-2.

Stomach surgery

Nutritional problems. Since the stomach is the first major food reservoir in the gastrointestinal tract, stomach surgery poses special problems in maintaining adequate nutrition. A number of these problems may develop immediately after the surgery, depending on the type of surgical procedure (Fig. 22-2) and the individual patient's response.[3] Other complications may occur later when the person begins to eat a regular diet.

Immediate postoperative period. Immediately after surgery, especially after a total gastrectomy, serious nutritional deficits may occur. If the gastric resection also involved a *vagotomy* (cutting of the vagus nerve, which supplies a major stimulus for gastric secretions), increased gastric fullness and distention may result. Lacking the normal nerve stimulus, the stomach becomes *atonic* (without normal muscle tone) and empties poorly. Food fermentation occurs, producing *flatus* or gas, as well as diarrhea. After extensive gastric surgery, weight loss is common. At least half these patients fail to regain weight to optimal levels.

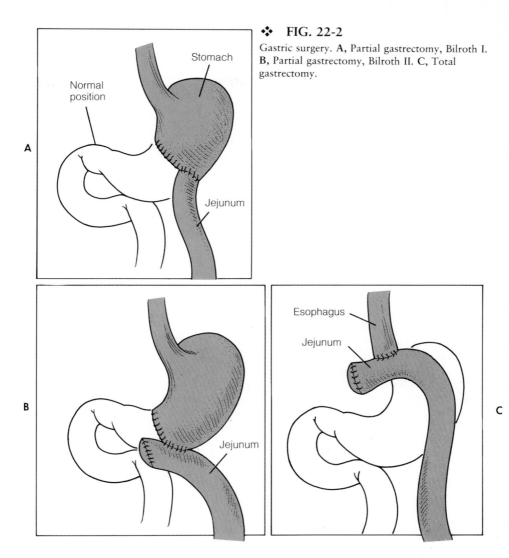

❖ **FIG. 22-2**

Gastric surgery. **A,** Partial gastrectomy, Bilroth I.
B, Partial gastrectomy, Bilroth II. **C,** Total
gastrectomy.

Generally, after surgery, frequent small oral feedings are resumed according
to the patient's tolerance. A typical pattern of simple dietary progression may
cover about a 2-week period. The basic principles of such general diet therapy
for the immediate postgastrectomy period involve: (1) size of meals—small
and frequent; and (2) nature of food—simple, easily digested, mild, low in
bulk. To cover this immediate postoperative nutritional need, however, after
the gastrectomy procedure surgeons are leaving a temporary catheter in place
with a *jejunostomy* (an opening to the jejunum), through which the patient
can be fed an elemental formula to ensure optimal nutritional support during
this important initial period.

Later "dumping syndrome." The so-called dumping syndrome is a frequently encountered complication following extensive gastric resection. After

---

BOX 22-2

❖ ——————— CLINICAL APPLICATION ——————— ❖

Case Study: John Has a Gastrectomy

After long experience with persistent peptic ulcer disease involving increasing amounts of gastric tissue, John Riley and his physician decided that surgery was needed. John then entered the hospital for a total gastrectomy. John withstood the surgery well and received some initial nutritional support from an elemental formula fed through a tube the surgeon had placed into his jejunum. After a few days the tube was removed and gradually over the next 2-week period John was able to take a soft diet in small oral feedings. Soon he recovered sufficiently to go home and gradually felt his strength returning. He was relieved to be free of his former ulcer pain and began to resume more of his usual activities, eating a regular diet of increasing volume and variety of foods.

As time went by, John began having more discomfort after meals. He felt a cramping sensation and increased heart beat. A wave of weakness would come with sweating and dizziness. Often he would become nauseated and vomit. As his anxiety increased he began to eat less and less. His weight began to drop; soon he was in a state of general malnutrition.

Finally John returned to seek medical help. The physician and clinical nutritionist outlined a change in his eating habits, and a special food plan was worked out for him. Although the diet seemed strange to him, John followed it faithfully because he had felt so ill. To his surprise, he soon found that his previous symptoms after eating had almost completely disappeared. Because he felt so much better on the new diet plan, he formed new eating habits around it. His weight gradually returned to normal and his state of nutrition markedly improved. He found that he would always fare better if he would "nibble" on food items throughout the day, rather than consume a large, heavy meal as he used to do.

Questions for Case Analysis

1. What were John's nutritional needs immediately after surgery and over the next 2 weeks? Why was it necessary for his feedings to be resumed cautiously?
2. Why was an emphasis given to postsurgical protein sources? How was this nutrient need provided?
3. Why do sufficient kcalories have to be consumed after surgery?
4. Why is fluid therapy of paramount importance after surgery?
5. What minerals and vitamins need special attention after surgery? Why?
6. When John began to feel better and resumed regular eating, why did he become ill? Describe his symptoms and give reasons for their development.
7. Outline the principles of the special diet the clinic provided to relieve John's symptoms. Plan a day's meal and snack pattern for John with basic instructions and suggestions you would discuss with him.

---

the initial recovery from surgery, when the patient begins to feel better and eats a regular diet in greater volume and variety, discomfort may be experienced about 15 minutes after meals. A cramping full feeling develops, the pulse becomes rapid, and a wave of weakness, cold sweating, and dizziness may follow. Often the person may become nauseated and vomit. These distressing reactions to food intake only increase anxiety. As a result, less and less food is eaten. Increasing weight loss and general malnutrition result.

❖

BOX 22-3
Diet for Postoperative Gastric Dumping Syndrome

General description
1. Five or six small meals daily
2. Relatively high fat content to retard passage of food and help maintain weight
3. High protein content (meat, egg, cheese) to rebuild tissue and maintain weight
4. Relatively low carbohydrate content to prevent rapid passage of quickly used foods
5. No milk; no sugar, sweets, or desserts; no alcohol or sweet carbonated beverages
6. Liquids between meals only; avoid fluids for at least 1 hour before and after meals
7. Relatively low-roughage foods; raw foods as tolerated

Meal pattern

Breakfast	2 scrambled eggs with 1 or 2 tbsp butter or margarine
	½-1 slice bread or small serving cereal with butter or margarine
	2 crisp bacon strips
	1 serving solid fruit*
Midmorning sandwich of:	1 slice bread with butter or margarine
	2 oz (56 g) lean meat
Lunch	4 oz (112 g) lean meat with 1 or 2 tbsp butter or margarine
	Green or colored vegetable† with butter or margarine
	½-1 slice bread with butter or margarine
	½ banana or other solid fruit*
Midafternoon	Same snack as midmorning
Dinner	4 oz (112 g) lean meat with 1 or 2 tbsp butter or margarine
	Green or colored vegetable† with butter or maragrine
	½-1 slice bread with butter or margarine (or small serving starchy vegetable substitute)
	1 serving solid fruit*
Bedtime	2 oz (56 g) meat or 2 eggs or 2 oz (56 g) cheese or cottage cheese
	1 slice bread or 5 crackers with butter or margarine

*Fruit choice: applesauce, baked apple, canned fruit (drained), banana, orange, or grapefruit sections.
†Vegetable choice: asparagus, spinach, green beans, squash, beets, carrots, green peas.

This complex of symptoms constitutes a shock syndrome that results when a meal containing a large proportion of readily soluble carbohydrate rapidly enters, "dumps" into, the small intestine. When the stomach has been removed, the food passes directly from the esophagus into the small intestine, as shown in Fig. 22-2. This rapidly entering food mass is a concentrated solution in relation to the surrounding circulation of blood. Thus, to achieve an osmotic balance, or a state of **isotonicity** (p. 114), water is drawn from the blood circulation into the intestine. This water shift causes a rapid shrinking of the vascular fluid volume. As a result, the blood pressure drops, and signs of rapid heart action to rebuild the blood volume appear: rapid pulse, sweating, weakness, and tremors. Later, in about 2 hours, a second sequence of events usually follows. The initial concentrated solution of carbohydrate has been rapidly digested and absorbed. In turn, the blood glucose rises rapidly and stimulates an overproduction of insulin. Eventually the blood sugar drops below normal levels, with symptoms of mild **hypoglycemia.** Dramatic relief from all these distressing symptoms, as well as gradual regaining of lost weight, follows careful control of the diet (Box 22-3). Later careful reintroduction of milk in small amounts may be used to test toleration. The patient may also find that eating slowly and lying down for 15 to 30 minutes after eating helps decrease the rate of gastric emptying.

Gallbladder surgery

For patients suffering from acute gallbladder disease, *cholecystitis,* or from gallstones, *cholelithiasis* (Fig. 22-3), the treatment is usually surgical removal

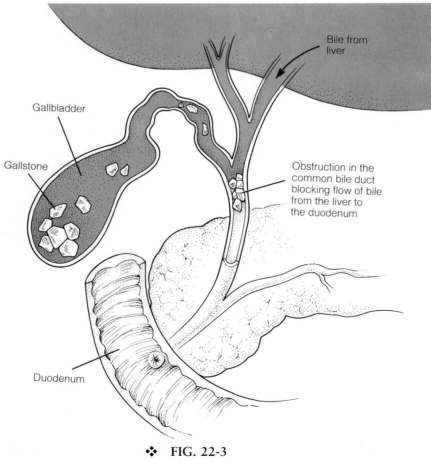

Bile from liver

Gallbladder

Gallstone

Obstruction in the common bile duct blocking flow of bile from the liver to the duodenum

Duodenum

❖ **FIG. 22-3**
Gallbladder with stones (cholelithiasis).

of the gallbladder, *cholecystectomy*. Since the function of the gallbladder is to concentrate and store bile, which aids in the digestion and absorption of fat, some moderation in dietary fat is usually indicated. After surgery, control of fat in the diet aids wound healing and comfort, since the hormonal stimulus for bile secretion (p. 127) would still be functional in the surgical area, causing pain with intake of fatty foods. Time is also needed for the body's readjustment to the more dilute supply of liver bile available to assist fat digestion and absorption. Depending on individual toleration and response, a relatively low-fat diet may be needed, such as the guide given previously for gallbladder disease (p. 286).

Intestinal surgery

In cases of intestinal disease involving lesions or obstructions, resection of the affected intestinal area may need to be done. In complicated cases involving large sections of the bowel and requiring surgical removal of most of the small intestine, nutritional support is difficult. In such cases TPN is used to supply major support with a small allowance of oral feeding for personal food desires. After general resection for less severe cases, a relatively low-residue diet, such as the general guide given for intestinal disease (p. 278), may be used to allow for healing and comfort. Sometimes the surgery requires making an opening in the abdominal wall to the outside from the intestine, a *stoma* (Fig 22-4), for the elimination of fecal waste materials. If the opening is in the area of the *ileum*, the first section of the large intestine, it is called an *ileostomy*. Here the

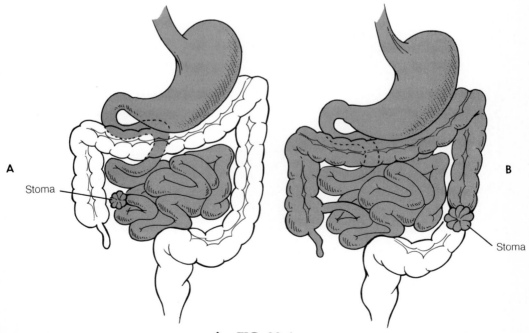

Stoma

A   B

Stoma

❖ **FIG. 22-4**
A, Ileostomy. **B,** Colostomy.

❖

BOX 22-4
Nonresidue Diet

General description
1. This diet includes only those foods free from fiber, seeds, and skins and with the minimum amount of residue.
2. Fruits and vegetables are omitted except for strained fruit juices.
3. Milk is omitted.
4. The diet is adequate in protein and calories, containing approximately 75 g protein, 100 g fat, 250 g carbohydrate, and 2260 calories. It is likely to be inadequate in vitamin A, calcium, and riboflavin.
5. If patients are to remain a long time on this diet, supplementary vitamins and minerals should be given.

Selection of foods

Foods	Allowed	Not allowed
Beverages	Carbonated beverages, coffee, tea	Milk, milk drinks
Bread	Crackers, melba or rusks	Whole-grain bread
Cereals	Refined as Cream of Wheat, Farina, fine cornmeal, Malt-o-Meal, pablum, rice, strained oatmeal, cornflakes, puffed rice, Rice Krispies	Whole-grain and other cereals
Cheese		None allowed
Desserts	Plain cakes and cookies, gelatin desserts, water ices, angel food cake, arrowroot cookies, tapioca puddings made with fruit juice only	Pastries, all others
Eggs	As desired, preferably hard cooked	Fried eggs
Fats	Butter or substitute, small amount cream	None
Fruits	Strained fruit juices	All others
Meat, fish, poultry	Tender beef, chicken, fish, lamb, liver, veal; crisp bacon	Fried or tough meat, pork
Potatoes or substitute	Only macaroni, noodles, spaghetti, refined rice	Potatoes, corn, hominy, unrefined rice
Soup	Bouillon and broth only	All others
Sweets	Hard candy, fondant, gumdrops, jelly, marshmallows, sugar, syrup, honey	Other candy, jam, marmalade
Vegetables	Tomato juice	All others
Miscellaneous	Salt	Pepper

Postsurgical nonresidue diet—general description
1. This diet is slightly higher in residue but has greater variety, including potatoes, white bread products, processed cheese, sauces, desserts made with milk, and cream for coffee and cereal.
2. The average daily menu will contain 85 g protein, 2300 calories, and is slightly higher in vitamins and minerals.

❖

BOX 22-4
Nonresidue Diet—cont'd

Selection of foods

To the selections listed on p. 362 add

  Cheese: Processed cheese, mild cream cheeses

  Potatoes: Prepared any way, no skin

  Bread: Any kind without bran, white bread, rolls, pancakes, waffles

  Fats: 2 oz cream or half-and-half per meal, cream sauce, cream gravy

  Desserts: All desserts except those containing fruit and nuts

  Condiments: As desired

NOTE: Fruit juice and hard candies may be taken between meals to increase caloric intake.

---

food mass is still fairly liquid and more problems are encountered in management. If the opening is further along the colon in the last part of the large intestine, it is called a *colostomy.* Here the water is largely reabsorbed by the large intestine, and the remaining feces is more formed, making management much easier. Coping with any "ostomy" is difficult at best and patients need much support and practical help in learning about self-care. Generally a relatively low-residue diet (p. 278) is helpful at first, but the aim is to advance as soon as possible to a regular diet. Progression to a regular diet is important both for nutritional value and for emotional support. Regular food provides much psychologic help to the patient, and dietary adjustments to individual tolerances for specific foods can easily be worked out. The person can revert to a low-residue intake occasionally when diarrhea occurs.

Rectal surgery

For a brief period after rectal surgery, or *hemorrhoidectomy,* a clear fluid or nonresidue diet (Box 22-4) may be indicated to reduce painful elimination and allow healing. In some cases a nonresidue commercial elemental formula such as Vivonex may be used to delay bowel movements until the surgical area has healed. Return to a regular diet is usually rapid.

SPECIAL NUTRITIONAL NEEDS FOR PATIENTS WITH BURNS
Nutritional support base

Treatment and prognosis. Each year more than 100,000 persons are burned severely enough to require special hospitalization and care.[4] Treatment of these extensive burns presents a tremendous nutritional challenge. In fact, nutritional care is often the determining factor in survival and healing. Several factors influence the plan of care and its outcome:

    1. Age. Elderly persons and very young children are more vulnerable.

    2. Health condition. Any preexisting health problems or the presence of other injuries complicate care.

    3. Burn severity. The location and severity of the burns and the time elapsed before treatment are highly significant.

Degree and extent of burns. The depth of the burn affects its treatment and healing process. *First-degree burns* involve cell damage only in the top layer of skin, the *epidermis*. *Second-degree burns* involve cell damage in both the top layer of skin and in the second skin layer, the *dermis*. *Third-degree burns* result in full-thickness skin loss, including the underlying fat layer. Second- and third-degree burns covering 15% to 20% or more of the total body surface, or even 10% loss in children and elderly persons, are serious and require extensive care. Burns of severe depth covering more than 50% of the body surface are often fatal. Patients with major burn injuries are usually transferred to a regional burn unit facility for specialized burn team care.

Stages of nutritional care

The nutritional care of the person with massive burns is constantly adjusted to individual needs and responses. At each stage critical attention is given to amino acid needs for tissue rebuilding, fluid-electrolyte balance, and energy (kcalories) support. Generally three periods of care occur during the immediate shock, recovery, and secondary feeding periods.

Immediate shock period. During the first hours after a burn until approximately the second day, massive flooding edema occurs at the burn site. Loss of protective skin leads to immediate losses of water; electrolytes, mainly sodium, and protein. As water is drawn from surrounding blood to replace the losses, general loss continues, blood volume and pressure drop, and urine output decreases. Cell dehydration follows. Immediate intravenous fluid therapy with a salt solution such as **lactated Ringer's solution** replaces water and electrolytes. After about 12 hours, when vascular permeability returns to normal and losses begin to decrease at the burn site, albumin solutions or plasma can be used to help restore blood volume. During this initial period no attempt is made to meet protein and kcalorie requirements because (1) infusion of glucose at this time may bring **hyperglycemia,** (2) amino acids would be lost at the burn site, and (3) **adynamic ileus** develops after the injury, making use of the gastrointestinal tract at this time impossible.

Recovery period. After about 48 to 72 hours, tissue fluids and electrolytes are gradually reabsorbed, balance is reestablished, and the pattern of massive tissue loss is reversed. A sudden **diuresis** occurs, indicating successful initial therapy. Usually the patient returns to preinjury weight by about the end of the first week. Constant attention to fluid intake and output, with checks for any signs of dehydration or overhydration, are essential.

Secondary feeding period. Toward the end of the first postburn week, adequate bowel function returns and a vigorous feeding program must begin. At this point, despite the patient's depression and lack of appetite, life itself may well depend on rigorous nutritional therapy. Three major reasons exist for these increased nutrient and energy demands:

1. *Tissue destruction.* has brought large losses of protein and electrolytes that must be replaced.

2. *Tissue catabolism.* has followed the injury with further loss of lean body mass and nitrogen.

3. *Increased metabolism.* brings added nutritional needs to cover the additional energy costs of infection or fever and the increased protein metabolism of tissue replacement and skin grafting.

Nutritional therapy. Successful nutritional therapy during this critical feeding period is based on vigorous protein and energy intake.

1. High protein. Individual protein needs will vary from 150 g/day to as high as 400 g/day, depending on the extent of the burn injury. Children require two to four times the normal RDAs of protein for age. In general, most adults need 2 to 3 g of protein/kg of body weight to achieve nitrogen balance.

2. High energy. For most adults, from 3500 to 4500 kcalories, or twice the usual basal metabolic rate, is necessary to spare protein essential for tissue rebuilding and to supply the greatly increased metabolic demands for energy. A liberal portion of the total kcalories should come from carbohydrate, with a moderate amount of fat supplying the remaining need.

3. High vitamin. Increased vitamin C, as much as 1 to 2 g/day, may be needed as a partner with amino acids for tissue rebuilding. Increased thiamin, riboflavin, and niacin are necessary for the increased energy and protein metabolism.

Dietary management. To meet these crucial nutrient demands, either enteral or parenteral methods of feeding may be used. For any method used, to achieve the increased nutritional goals indicated, a careful intake record must be maintained to measure progress toward these goals.

1. Enteral feeding. Oral feedings are desired if tolerated. Concentrated liquids are given using added protein or amino acids. Commercial formulas such as Ensure may be used as added interval nourishment. Solid foods based on individual preferences are usually tolerated by about the second week. Some patients may require calculated tube feedings to ensure adequate intake in correct nutrient proportions.[4] In this case low-bulk, defined formula solutions are given through small-bore feeding tubes. In either case, continuous support and encouragement are necessary, with food as attractive and appetizing as possible, supplying well-liked items and avoiding disliked ones.

2. Parenteral feeding. For some patients, oral intake and tube feedings may be inadequate to meet the increased nutritional demands, or enteral feeding may be impossible because of associated injuries or complications. In such cases parenteral feeding can provide essential nutritional support.

Follow-up reconstruction

Continued nutritional support is essential to maintain tissue strength for successful skin grafting or reconstructive plastic surgery. The patient will need not only physical rebuilding of body resources any surgery would require, but also much personal support to rebuild the human will and spirit, since disfigurement or disability is possible. Health team members can do much to help instill courage and confidence to face the future again. Optimal physical stamina gained through persistent supportive medical, nutritional, and nursing care will help the patient rebuild the personal resources needed to cope.

SUMMARY

The nutritional demands of surgery begin before the patient reaches the operating table. Before surgery the task is to correct any existing deficiencies and build nutritional reserves to meet surgical demands. After surgery the goal is to replace losses and support recovery. The additional task of encouraging eating is often required during this period of healing.

Postsurgical feedings are given in a variety of ways. The oral route is always preferred. Inability to eat or damage to the intestinal tract, however, may require feeding through a tube or into veins. Special formulas are used for such alternate means of nourishment and are designed to meet specific individual needs. For patients undergoing surgery on the gastrointestinal tract, special diets are modified according to the surgical procedure performed. For patients with massive burns, greatly increased nutritional support is required in successive stages of response to the burn injury and to the continuing tissue rebuilding requirements.

❖ REVIEW QUESTIONS

1. Describe the general impact of imbalances of the following nutritional factors through the pre-, immediate post-, and postoperative periods: protein, kcalories, vitamins and minerals, and fluids.
2. Describe the major surgical effects for which nutritional therapy must be planned following these procedures: mouth, throat, or neck surgery; gastric resection; cholecystectomy; and rectal surgery.
3. Write a 1-day meal plan for a person experiencing the postgastrectomy "dumping syndrome." What general dietary guidelines are used?
4. How do an ileostomy and a colostomy differ? What are the dietary needs of each one?
5. Outline the nutritional care of a burn patient from treatment for immediate shock through recovery and tissue reconstruction.

❖ SELF-TEST QUESTIONS

True-false
For each item you answer "false," write the correct statement.

1. Usually nothing is given by mouth for at least 8 hours before surgery to avoid food aspiration during anesthesia.
2. The most common nutrient deficiency related to surgery is that of protein.
3. Negative nitrogen is a rare finding after surgery.
4. Extensive drainage in complicated surgery cases increases water loss to dangerous levels if constant replacement is not provided.
5. Vitamin D is essential to wound healing since it provides a cementing substance to build strong connective tissue.
6. Oral liquid feedings usually provide little nourishment regardless of the type.
7. Tube feedings can only be prepared successfully from complete commercial preparations.
8. A postgastrectomy patient can usually return to regular eating within a few days.
9. After the diseased gallbladder is removed surgically, the patient can now tolerate freely any foods containing fats.
10. A careful diet record of the total food and liquid intake is important for a burn patient to ensure that increased nutrient and energy demands are met.

Multiple choice
1. Postsurgical edema develops at the wound site as a result of:
   a. Decreased plasma protein levels
   b. Excess water intake
   c. Excess sodium intake
   d. Lack of early ambulation and physical exercise

2. In a postoperative orthopedic patient's diet, protein is essential to:
   a. Provide extra energy needed to regain strength
   b. Provide a matrix to anchor mineral matter and form bone
   c. Control the basal metabolic rate
   d. Give more taste to the diet and thus increase appetite
3. Complete high-quality protein is essential to wound healing because it:
   a. Supplies the essential amino acids needed for tissue synthesis
   b. Spares carbohydrate to supply the increased energy demands
   c. Is easily digested and does not cause gastrointestinal problems
   d. Provides the most concentrated source of kcalories
4. A diet for the postgastrectomy "dumping syndrome" should include:
   (1) Small frequent meals   (4) High-protein content
   (2) No liquid with meals   (5) Relatively high-fat content
   (3) No milk, sugar, sweets, or desserts
        a. 1, 4, and 5   c. All of these
        b. 1, 2, and 3   d. 3, 4, and 5
5. A diet high in protein and kcalories is essential for a burn patient to:
   (1) Replace the extensive loss of tissue protein at the burn sites
   (2) Provide essential amino acids for extensive tissue healing
   (3) Counteract the negative nitrogen balance from loss of lean body mass
   (4) Meet added metabolic demands of infection or fever
        a. 1 and 2   c. 1 and 3
        b. All of these   d. 1 and 4

❖ SUGGESTIONS FOR ADDITIONAL STUDY

Individual or group project: commercial formula products
Make a survey to discover as many of the commercial products available for both oral and tube feeding as possible. Include both complete defined formulas such as Ensure and elemental formulas such as Vivonex. To gather information, with a taste-testing session if possible, interview a clinical nutritionist who is involved in their use. Visit a pharmacy, survey the products available, and discuss each one with the pharmacist. Also survey advertisements in the dietetic, nursing, and medical journals. From all your sources, compare these products regarding nutritional composition, uses, and cost. Prepare a report of your findings and conclusions to discuss in class.

References
1. Baptista RJ and others: The cost of home total parenteral nutrition, Nutr Clin Prac 2(1):14, 1987.
2. Palacio JC and Rombeau JL: Dietary fiber: a brief review and potential application to enteral nutrition, Nutr Clin Prac 5(3):99, 1990.
3. Miholic J and others: Nutritional consequences of total gastrectomy: the relationship between mode of reconstruction, postprandial symptoms, and body composition, Surgery 108:488, Sept 1990.
4. Ireton-Jones CS and Baxter CR: Nutrition for adult burn patients: a review, Nutr Clin Prac 6(1):3, 1991.

Further reading
Skipper A and Rotman N: A survey of the role of the dietitian in preparing patients for home enteral feeding, J Am Diet Assoc 90:939, 1990.
  This article describes the roles of both dietitian and nurse in teaching patients self-care skills needed for using tube feeding at home.
Slavin J: Commercially available enteral formulas with fiber and bowel function measures, Nutr Clin Prac 5(6):247, 1990.
  This article reviews the types of commercial enteral formulas that contain dietary fiber and provides guidelines for evaluating commercial products according to type of fiber contained, potential problems with high-fiber intakes, and which patients are good candidates for their use.

23

❖

Nutrition and cancer

KEY CONCEPTS

Environmental agents, genetic factors, and the strength of the body's immune system relate to the development of cancer.

The strength of the body's immune system relates to its overall nutritional status.

Nutritional problems in the care of cancer relate to the nature of the disease process and to the medical treatment methods.

*O*ver the past few years, with accumulating environmental problems and changing life-styles, cancer has become an increasing health problem. The American Cancer Society estimates that approximately 440,000 Americans die of cancer each year, with about 30% dying of lung cancer, which has been directly linked to smoking. Overall, cancer now ranks second, after heart disease, as a leading cause of death in the United States, accounting for about 20% of the total number of deaths each year. Since cancer is generally associated with the aging process, the increasing life expectancy has contributed in some measure to this increasing incidence.

In this chapter, we look at the relationships between cancer and nutrition. We see that important nutritional connections exist in two main areas: (1) *prevention*, related to the environment and the body's defense system; and (2) *therapy*, related to nutrition support for medical treatment and rehabilitation.

PROCESS OF CANCER DEVELOPMENT
The nature of cancer

Multiple forms. One of the problems in the study and treatment of cancer is that it is not a single problem. It has a highly varying nature and expresses itself in multiple forms. The general term *cancer* is used to designate a malignant tumor or **neoplasm**, meaning *new growth*. However, many forms of cancer vary worldwide and change with population migrations to different environments. It would be more correct, therefore, to use the plural term *cancers* in discussing this great variety of neoplasms.

Nutrition relationships. For these reasons no one specific treatment or "special diet" for cancer exists, despite various fad diets and claims. Rather, relationships of nutrition and cancer care center on two fundamental areas: (1) *prevention* in relation to the environment and the body's natural defense system, and (2) *therapy* in relation to nutritional support for medical treatment and rehabilitation.

The normal cell. Human life results from the process of individual cell growth and reproduction. This process goes on repeatedly, almost without error, guided by the cell's **genes**. In adults, approximately 3 to 4 million cells complete the life-sustaining process of cell division every second, largely without mistake, guided by the "genetic code" contained in the specific cell nucleus material in each gene, *deoxyribonucleic acid (DNA)*, which is the controlling agent. Each gene carries specific genetic information that controls synthesis of specific proteins and transmits genetic inheritance. Thus cells arise only from preexisting cells by cell division and carry the cell's genetic pattern. Normal cell structures and functions operate in an orderly manner under gene control, directing the cell's specific processes of protein synthesis, with "regulatory genes" switching on and off as needed to control normal cell activities.

The cancer cell. This orderly cell operation can be lost, however, with **mutation** or changes in the genes, especially the regulatory genes. A cell may become malignant and start a tumor when its normal gene control is lost. This "misguided cell" and its tumor tissue represent normal cell growth that has "gone wild." The types of cancer tumors are identified by their primary site of origin and by their stage of growth. *Sarcomas* arise from connective tissue; *carcinomas* arise from epithelial tissue. Stages of tumor development depend on its rate of growth, its degree of functional self-control, and its amount of penetration or spread into surrounding tissue. Also, since the incidence of cancer increases with age, a relationship exists between cancer cell development and the aging process in cells, tissues, and organ systems.

Causes of cancer cell development

The underlying cause of cancer is thus the fundamental loss of cell control over normal cell reproduction. Several factors, however, may contribute to this loss and change a normal cell into a cancer cell.

Mutations. As indicated, mutations, or changes in a cell's genes, are caused by loss of one or more of the regulatory genes in the cell nucleus or damage to a specific gene controlling a specific function. Such a mutant gene may be inherited. Some cancers have strong genetic causes and tend to run in families, as research indicates in the case of colon cancer.[1]

Chemical carcinogens. Agents that cause cancer are called *carcinogens*. Several chemical substances can interfere with the structure or function of regulatory genes. Exposure to such agents may be by individual choice, as in cigarette smoking, or by general exposure to environmental contaminants such as pesticides and industrial chemicals. Actions of such substances may result in gene mutation, damage to gene regulation, or activation of a dormant virus.

Radiation. Radiation damage to genes may come from x-rays, radioactive materials, atomic exhausts or wastes, or from sunlight. The overexposure to sunlight is related to skin cancer, rapidly on the rise in the United States and Europe, afflicting younger and younger persons. Common forms on the head and neck are usually basal cell carcinoma and are easily cured by surgical removal. However, a far more lethal form, *malignant melanoma*, strikes more than 15,000 Americans a year, killing some 45% of them.

Viruses. *Oncogenic*, tumor-inducing, viruses that interfere with function of regulatory genes have been identified in animals and are the focus of much current research. Although oncogenes were first found in viruses, their history indicates that they also function in normal vertebrate cells. A virus is little more than a packet of a few genes, usually fewer than five, whereas cells of complex organisms such as humans have thousands. Disease viruses act as parasites, taking over the cell machinery to reproduce themselves.

Epidemiologic factors. *Epidemiology* is the study of disease incidence in populations. Studies of cancer distribution involve factors such as race, region, age, heredity, occupation, and diet. Racial incidence changes as population groups migrate to new environments, which have their different distinct contaminants and diets and life-styles, and then acquire the cancer characteristics of the new population. The American incidence of breast cancer, for example, has been used as a model for the diet-cancer connection in relation to obesity and the American high-fat diet.[2,3]

Stress factors. Stress is an increasing disease factor in our complex society, especially in high-risk populations that lack social and economic supports. Psychic trauma, especially the loss of central personal relationships, takes its toll. Studies of people under stress have shown measured reduction of immune response to disease, especially in response of "natural killer cells" of the immune system.[4] Such stressful states make a person more vulnerable to other cancer-producing factors through their influence on the integrity of the immune system, food behaviors, and nutritional status.

The body's defense system

The human body's defense system is remarkably efficient and complex. Special cells protect us, not only against external invaders such as bacteria and viruses, but also against internal "aliens" such as cancer cells.

Defensive cells of the immune system. Two major cell populations provide the immune system's primary "search and destroy" defense for detecting and killing alien "nonself" substances that carry potential disease, including cancer cells that may arise daily in the body. These two populations of *lymphocytes*, a special type of white blood cell, develop early in life from a common stem cell in the bone marrow. The two types are called *T cells*, derived from thymus cells, and *B cells*, derived from bursal intestinal cells (Fig. 23-1).

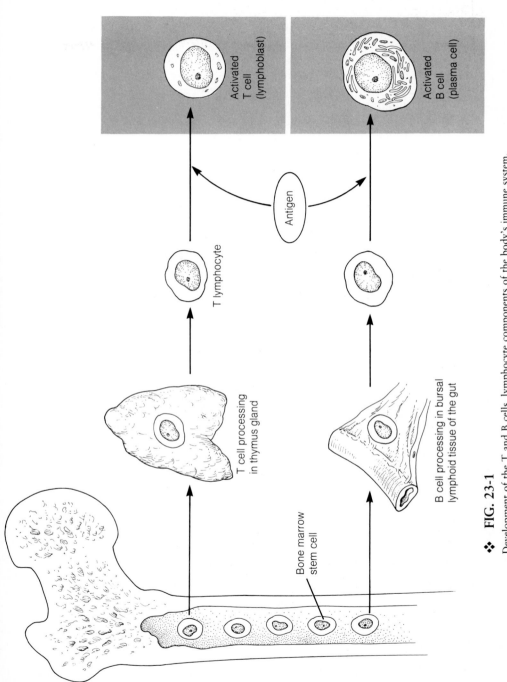

❖ **FIG. 23-1**

Development of the T and B cells, lymphocyte components of the body's immune system.

A major function of T cells is to activate the *phagocytes*, special cells that destroy invaders, and to act themselves as special killer cells that attack and kill disease-carrying **antigens**. A major function of B cells is to produce specialized protein known as **antibodies**, which in turn also kill antigens. Specially tailored proteins called *monoclonal antibodies* have been grown in laboratory mice from specific single-cell *clones* of original antibodies, giving medical researchers a tool to diagnose and treat several diseases, including cancer.

Relation of nutrition to immunity. Nutritional support is necessary to maintain the integrity of the human immune system. Severely malnourished persons show changes in the structure and function of the immune system. These changes are due to **atrophy** or losses in basic tissues involved: liver, bowel wall, bone marrow, spleen, and lymphoid tissue. The role of nutrition in maintaining normal immunity and combating sustained attacks of disease such as cancer is fundamental.[2]

The healing process and nutrition. The strength of any body tissue is maintained through constant synthesis of tissue protein, building and rebuilding. Such strong tissue is a front line of the body's defense. This process of tissue building and healing requires optimal nutritional intake. Specific nutrients, protein and key vitamins and minerals, as well as nonprotein energy sources, must constantly be supplied in the diet. Wise and early use of vigorous nutritional support for cancer patients has been shown to provide recovery of normal nutritional status, including **immunocompetence**, thus improving their response to therapy and prognosis.[5]

NUTRITIONAL SUPPORT FOR CANCER TREATMENT

Three major forms of therapy are used today as medical treatment for cancer: (1) surgery, (2) radiation, and (3) chemotherapy. Each one requires nutritional support.

Surgery

Any surgery, as discussed in Chapter 22, requires nutritional support for the healing process. This is particularly true for patients with cancer because their general condition is often weakened by the disease process and its drain on the body's resources. With early diagnosis and sound nutritional support before and after surgery, many tumors can successfully be removed, and recovery is often ensured. Nutritional therapy will also include any needed modifications in food texture or in specific nutrients, depending on the site of the surgery or the function of the organ involved. Various methods of feeding patients after surgery may be reviewed in Chapter 22.

Radiation

The site and intensity of the radiation treatment (Fig. 23-2) determine the nature of nutritional problems the patient may experience. For example, radiation to the area of the head, neck, or esophagus affects the oral mucosa and salivary secretions. This will affect taste sensations and sensitivity to food texture and temperature. Similarly, radiation to the abdominal area affects the intestinal mucosa. This causes loss of villi and absorbing surface; thus malabsorption problems may follow. Also, ulcers or inflammation and obstruction

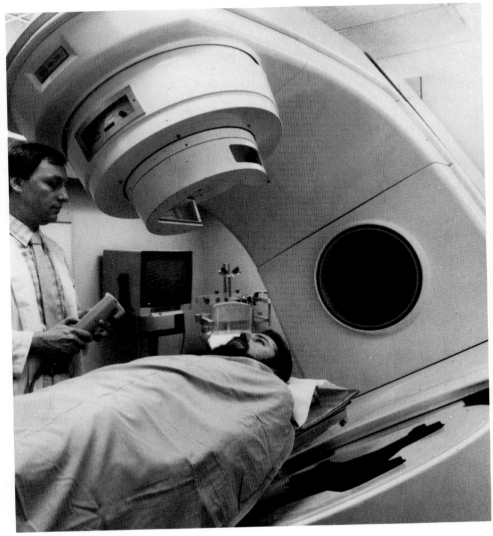

❖ **FIG. 23-2**
Cancer patient undergoing radiation treatment.

or *fistulas* may develop from the tissue breakdown. A fistula, from the Latin word for "pipe," is an abnormal opening or passageway within the body or to the outside. As such, it interferes with normal functioning of the involved tissue. The general malabsorption problem may be further compounded by lack of food intake resulting from loss of appetite and nausea.

Chemotherapy

Several drugs have been developed to combat various cancers. They are often used in combinations to achieve a desired effect in killing the cancer cells. Because these drugs are highly toxic, however, they have similar effects on

❖

BOX 23-1
Tyramine-Restricted Diet

General directions

- Designed for patients on monoamine oxidase (MAO) inhibitors, drugs that have been reported to cause hypertensive crises when used with tyramine-rich foods. These include foods in which aging, protein breakdown, and putrefaction are used to increase flavor. Studies indicate that as little as 5 to 6 mg tyramine can produce a response, and 25 mg is a danger dose.
- Food sources of other pressor amines such as histamine, dihydroxyphenylalanine, and hydroxytyramine are also avoided.
- Avoid all foods listed. Limited amounts of foods with a lower tyramine amount such as yeast bread may be included in a specific diet.
- Avoid over-the-counter drugs such as decongestants, cold remedies, and antihistamines.

Foods to avoid	Representative tyramine values (μg/g or ml)	Additional foods to avoid
Cheeses		Other aged cheeses
N.Y. state cheddar	1416	Blue
Gruyére	516	Boursault
Stilton	466	Brick
Emmenthaler	225	Cheddars (other)
Brie	180	Gouda
Camembert	86	Mozzarella
Processed American	50	Parmesan
Wines		Provolone
Chianti	25.4	Romano
Sherry	3.6	Roquefort
Riesling	0.6	Yeast and products made with
Sauterne	0.4	yeast
Beer, ale—varies with brand		Homemade bread
Highest	4.4	Yeast extracts such as soup
Average	2.3	cubes, canned meats, and marmite
Least	1.8	Italian broad beans with pod (fava beans)
		Meat
		Aged game
		Liver
		Canned meats with yeast extracts
		Fish (salted dried)
		Herring, cod, capelin
		Pickled herring
		Other
		Cream, especially sour
		Yogurt
		Soy sauce, vanilla, chocolate
		Salad dressings

normal cells and have to be regulated carefully. This accounts for their side effects on such rapidly growing tissues as those of the bone marrow, gastrointestinal tract, and hair and for problems in nutritional management. Other problems may relate to use of pretreatment antidepressant drugs that have special blood pressure effects when used with certain tyramine-rich foods. These drugs are the *monoamine oxidase (MAO)* inhibitors. Their use would require a tyramine-restricted diet (Box 23-1).

Gastrointestinal effects. Numerous problems may develop that interfere with food tolerance: nausea and vomiting, loss of normal taste sensations and lack of appetite, diarrhea, ulcers, malabsorption, or *stomatitis*, an inflammation of the tissues around the mouth.

Bone marrow effects. Interference with the production of specific blood factors causes related problems: reduced red blood cells causing anemia, reduced white blood cells causing lowered resistance to infections, and reduced blood platelets causing bleeding.

Hair follicle effects. Interference with normal hair growth results in general hair loss or baldness.

NUTRITIONAL THERAPY
Problems related to the disease process

General feeding problems pose a great challenge to the nutritionist who is planning care and the nurse who is providing important supportive assistance. These problems relate to the overall systemic effects of the cancer itself and to the specific individual responses to the type of cancer involved.

General systemic effects. The disease process of cancer causes three basic systemic effects: (1) anorexia, or loss of appetite, (2) increased metabolism, and (3) negative nitrogen balance. These effects result in poor food intake, increased nutrient and energy needs, and more *catabolism* or breaking down of body tissues. A continuing weight loss ensues. The extent of these effects may vary widely with individual patients, from mild response to extreme forms of debilitating **cachexia** seen in advanced disease. This extreme weight loss and weakness is caused by abnormalities in glucose metabolism so that the patient's body feeds off its own tissue protein.

Specific effects related to type of cancer. In addition to the primary nutritional problems caused by the disease process itself, secondary problems in eating or use of nutrients relate to specific tumors that cause obstructions or lesions in the gastrointestinal tract or adjacent tissue. Such conditions limit food intake and digestion, as well as absorption of nutrients. Depending on the nature and location of the tumor, as well as its medical treatment, a variety of individual nutritional problems may occur and require personal attention.

Basic objectives of nutritional therapy

Prevention of catabolism. Every effort is made to meet the increased metabolic demands of the disease process and thus prevent extensive catabolic effects in tissue breakdown. It is far easier to maintain nutrition from the beginning than to rebuild the body after extensive malnutrition. This catabolic effect may be increased by the medical treatment.

Relief of symptoms. The symptoms of the disease or side effects of the treatment can be devastating for the patient. Relief for the patient requires much individual and family counseling to devise ways of meeting needs and helping the patient to eat. The types of foods used, their preparation and service, or the process of feeding may have to be changed according to individual situations or responses and needs.

Although the clinical nutritionist and the physician have the primary responsibility for planning and managing the nutritional therapy program, a tremendous contribution is made by the nursing staff and other health care personnel in the day-to-day support and counsel in helping the patient to eat. It is often just this kind of constant care and support that makes the difference in combating the course of the disease and in ensuring the comfort and well-being of the patient.

Principles of nutritional care

Two basic principles underlie all sound patient care, as discussed in Chapter 17: identifying needs and planning care based on these needs. Only then can one determine if real needs are being met. Thus nutrition assessment and nutritional care planning are primary concerns.

Nutrition assessment. Determining and monitoring the nutritional status of each patient is the primary responsibility of the clinical nutritionist, but other support staff in nursing often assist. Procedures used include body measurements and calculations of body composition, laboratory tests and interpretation of results, physical examination and clinical observations, and complete dietary analyses. These procedures may be reviewed in Chapter 17.

Personal care plan. Based on the detailed information gathered about each patient, including living situation and other personal and social needs, the clinical nutritionist, in consultation with the physician, develops a personal plan of nutritional therapy for each patient. This outline can then be incorporated into the nursing care plan, since the nutritionist works with the nursing staff to carry it out. The day-to-day plan is constantly checked with the patient and family, and changed as needed to meet the nutritional demands of the patient's condition and the person's individual desires and tolerances.

Nutritional needs

Although individual needs vary, guidelines for nutritional therapy must meet specific nutrient needs and goals related to the accelerated metabolism, which demands increased protein tissue synthesis and energy production.

Energy. The hypermetabolic nature of the disease and its healing requirements place great energy demands on the cancer patient. Sufficient fuel from carbohydrate, and to a lesser extent from fat, must be available to spare protein for vital tissue building. An adult patient with good nutritional status will need about 2000 kcalories, or 25 to 30 kcal/kg, for maintenance requirements. More kcalories may be needed according to the degree of individual stress or amount of weight gain needed. A malnourished patient will require 2500 to 3500 kcalories, or 35 to 40 kcal/kg, depending on the degree of malnutrition or extent of tissue injury.

Protein. Necessary tissue building for healing and to offset tissue break-down by the disease requires essential amino acids and nitrogen. Efficient protein use depends on an optimal protein/kcalorie ratio to promote tissue building and prevent tissue catabolism. An adult patient with good nutritional status will need approximately 80 to 100 g of high-quality protein to meet maintenance requirements. A malnourished patient will need between 100 to 150 g to replenish deficits and restore positive nitrogen balance.

Vitamins and minerals. Key vitamins and minerals control protein and energy metabolism through their co-enzyme roles in specific cell enzyme path-ways. (See Chapters 6 and 7.) They also play important roles in building and maintaining strong tissue. Thus an optimal intake of vitamins and minerals, at least to the RDA standards but more frequently to higher therapeutic levels. Supplements to the dietary sources are usually indicated.

Fluid. Adequate fluid intake must be ensured for two reasons: (1) to replace gastrointestinal losses from fever, infection, vomiting, or diarrhea; and (2) to help the kidneys dispose of metabolic breakdown products from destroyed cancer cells and from toxic drugs used in chemotherapy. Some of these drugs, such as cyclophosphamide (Cytoxin), require as much as 2 to 3 L of forced fluids daily to prevent hemorrhagic cystitis.

Nutritional management

Achieving these nutritional objectives and needs, in the face of frequent poor food tolerance or inability to eat, presents a great challenge to the nutrition support team. The specific method of feeding depends on the patient's con-dition. However, four basic methods are available to the clinical nutritionist and physician in managing a particular patient's nutritional care. Two of these are **enteral**, using the gastrointestinal tract; two are *parenteral*, using a vein.

Enteral: oral diet with nutrient supplementation. An oral diet with supple-mentation is the most desired form of feeding whenever possible. A personal food plan must be worked out with the patient and family, based on the nutrition assessment information gathered. It must include adjustments in food texture and temperature, food choices, and tolerances. It should provide as much caloric and nutrient density as possible in smaller volumes of food. It must give special attention to eating problems with loss of appetite, mouth problems, and gastrointestinal problems.

1. Loss of appetite. Anorexia is a major problem that curtails food intake when it is needed most. It often sets up a vicious cycle that can lead to the gross malnutrition of *cancer cachexia* if not countered by much effort. A vigorous program of eating, *not dependent on appetite for stimulus*, must be planned with the patient and family. The overall goal is to provide food with as much *nutrient density* as possible so that "every bite will count."

2. Mouth problems. Various problems contributing to eating difficulties may stem from sore mouth, stomatitis, or taste changes. Sore mouth often results from chemotherapy or radiation to the head and neck area. Frequent small snacks, soft and bland in nature and cool or cold in temperature, are often better tolerated. Often the treatment may alter the tongue's taste buds, causing taste distortion, "taste blindness," and inability to distinguish the basic tastes of sweet, sour, salt, or bitter, bringing more food aversions. Strong food

❖

BOX 23-2
Controlling Nausea and Vomiting in Patients Receiving Chemotherapy

Chemotherapy creates an almost "catch-22" situation in terms of the nutritional management of patients with cancer. On the one hand, it works best in the patient who is well nourished. On the other hand, it often triggers nausea and vomiting to such a degree that the patient cannot consume enough food to be well nourished. The resulting course of malnutrition may be further aggravated by alterations in taste acuity. To help prevent this problem of malnutrition, the health care provider can take several actions:

- *Obtain a detailed history of emesis.* Include data about onset, duration, and severity. Estimate the severity by degree of weight loss, electrolyte depletion, and retching. Also record factors aggravating or relieving emesis.
- *Limit food intake.* Do this selectively and carefully to avoid taste aversions to foods previously enjoyed by the patient.
- *Evaluate emetic effect of antiemetic drugs.* Note drugs used in patient's medical chemotherapy, anticipating possible emetic effects, as well as effectiveness of any antiemetic drugs being used to control the nausea. Relate personal food plan and support counseling with patient and family about these effects.
- *Identify potential psychogenic causes.* These are suspected when emesis occurs before the drug is administered or just as it is administered. Anticipatory nausea and vomiting have also been associated with the office or clinic visit, a person (physician, nurse), or an event associated with treatment. This is most often seen in patients on chemotherapy for more than 6 months.
- *Identify other illnesses.* Congestive heart failure, influenza, and bowel obstruction may also be responsible for nausea and vomiting.
- *Identify other drugs, treatments.* Use of other emetic drugs (antibiotics, digitalis, narcotics) or radiation therapy may aggravate nausea and vomiting during chemotherapy.

---

seasonings and high-protein liquid drinks may be helpful. Because the treatment may also alter salivary secretions, foods with a high liquid content should be used. Solid foods may be swallowed more easily with use of sauces, gravies, broth, yogurt, or salad dressings. A food processor or blender can render foods in semisolid or liquid forms for easier swallowing. Any dental problems should be corrected to help with chewing.

3. *Gastrointestinal problems.* Chemotherapy often causes nausea and vomiting that need special individual attention (Box 23-2). Food that is hot, sweet, fatty, or spicy sometimes enhances nausea and can be avoided according to individual tolerances. Small, frequent feedings of soft to liquid cold foods, eaten slowly with rests in between, may be helpful. The physician's use of antinausea drugs (such as Compazine) may help with food tolerances. Special surgical treatment involving the gastrointestinal tract will require related dietary modifications, as discussed in Chapter 22. Chemotherapy or radiation treatment can affect the mucosal cells secreting lactase and thus create lactose intolerance. In such cases a nonmilk-base nutrient supplement such as Ensure, which is a soy-base product, may be used.

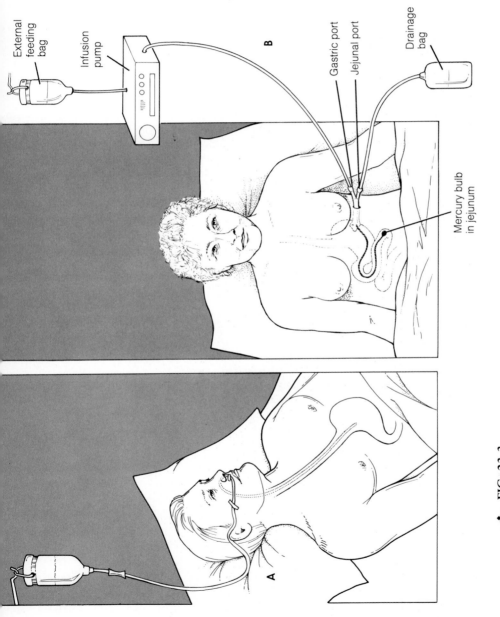

External feeding bag

Infusion pump

B

Gastric port
Jejunal port

Drainage bag

Mercury bulb in jejunum

A

❖ **FIG. 23-3**

Types of tube feeding. **A,** Common nasogastric feeding tube. **B,** Gastrostomy-jejunal enteral feeding tube.

Enteral: tube feeding. When the gastrointestinal tract can still be used but the patient is unable to eat and requires more assistance to achieve essential intake goals, tube feeding may be indicated. Fig. 23-3 illustrates the placement of different types of feeding tubes. Many patients have negative feelings about tube feeding, however, especially use of a nasogastric tube. Table 23-1 lists some helpful procedures with such patients. On the other hand, some highly motivated patients have even learned to pass their small-caliber tubes themselves. In some instances patients can be fed by pump-monitored slow drip during the night and be freed from the tube during the day. The use of special formulas and delivery system equipment has also made home enteral nutrition possible and practical. Commercial formulas are used in hospitals because of many uncontrolled factors and health regulations. However, less costly blended food formulas may be used at home if strict sanitation rules are observed, as described in Chapter 22; a sample formula appears in Table 23-2. Table 23-2 lists additional examples of blended tube feedings.

Parenteral: peripheral vein feeding. When the gastrointestinal tract cannot

❖ **TABLE 23-1**   *Problem-solving tips for patients receiving enteral nutrition*

Problem	Suggested solutions
Thirst, oral dryness	Lubricate lips
	Chew sugarless gum
	Brush teeth
	Rinse mouth frequently
	CAUTION: Use lemon drops sparingly because of cariogenic effects
Tube discomfort	Gargle with a mixture of warm water and mouthwash
	Gently blow nose
	Clean tube regularly with water or water-soluble lubricant
	If persistent, pull tube out gently, clean it, and reinsert
	Request smaller tube
Tension, fullness	Relax, breathe deeply after each feeding
Loud stomach noises	Take feedings in private
Limited mobility	Change positions in bed or chair
	Walk around the house or hospital corridor
Gustatory distress	
General dissatisfaction with feeding	Warm or chill feedings
	CAUTION: Feedings that are too cold may cause diarrhea
	Serve favorite foods that have been liquified
Persistent hunger	Chew a favorite food, then spit it out
	Chew gum
	Suck lemon drops (sparingly)
Inability to drink	Rinse mouth frequently with water and other liquids

❖ **TABLE 23-2** *Types of tube feedings*

Ingredients	Calories	Protein (g)	Fat (g)	Carbohydrates (g)
Regular tube feeding				
6 eggs	452	36.6	33.0	—
1 L homogenized milk	666	34.2	38.1	47.8
1 cup nonfat milk solids	434	42.7	1.2	121.3
½ cup Karo syrup	469			62.4
1 tablet brewer's yeast				
75 mg ascorbic acid				
¼ tsp salt				
1500 ml				
TOTAL	2021	113.5	72.3	231.5
Sustagen				
3 cups Sustagen	1755	105.0	15.0	300.0
4 cups water				
1200 ml				
600 g Sustagen (4 cups)	2300	140.0	20.0	400.0
1200 ml water				
1400 ml				
Add for banana Sustagen:				
2 tsp banana flakes	88	1.2	—	23.0
or				
1 mashed banana				
Low-calcium tube feeding				
6 cans strained meat	540	80.4	25.2	0
1 L fruit juice	432	0	2.0	108.0
¼ cup Karo syrup	234			61.0
Ascorbic acid				
Brewer's yeast				
1800 ml				
TOTAL:	1206	80.4	27.2	169.0
Low-sodium tube feeding				
1 L low-sodium milk	666	34.2	38.1	47.8
Casec 90 g—3 oz 18 tbsp	306	75.0		
¼ cup Karo syrup	234			61.0
1000 ml				
TOTAL:	1206	109.2	38.1	108.8

be used and nutritional support is vital, intravenous feeding must be initiated. For brief periods—in cases requiring less concentrated intakes of energy and nutrients— solutions of dextrose, amino acids, vitamins, and minerals, with concurrent use of lipid emulsions, may be fed into smaller peripheral veins. This use of smaller peripheral veins carries less risk than use of a larger central vein, and can supply necessary support when nutrient needs are not excessive. Peripheral vein feeding is combined with tube feeding to supply additional needs in some cases, avoiding the use of a central vein.

Parenteral: central vein feeding. When nutritional needs are greater and must continue over an extended period of time, central vein feeding has often provided a life-saving alternative.[5] This *total parenteral nutrition (TPN)* process requires surgical placement of the catheter (see Fig. 22-1), along with careful assessment, monitoring, and administration. These procedures are discussed in Chapter 22. Although it does carry risks and thus requires skilled team management, this hyperalimentation process has provided a significant means of turning cancer patients' metabolic status from catabolism to anabolism, often avoiding the serious development of cancer cachexia.

CONCLUSIONS: CANCER THERAPY AND PREVENTION

As indicated in the beginning of this chapter, relationships of nutrition and cancer center on therapy and prevention.

Therapy

Ample evidence at this point indicates that vigorous nutritional support increases the chances for success of medical treatments in the care of cancer. The fundamental reasons for this improved possible outcome have been reviewed here briefly. It is also evident that much effort on the part of the health care team, the patient, and the family, all working together, is absolutely necessary for this vigorous nutritional support to become a reality.

Prevention

On the basis of studies concerning possible associations of nutritional factors and food forms with cancer, the National Research Council Committee on Diet, Nutrition, and Cancer has issued guidelines for the public to help persons make generally healthy food choices to reduce risks. The committee indicated that these statements were intended to serve as interim guidelines until more information is available, but that they are consistent with good nutrition and health practices and are likely to reduce the risk of cancer. These six guidelines follow:

1. *Fat.* Reduce fat intake from the usual American average of 40% of total kcalories to 30% to reduce the risk of breast and colon cancer associated with high-fat diets.

2. *Fiber.* Increase the use of a variety of fruits, vegetables, legumes, and whole-grain cereal products to ensure sufficient amount and type of dietary fiber to reduce the risk of colon cancer.

3. *Vitamins A and C.* Emphasize the use of citrus fruits, carotene-rich vegetables and fruits, and vegetables of the *Cruciferae* (cabbage) family.

4. *Processed meats.* Minimize consumption of salt-cured, pickled, or smoked foods, including smoked sausages, hot dogs, ham, and smoked fish. These smoke-cured foods have been associated with cancer in some populations.

5. *Food pesticides and additives.* Minimize contamination of foods by carcinogens from any source, agricultural or food industry, whether avoidable or unavoidable. Intentional food pesticides and additives, direct or indirect, should continue to be evaluated for carcinogenic activity before they are approved for use in the food supply.

6. *Alcohol.* Moderate the use of alcoholic beverages, if they are used at all.

Of these six guidelines, the first four can be directly controlled by individual food choices. The fifth one requires action by the agricultural and food processing industries, but consumers can exercise influence through their food buying habits and support of reforms in pesticide laws (p. 181). The final guideline relates to personal attitudes and habits concerning use of alcohol. Here, as is often the case in health habits in general, moderation is the key.

SUMMARY

The general term *cancer* is given to various abnormal, malignant tumors in different tissue sites. The cancer cell is derived from a normal cell that loses control over its cell growth and reproduction. Cancer cell development occurs via mutation of regulatory genes and is influenced by environmental chemical carcinogens, radiation, and special viruses. Other associated factors include diet, excessive alcohol use, and smoking, as well as physical and psychologic stress. These effects and cell development are mediated by the body's immune system, primarily through its two types of special white blood cells: T cells that can kill invading disease-causing agents, and B cells that can make specific antibodies to attack these agents.

Cancer therapy consists primarily of surgery, radiation, and chemotherapy with specific toxic drugs. Supportive nutritional care must be highly individualized according to body responses to the disease and its treatment. It is based on nutrition assessment and provided by a number of routes: oral, tube feeding, peripheral vein, and TPN through a large central vein. In any case, nutritional management must meet specific physical and psychologic needs of individual patients.

❖ REVIEW QUESTIONS

1. What is cancer? Describe several major causes of cancer cell formation. Why is cancer an increasing health problem?
2. In what two main ways does nutrition relate to cancer? Give examples of each.
3. Describe the major types of defense cells that make up the body's major components of its immune system. How does nutrition relate to immunity?
4. Describe nutritional problems associated with each of the three medical treatments of cancer.
5. Outline the general procedure for the nutritional management of a cancer patient.
6. List and describe the National Research Council's dietary guidelines for reducing the risk of cancer.

❖ SELF-TEST QUESTIONS

True-false
For each item you answer "false," write the correct statement.
1. A cancer cell is unrelated to a normal cell.
2. Genes consist of cell nucleus material that controls protein synthesis and transmits hereditary information.
3. Chemical carcinogens are substances that can cause the development of cancer.
4. The incidence of cancer is not related to age.
5. Cancer-causing mutant genes may be inherited, making a person more susceptible to the influence of some added environmental agent.
6. Antigens are specialized protein components of our immune systems that protect us against disease.
7. Head and neck surgery for cancer seldom requires diet modification in texture of foods.

8. A cancer patient treated with a MAO inhibitor drug for depression would require a special low-tyramine diet.

Multiple choice

1. Special blood cells that are major components of the immune system are:
   a. Erythrocytes
   b. Lymphocytes
   c. Antibodies
   d. Platelets
2. A serious primary problem resulting from prolonged vomiting from cancer chemotherapy relates to:
   a. Nitrogen balance
   b. Calcium balance
   c. Fluid and electrolyte balance
   d. Glucose balance
3. Side effects of cancer chemotherapy that reflect the toxic effect of the drugs on rapidly reproducing cells include:
   a. Severe headaches
   b. Gastrointestinal symptoms
   c. Increased urination
   d. Decreased appetite
4. Adequate high-quality protein is essential in a cancer patient's diet to:
   a. Prevent catabolism
   b. Meet increased energy demands
   c. Prevent anabolism
   d. Stimulate hypermetabolism
5. Small amounts of which of the following types of food would most likely help treat the nausea caused by cancer chemotherapy?
   a. Hot liquids
   b. Dry, spicy foods
   c. Warm, fat-seasoned foods
   d. Soft, cold foods

❖ SUGGESTIONS FOR ADDITIONAL STUDY

Individual project: analysis of a cancer patient's diet

Interview a cancer patient being treated by chemotherapy. Collect and analyze the following data:

1. Specific drugs used, their specific main action and side effects
2. Symptoms experienced by the patient
3. Total food intake for 1 day
4. Efforts made by the patient to deal with any eating difficulties such as mouth problems, gastrointestinal problems, or loss of appetite
5. Any nutrient or food supplements used

Calculate the protein and kcalories in the day's food intake. Evaluate the protein/kcalorie ratio in terms of the need to prevent protein use for energy. On the basis of your findings, outline a personal food plan for the patient. Also, make a list of suggestions for helping a patient with nausea and other eating problems as a result of cancer therapy. If possible, discuss the food plan with the patient.

Individual or group project: cancer education

Make a list of all the possible community resources for educating persons about cancer. These resources can be programs, persons, and materials designed to meet needs of both those with cancer and the general public. Content of such resources may include any aspect of cancer, including the nature of the disease process, types and incidence of various forms of cancer, risk factors and their reduction, signs that may point to potential problems and need medical evaluation, cancer treatment and its effects, or nutrition.

Include as a primary resource the local chapter office of the American Cancer Society.

Make an appointment to visit the office and interview a staff member about the society's work. Obtain any educational materials available. Make similar visits to community clinical facilities, hospitals, public health agencies, private practitioners, and interview any professional persons involved in cancer care and education. These persons may include nurses, clinical nutritionists and dietitians, health educators, or physicians.

Evaluate your findings and compare them with those of other students in a full class discussion.

Individual or group project: total parenteral nutrition (TPN)
Interview a hospital clinical dietitian working with a nutrition support team. Discuss the program and general protocol for use of TPN. What type of solutions are used? If possible, observe the mixing of the formula by the pharmacist. Accompany the clinical dietitian and nurse on a visit to a patient who is receiving TPN. Observe the nutrition assessment and formula administration. Write a report of your findings and discuss them in class, comparing your information with that gathered by other members of the class at other facilities. If a person receiving home TPN is available, make a home visit and discuss the procedures used by the patient and family. What is the process for educating the patient and family about using home TPN? What plan is made for obtaining the necessary formula solutions prescribed? What records are kept? What monitoring procedures are used? Report your findings in class for discussion.

References
1. Gormon C: New clues in detecting a killer, Time 130(8):47, 1987.
2. Havas S: Macronutrients and cancer, Clin Nutr 9(2):49, 1990.
3. Lane HW and Carpenter JT Jr: Breast cancer: incidence, nutritional concerns, and treatment approaches, J Am Diet Assoc 87(6):765, 1987.
4. Berdanier CD: The many faces of stress, Nutr Today 22(2):12, 1987.
5. Bozzetti F: Effects of artificial nutrition on the nutritional status of cancer patients, J Parenter Enteral Nutr 13:406, 1989.

Further reading
Blonston G: Cancer—cut the risk in half, Am Health VI(3):42, 1987.

This author makes a good case for cancer risk reduction with reduced fat intake and increased dietary fiber, weight control and increased exercise, and stopping smoking.

Burros M: Freshness and light, Am Health V(6):64, 1986.

This article presents a buyer's guide for fresh produce, with special focus on helping prevent skin cancer.

Hackman E, Barnett R, and Chobanian L: Surprise nutrients: the secret life of summer fruits, Am Health VI(6):121, 1987.

This article presents an interesting review of high-nutrient fruits, helpful in increasing dietary sources of vitamins and fiber in relation to reducing risks for diseases such as cancer, complete with many excellent illustrations, nutrient charts, and recipes.

APPENDIX A
Nutritive values of the edible parts of food

Foods, Approximate Measures, Units, and Weight		(g)	Water (%)	Food Energy (cal)	Protein (g)	Fat (g)	Saturated (total) (g)	Unsaturated Oleic (g)	Unsaturated Linoleic (g)
Dairy Products (Cheese, Cream, Imitation Cream, Milk; Related Products)									
Cheese:									
Natural:									
Blue	1 oz	28	42	100	6	8	5.3	1.9	.2
Camembert (3 wedges per 4 oz container)	1 wedge	38	52	115	8	9	5.8	2.2	.2
Cheddar:									
Cut pieces	1 oz	28	37	115	7	9	6.1	2.1	.2
	1 cu in	17.2	37	70	4	6	3.7	1.3	.1
Shredded	1 cup	113	37	455	28	37	24.2	8.5	.7
Cottage (curd not pressed down):									
Creamed (cottage cheese, 4% fat):									
Large curd	1 cup	225	79	235	28	10	6.4	2.4	.2
Small curd	1 cup	210	79	220	26	9	6.0	2.2	.2
Low fat (2%)	1 cup	226	79	205	31	4	2.8	1.0	.1
Low fat (1%)	1 cup	226	82	165	28	2	1.5	.5	.1
Uncreamed (cottage cheese dry curd, less than ½% fat)	1 cup	145	80	125	25	1	.4	.1	Tr
Cream	1 oz	28	54	100	2	10	6.2	2.4	.2
Mozzarella, made with—									
Whole milk	1 oz	28	48	90	6	7	4.4	1.7	.2
Part skim milk	1 oz	28	49	80	8	5	3.1	1.2	.1
Parmesan, grated:									
Cup, not pressed down	1 cup	100	18	455	42	30	19.1	7.7	.3
Tablespoon	1 tbsp	5	18	25	2	2	1.0	.4	Tr
Ounce	1 oz	28	18	130	12	9	5.4	2.2	.1
Provolone	1 oz	28	41	100	7	8	4.8	1.7	.1
Ricotta, made with—									
Whole milk	1 cup	246	72	430	28	32	20.4	7.1	.7
Part skim milk	1 cup	246	74	340	28	19	12.1	4.7	.5
Romano	1 oz	28	31	110	9	8	—	—	—
Swiss	1 oz	28	37	105	8	8	5.0	1.7	.2
Pasteurized process cheese:									
American	1 oz	28	39	105	6	9	5.6	2.1	.2
Swiss	1 oz	28	42	95	7	7	4.5	1.7	.1
Pasteurized process cheese food, American	1 oz	28	43	95	6	7	4.4	1.7	.1
Pasteurized process cheese spread, American	1 oz	28	48	80	5	6	3.8	1.5	.1
Cream, sweet:									
Half-and-half (cream and milk)	1 cup	242	81	315	7	28	17.3	7.0	.6
	1 tbsp	15	81	20	Tr	2	1.1	.4	Tr
Light, coffee, or table	1 cup	240	74	470	6	46	28.8	11.7	1.0
	1 tbsp	15	74	30	Tr	3	1.8	.7	.1
Whipping, unwhipped (volume about double when whipped):									
Light	1 cup	239	64	700	5	74	46.2	18.3	1.5
	1 tbsp	15	64	45	Tr	5	2.9	1.1	.1
Heavy	1 cup	238	58	820	5	88	54.8	22.2	2.0
	1 tbsp	15	58	80	Tr	6	3.5	1.4	.1
Whipped topping (pressurized)	1 cup	60	61	155	2	13	8.3	3.4	.3
	1 tbsp	3	61	10	Tr	1	.4	.2	Tr
Cream, sour	1 cup	230	71	495	7	48	30.0	12.1	1.1
	1 tbsp	12	71	25	Tr	3	1.6	.6	.1

From Adams, C.F., and Richardson, M.: Nutritive value of foods, Home and Garden Bulletin No. 72, U.S. Department of Agriculture, Washington, D.C., 1981, U.S. Government Printing Office.
Blanks indicate no data available.
Tr, Trace.
For notes, see end of table.

| | | | | | Nutrients in Indicated Quantity | | | | |

Carbohydrate (g)	Calcium (mg)	Phosphorus (mg)	Iron (mg)	Potassium (mg)	Vitamin A Value (IU)	Thiamin (mg)	Riboflavin (mg)	Niacin (mg)	Ascorbic Acid (mg)
1	150	110	.1	73	200	.01	.11	.3	0
Tr	147	132	.1	71	350	.01	.19	.2	0
Tr	204	145	.2	28	300	.01	.11	Tr	0
Tr	124	88	.1	17	180	Tr	.06	Tr	0
1	815	579	.8	111	1200	.03	.42	.1	0
6	135	297	.3	190	370	.05	.37	.3	Tr
6	126	277	.3	177	340	.04	.34	.3	Tr
8	155	340	.4	217	160	.05	.42	.3	Tr
6	138	302	.3	193	80	.05	.37	.3	Tr
3	46	151	.3	47	40	.04	.21	.2	0
1	23	30	.3	34	400	Tr	.06	Tr	0
1	163	117	.1	21	260	Tr	.08	Tr	0
1	207	149	.1	27	180	.01	.10	Tr	0
4	1376	807	1.0	107	700	.05	.39	.3	0
Tr	69	40	Tr	5	40	Tr	.02	Tr	0
1	390	229	.3	30	200	.01	.11	.1	0
1	214	141	.1	39	230	.01	.09	Tr	0
7	509	389	.9	257	1210	.03	.48	.3	0
13	669	449	1.1	308	1060	.05	.46	.2	0
1	302	215	—	—	160	—	.11	Tr	0
1	272	171	Tr	31	240	.01	.10	Tr	0
Tr	174	211	.1	46	340	.01	.10	Tr	0
1	219	216	.2	61	230	Tr	.08	Tr	0
2	163	130	.2	79	260	.01	.13	Tr	0
2	159	202	.1	69	220	.01	.12	Tr	0
10	254	230	.2	314	260	.08	.36	.2	2
1	16	14	Tr	19	20	.01	.02	Tr	Tr
9	231	192	.1	292	1730	.08	.36	.1	2
1	14	12	Tr	18	110	Tr	.02	Tr	Tr
7	166	146	.1	231	2690	.06	.30	.1	1
Tr	10	9	Tr	15	170	Tr	.02	Tr	Tr
7	154	149	.1	179	3500	.05	.26	.1	1
Tr	10	9	Tr	11	220	Tr	.02	Tr	Tr
7	61	54	Tr	88	550	.02	.04	Tr	0
Tr	3	3	Tr	4	30	Tr	Tr	Tr	0
10	268	195	.1	331	1820	.08	.34	.2	2
1	14	10	Tr	17	90	Tr	.02	Tr	Tr

			Nutrients in Indicated Quantity					
							Fatty Acids	
								Unsaturated	
				Food			Saturated		
		Water	Energy	Protein	Fat	(total)	Oleic	Linoleic
Foods, Approximate Measures, Units, and Weight	(g)	(%)	(cal)	(g)	(g)	(g)	(g)	(g)
Cream products, imitation (made with vegetable fat):								
Sweet:								
Creamers:								
Liquid (frozen)	1 cup	245	77	335	2	24	22.8	.3	Tr
	1 tbsp	15	77	20	Tr	1	1.4	Tr	0
Powdered	1 cup	94	2	515	5	33	30.6	.9	Tr
	1 tsp	2	2	10	Tr	1	.7	Tr	0
Whipped topping:								
Frozen	1 cup	75	50	240	1	19	16.3	1.0	.2
	1 tbsp	4	50	15	Tr	1	.9	.1	Tr
Powdered, made with whole milk	1 cup	80	67	150	3	10	8.5	.6	.1
	1 tbsp	4	67	10	Tr	Tr	.4	Tr	Tr
Pressurized	1 tbsp	4	60	10	Tr	1	.8	.1	Tr
Sour dressing (imitation sour cream) made with	1 cup	235	75	415	8	39	31.2	4.4	1.1
nonfat dry milk	1 tbsp	12	75	20	Tr	2	1.6	.2	.1
Milk:								
Fluid:								
Whole (3.3% fat)	1 cup	244	88	150	8	8	5.1	2.1	.2
Lowfat (2%):								
No milk solids added	1 cup	244	89	120	8	5	2.9	1.2	.1
Lowfat (1%):								
No milk solids added	1 cup	244	90	100	8	3	1.6	.7	.1
Nonfat (skim):								
No milk solids added	1 cup	245	91	85	8	Tr	.3	.1	Tr
Buttermilk	1 cup	245	90	100	8	2	1.3	.5	Tr
Canned:								
Evaporated, unsweetened:								
Whole milk	1 cup	252	74	340	17	19	11.6	5.3	0.4
Skim milk	1 cup	255	79	200	19	1	.3	.1	Tr
Sweetened, condensed	1 cup	306	27	980	24	27	16.8	6.7	.7
Dried:								
Buttermilk	1 cup	120	3	465	41	7	4.3	1.7	.2
Nonfat instant:								
Envelope, net wt, 3.2 oz[5]	1 envelope	91	4	325	32	1	.4	.1	Tr
Cup[7]	1 cup	68	4	245	24	Tr	.3	.1	Tr
Milk beverages:								
Chocolate milk (commercial):								
Regular	1 cup	250	82	210	8	8	5.3	2.2	.2
Lowfat (2%)	1 cup	250	84	180	8	5	3.1	1.3	.1
Lowfat (1%)	1 cup	250	85	160	8	3	1.5	.7	.1
Eggnog (commercial)	1 cup	254	74	340	10	19	11.3	5.0	.6
Malted milk, home-prepared with 1 cup of whole milk and 2 to 3 heaping tsp of malted milk powder (about ¾ oz):								
Chocolate	1 cup of milk plus ¾ oz of powder	265	81	235	9	9	5.5	—	—
Natural	1 cup of milk plus ¾ oz of powder	265	81	235	11	10	6.0	—	—
Shakes, thick:[8]								
Chocolate, container, net wt, 10.6 oz	1 container	300	72	355	9	8	5.0	2.0	.2
Vanilla, container, net wt, 11 oz	1 container	313	74	350	12	9	5.9	2.4	.2
Milk desserts, frozen:								
Ice cream:								
Regular (about 11% fat):								
Hardened	½ gal	1064	61	2155	38	115	71.3	28.8	2.6
	1 cup	133	61	270	5	14	8.9	3.6	.3
	3 fl oz container	50	61	100	2	5	3.4	1.4	.1
Soft serve (frozen custard)	1 cup	173	60	375	7	23	13.5	5.9	.6
Rich (about 16% fat), hardened	½ gal	1188	59	2805	33	190	118.3	47.8	4.3
	1 cup	148	59	350	4	24	14.7	6.0	.5
Ice milk:								
Hardened (about 4.3% fat)	½ gal	1048	69	1470	41	45	28.1	11.3	1.0
	1 cup	131	69	185	5	6	3.5	1.4	.1
Soft serve (about 2.6% fat)	1 cup	175	70	225	8	5	2.9	1.2	0.1
Sherbet (about 2% fat)	½ gal	1542	66	2160	17	31	19.0	7.7	.7
	1 cup	193	66	270	2	4	2.4	1.0	.1

For notes, see end of table.

Nutrients in Indicated Quantity

Carbohydrate (g)	Calcium (mg)	Phosphorus (mg)	Iron (mg)	Potassium (mg)	Vitamin A Value (IU)	Thiamin (mg)	Riboflavin (mg)	Niacin (mg)	Ascorbic Acid (mg)
28	23	157	.1	467	220[1]	0	0	0	0
2	1	10	Tr	29	10[1]	0	0	0	0
52	21	397	.1	763	190[1]	0	.16[1]	0	0
1	Tr	8	Tr	16	Tr[1]	0	Tr[1]	0	0
17	5	6	.1	14	650[1]	0	0	0	0
1	Tr	Tr	Tr	1	30[1]	0	0	0	0
13	72	69	Tr	121	290[1]	.02	.09	Tr	1
1	4	3	Tr	6	10[1]	Tr	Tr	Tr	Tr
1	Tr	1	Tr	1	20[1]	0	0	0	0
11	266	205	.1	380	20[1]	.09	.38	.2	2
1	14	10	Tr	19	Tr	.01	.02	Tr	Tr
11	291	228	.1	370	310[2]	.09	.40	.2	2
12	297	232	.1	377	500	.10	.40	.2	2
12	300	235	.1	381	500	.10	.41	.2	2
12	302	247	.1	406	500	.09	.34	.2	2
12	285	219	.1	371	80[3]	.08	.38	.1	2
25	657	510	.5	764	610[3]	.12	.80	.5	5
29	738	497	.7	845	1000[4]	.11	.79	.4	3
166	868	775	.6	1136	1000[3]	.28	1.27	.6	8
59	1421	1119	.4	1910	260[3]	.47	1.90	1.1	7
47	1120	896	.3	1552	2160[6]	.38	1.59	.8	5
35	837	670	.2	1160	1610[6]	.28	1.19	.6	4
26	280	251	.6	417	300[3]	.09	.41	.3	2
26	284	254	.6	422	500	.10	.42	.3	2
26	287	257	.6	426	500	.10	.40	.2	2
34	330	278	.5	420	890	.09	.48	.3	4
29	304	265	.5	500	330	.14	.43	.7	2
27	347	307	.3	529	380	.20	.54	1.3	2
63	396	378	.9	672	260	.14	.67	.4	0
56	457	361	.3	572	360	.09	.61	.5	0
254	1406	1075	1.0	2052	4340	.42	2.63	1.1	6
32	176	134	.1	257	540	.05	.33	.1	1
12	66	51	Tr	96	200	.02	.12	.1	Tr
38	236	199	.4	338	790	.08	.45	.2	1
256	1213	927	.8	1771	7200	.36	2.27	.9	5
32	151	115	.1	221	900	.04	.28	.1	1
232	1409	1035	1.5	2117	1710	.61	2.78	.9	6
29	176	129	.1	265	210	.08	.35	.1	1
38	274	202	.3	412	180	.12	.54	.2	1
469	827	594	2.5	1585	1480	.26	.71	1.0	31
59	103	74	.3	198	190	.03	.09	.1	4

| | | | | | | Fatty Acids | | |
| | | | | | | | Unsaturated | |
Foods, Approximate Measures, Units, and Weight		Water (%)	Food Energy (cal)	Protein (g)	Fat (g)	Saturated (total) (g)	Oleic (g)	Linoleic (g)
	(g)							
Milk desserts, other:								
Custard, baked	1 cup	265	77	305	14	15	6.8	5.4	.7
Puddings:								
From home recipe:								
Starch base:								
Chocolate	1 cup	260	66	385	8	12	7.6	3.3	.3
Vanilla (blancmange)	1 cup	255	76	285	9	10	6.2	2.5	.2
Tapioca cream	1 cup	165	72	220	8	8	4.1	2.5	.5
From mix (chocolate) and milk:								
Regular (cooked)	1 cup	260	70	320	9	8	4.3	2.6	.2
Instant	1 cup	260	69	325	8	7	3.6	2.2	.3
Yogurt:								
With added milk solids:								
Made with lowfat milk:								
Fruit-flavored[9]	1 container, net wt 8 oz	227	75	230	10	3	1.8	.6	.1
Plain	1 container, net wt 8 oz	227	85	145	12	4	2.3	.8	.1
Made with nonfat milk	1 container, net wt 8 oz	227	85	125	13	Tr	.3	.1	Tr
Without added milk solids:								
Made with whole milk	1 container, net wt 8 oz	227	88	140	8	7	4.8	1.7	.1
Eggs								
Eggs, large (24 oz per dozen):								
Raw:								
Whole, without shell	1 egg	50	75	80	6	6	1.7	2.0	.6
White	1 white	33	88	15	3	Tr	0	0	0
Yolk	1 yolk	17	49	65	3	6	1.7	2.1	.6
Cooked:								
Fried in butter	1 egg	46	72	85	5	6	2.4	2.2	.6
Hard-cooked, shell removed	1 egg	50	75	80	6	6	1.7	2.0	.6
Poached	1 egg	50	74	80	6	6	1.7	2.0	.6
Scrambled (milk added) in butter; also omelet	1 egg	64	76	95	6	7	2.8	2.3	.6
Fats, Oils; Related Products								
Butter:								
Regular (1 brick or 4 sticks per lb):								
Stick (½ cup)	1 stick	113	16	815	1	92	57.3	23.1	2.1
Tablespoon (about ⅛ stick)	1 tbsp	14	16	100	Tr	12	7.2	2.9	.3
Pat (1-in square, ⅓ in high; 90 per lb)	1 pat	5	16	35	Tr	4	2.5	1.0	.1
Whipped (6 sticks or two 8 oz containers per lb)								
Stick (½ cup)	1 stick	76	16	540	1	61	38.2	15.4	1.4
Tablespoon (about ⅛ stick)	1 tbsp	9	16	65	Tr	8	4.7	1.9	.2
Pat (1¼ in square, ⅓ in high; 120 per lb)	1 pat	4	16	25	Tr	3	1.9	.8	.1
Fats, cooking (vegetable shortenings)	1 cup	200	0	1770	0	200	48.8	88.2	48.4
	1 tbsp	13	0	110	0	13	3.2	5.7	3.1
Lard	1 tbsp	13	0	115	0	13	5.1	5.3	1.3
Margarine:								
Regular (1 brick or 4 sticks per lb):								
Stick (½ cup)	1 stick	113	16	815	1	92	16.7	42.9	24.9
Tablespoon (about ⅛ stick)	1 tbsp	14	16	100	Tr	12	2.1	5.3	3.1
Pat (1-in square, ⅓ in high; 90 per lb)	1 pat	5	16	35	Tr	4	.7	1.9	1.1
Soft, two 8 oz containers per lb	1 container	227	16	1635	1	184	32.5	71.5	65.4
	1 tbsp	14	16	100	Tr	12	2.0	4.5	4.1
Whipped (6 sticks per lb):								
Stick (½ cup)	1 stick	76	16	545	Tr	61	11.2	28.7	16.7
Tablespoon (about ⅛ stick)	1 tbsp	9	16	70	Tr	8	1.4	3.6	2.1
Oils, salad or cooking:								
Corn	1 cup	218	0	1925	0	218	27.7	53.6	125.1
	1 tbsp	14	0	120	0	14	1.7	3.3	7.8
Olive	1 cup	216	0	1910	0	216	30.7	154.4	17.7
	1 tbsp	14	0	120	0	14	1.9	9.7	1.1
Peanut	1 cup	216	0	1910	0	216	37.4	98.5	67.0
	1 tbsp	14	0	120	0	14	2.3	6.2	4.2
Safflower	1 cup	218	0	1925	0	218	20.5	25.9	159.8
	1 tbsp	14	0	120	0	14	1.3	1.6	10.0
Soybean oil, hydrogenated	1 cup	218	0	1925	0	218	31.8	93.1	75.6
(partially hardened)	1 tbsp	14	0	120	0	14	2.0	5.8	4.7

For notes, see end of table.

Nutrients In Indicated Quantity

Carbohydrate (g)	Calcium (mg)	Phosphorus (mg)	Iron (mg)	Potassium (mg)	Vitamin A Value (IU)	Thiamin (mg)	Riboflavin (mg)	Niacin (mg)	Ascorbic Acid (mg)
29	297	310	1.1	387	930	.11	.50	.3	1
67	250	255	1.3	445	390	.05	.36	.3	1
41	298	232	Tr	352	410	.08	.41	.3	2
28	173	180	.7	223	480	.07	.30	.2	2
59	265	247	.8	354	340	.05	.39	.3	2
63	374	237	1.3	335	340	.08	.39	.3	2
42	343	269	.2	439	120[10]	.08	.40	.2	1
16	415	326	.2	531	150[10]	.10	.49	.3	2
17	452	355	.2	579	20[10]	.11	.53	.3	2
11	274	215	.1	351	280	.07	.32	.2	1
1	28	90	1.0	65	260	.04	.15	Tr	0
Tr	4	4	Tr	45	0	Tr	.09	Tr	0
Tr	26	86	.9	15	310	.04	.07	Tr	0
1	26	80	.9	58	290	.03	.13	Tr	0
1	28	90	1.0	65	260	.04	.14	Tr	0
1	28	90	1.0	65	260	.04	.13	Tr	0
1	47	97	.9	85	310	.04	.16	Tr	0
Tr	27	26	.2	29	3470[11]	.01	.04	Tr	0
Tr	3	3	Tr	4	430[11]	Tr	Tr	Tr	0
Tr	1	1	Tr	1	150[11]	Tr	Tr	Tr	0
Tr	18	17	.1	20	2310[11]	Tr	.03	Tr	0
Tr	2	2	Tr	2	290[11]	Tr	Tr	Tr	0
Tr	1	1	Tr	1	120[11]	0	Tr	Tr	0
0	0	0	0	0	—	0	0	0	0
0	0	0	0	0	—	0	0	0	0
0	0	0	0	0	0	0	0	0	0
Tr	27	26	.2	29	3750[12]	.01	.04	Tr	0
Tr	3	3	Tr	4	470[12]	Tr	Tr	Tr	0
Tr	1	1	Tr	1	170[12]	Tr	Tr	Tr	0
Tr	53	53	.4	59	7500[12]	.01	.08	.1	0
Tr	3	3	Tr	4	470[12]	Tr	Tr	Tr	0
Tr	18	17	.1	20	2500[12]	Tr	.03	Tr	0
Tr	2	2	Tr	2	310[12]	Tr	Tr	Tr	0
0	0	0	0	0	—	0	0	0	0
0	0	0	0	0	—	0	0	0	0
0	0	0	0	0	—	0	0	0	0
0	0	0	0	0	—	0	0	0	0
0	0	0	0	0	—	0	0	0	0
0	0	0	0	0	—	0	0	0	0
0	0	0	0	0	—	0	0	0	0
0	0	0	0	0	—	0	0	0	0
0	0	0	0	0	—	0	0	0	0

Foods, Approximate Measures, Units, and Weight		(g)	Water (%)	Food Energy (cal)	Protein (g)	Fat (g)	Saturated (total) (g)	Oleic (g)	Linoleic (g)
Soybean-cottonseed oil blend,	1 cup	218	0	1925	0	218	38.2	63.0	99.6
hydrogenated	1 tbsp	14	0	120	0	14	2.4	3.9	6.2
Salad dressings:									
Commercial:									
Blue cheese:									
Regular	1 tbsp	15	32	75	1	8	1.6	1.7	3.8
Low calorie (5 cal per tsp)	1 tbsp	16	84	10	Tr	1	.5	.3	Tr
French:									
Regular	1 tbsp	16	39	65	Tr	6	1.1	1.3	3.2
Low calorie (5 cal per tsp)	1 tbsp	16	77	15	Tr	1	.1	.1	.4
Italian:									
Regular	1 tbsp	15	28	85	Tr	9	1.6	1.9	4.7
Low calorie (2 cal per tsp)	1 tbsp	15	90	10	Tr	1	.1	.1	.4
Mayonnaise	1 tbsp	14	15	100	Tr	11	2.0	2.4	5.6
Mayonnaise type:									
Regular	1 tbsp	15	41	65	Tr	6	1.1	1.4	3.2
Low calorie (8 cal per tsp)	1 tbsp	16	81	20	Tr	2	.4	.4	1.0
Tartar sauce, regular	1 tbsp	14	34	75	Tr	8	1.5	1.8	4.1
Thousand Island:									
Regular	1 tbsp	16	32	80	Tr	8	1.4	1.7	4.0
Low calorie (10 cal per tsp)	1 tbsp	15	68	25	Tr	2	.4	.4	1.0
From home recipe:									
Cooked type[13]	1 tbsp	16	68	25	1	2	.5	.6	.3
Fish, Shellfish, Meat, Poultry, Related Products									
Fish and shellfish:									
Bluefish, baked with butter or margarine	3 oz	85	68	135	22	4	—	—	—
Clams:									
Raw, meat only	3 oz	85	82	65	11	1	—	—	—
Canned, solids and liquid	3 oz	85	86	45	7	1	.2	Tr	Tr
Crabmeat (white or king), canned, not pressed down	1 cup	135	77	135	24	3	.6	0.4	0.1
Fish sticks, breaded, cooked, frozen (stick, 4 × 1 × ½ in)	1 fish stick or 1 oz	28	66	50	5	3	—	—	—
Haddock, breaded, fried[14]	3 oz	85	66	140	17	5	1.4	2.2	1.2
Ocean perch, breaded, fried[14]	1 fillet	85	59	195	16	11	2.7	4.4	2.3
Oysters, raw, meat only (13-19 medium Selects)	1 cup	240	85	160	20	4	1.3	.2	.1
Salmon, pink, canned, solids and liquid	3 oz	85	71	120	17	5	.9	.8	.1
Sardines, Atlantic, canned in oil, drained solids	3 oz	85	62	175	20	9	3.0	2.5	.5
Scallops, frozen, breaded, fried, reheated	6 scallops	90	60	175	16	8	—	—	—
Shad, baked with butter or margarine, bacon	3 oz	85	64	170	20	10	—	—	—
Shrimp:									
Canned meat	3 oz	85	70	100	21	1	.1	.1	Tr
French fried[16]	3 oz	85	57	190	17	9	2.3	3.7	2.0
Tuna, canned in oil, drained solids	3 oz	85	61	170	24	7	1.7	1.7	.7
Tuna salad[17]	1 cup	205	70	350	30	22	4.3	6.3	6.7
Meat and meat products:									
Bacon (20 slices per lb, raw), broiled or fried, crisp	2 slices	15	8	85	4	8	2.5	3.7	.7
Beef, cooked:[18]									
Cuts braised, simmered, or pot roasted:									
Lean and fat (piece, 2½ × 2½ × ¾ in)	3 oz	85	53	245	23	16	6.8	6.5	.4
Lean only from item directly above	2.5 oz	72	62	140	22	5	2.1	1.8	.2
Ground beef, broiled:									
Lean with 10% fat	3 oz or patty 3 × ⅝ in	85	60	185	23	10	4.0	3.9	.3
Lean with 21% fat	2.9 oz or patty 3 × ⅝ in	82	54	235	20	17	7.0	6.7	.4
Roast, oven cooked, no liquid added:									
Relatively fat, such as rib:									
Lean and fat (2 pieces, 4⅛ × 2¼ × ¼ in)	3 oz	85	40	375	17	33	14.0	13.6	.8
Lean only	1.8 oz	51	57	125	14	7	3.0	2.5	.3
Relatively lean, such as heel of round:									
Lean and fat (2 pieces, 4⅛ × 2¼ × ¼ in)	3 oz	85	62	165	25	7	2.8	2.7.	.2
Lean only	2.8 oz	78	65	125	24	3	1.2	1.0	0.1

For notes, see end of table.

Nutrients in Indicated Quantity

Carbohydrate (g)	Calcium (mg)	Phosphorus (mg)	Iron (mg)	Potassium (mg)	Vitamin A Value (IU)	Thiamin (mg)	Riboflavin (mg)	Niacin (mg)	Ascorbic Acid (mg)
0	0	0	0	0	—	0	0	0	0
0	0	0	0	0	—	0	0	0	0
1	12	11	Tr	6	30	Tr	.02	Tr	Tr
1	10	8	Tr	5	30	Tr	.01	Tr	Tr
3	2	2	.1	13	—	—	—	—	—
2	2	2	.1	13	—	—	—	—	—
1	2	1	Tr	2	Tr	Tr	Tr	Tr	—
Tr	Tr	1	Tr	2	Tr	Tr	Tr	Tr	—
Tr	3	4	.1	5	40	Tr	.01	Tr	—
2	2	4	Tr	1	30	Tr	Tr	Tr	—
2	3	4	Tr	1	40	Tr	Tr	Tr	—
1	3	4	.1	11	30	Tr	Tr	Tr	Tr
2	2	3	.1	18	50	Tr	Tr	Tr	Tr
2	2	3	.1	17	50	Tr	Tr	Tr	Tr
2	14	15	.1	19	80	.01	.03	Tr	Tr
0	25	244	.6	—	40	.09	.08	1.6	—
2	59	138	5.2	154	90	.08	.15	1.1	8
2	47	116	3.5	119	—	.01	.09	.9	—
1	61	246	1.1	149	—	.11	.11	2.6	—
2	3	47	.1	—	0	.01	.02	.5	—
5	34	210	1.0	296	—	.03	.06	2.7	2
6	28	192	1.1	242	—	.10	.10	1.6	—
8	226	343	13.2	290	740	.34	.43	6.0	—
0	167[15]	243	.7	307	60	.03	.16	6.8	—
0	372	424	2.5	502	190	.02	.17	4.6	—
9	—	—	—	—	—	—	—	—	—
0	20	266	.5	320	30	.11	.22	7.3	—
1	98	224	2.6	104	50	.01	.03	1.5	—
9	61	162	1.7	195	—	.03	.07	2.3	—
0	7	199	1.6	—	70	.04	.10	10.1	—
7	41	291	2.7	—	590	.08	.23	10.3	2
Tr	2	34	.5	35	0	.08	.05	.8	—
0	10	114	2.9	184	30	.04	.18	3.6	—
0	10	108	2.7	176	10	.04	.17	3.3	—
0	10	196	3.0	261	20	.08	.20	5.1	—
0	9	159	2.6	221	30	.07	.17	4.4	—
0	8	158	2.2	189	70	.05	.13	3.1	—
0	6	131	1.8	161	10	.04	.11	2.6	—
0	11	208	3.2	279	10	.06	.19	4.5	—
0	10	199	3.0	268	Tr	.06	.18	4.3	—

						Fatty Acids		
						Saturated (total) (g)	Unsaturated	
							Oleic (g)	Linoleic (g)
Foods, Approximate Measures, Units, and Weight		(g)	Water (%)	Food Energy (cal)	Protein (g)	Fat (g)		
Steak:								
Relatively fat sirloin, broiled:								
Lean and fat (piece, 2½ × 2½ × ¾ in)	3 oz	85	44	330	20	27	11.3	11.1	.6
Lean only	2.0 oz	56	59	115	18	4	1.8	1.6	.2
Relatively lean-round, braised:								
Lean and fat (piece, 4⅛ × 2¼ × ½ in)	3 oz	85	55	220	24	13	5.5	5.2	.4
Lean only	2.4 oz	68	61	130	21	4	1.7	1.5	.2
Beef, canned:								
Corned beef	3 oz	85	59	185	22	10	4.9	4.5	.2
Corned beef hash	1 cup	220	67	400	19	25	11.9	10.9	.5
Beef, dried, chipped	2½ oz jar	71	48	145	24	4	2.1	2.0	.1
Beef and vegetable stew	1 cup	245	82	220	16	11	4.9	4.5	.2
Beef potpie (home recipe), baked (piece, ⅓ of 9-in diameter pie)[19]	1 piece	210	55	515	21	30	7.9	12.8	6.7
Chili con carne with beans, canned	1 cup	255	72	340	19	16	7.5	6.8	.3
Chop suey with beef and pork (home recipe)	1 cup	250	75	300	26	17	8.5	6.2	.7
Heart, beef, lean, braised	3 oz	85	61	160	27	5	1.5	1.1	.6
Lamb, cooked:								
Chop, rib (cut 3 per lb with bone), broiled:								
Lean and fat	3.1 oz	89	43	360	18	32	14.8	12.1	1.2
Lean only	2 oz	57	60	120	16	6	2.5	2.1	.2
Leg, roasted:								
Lean and fat (2 pieces, 4⅛ × 2¼ × ¼ in)	3 oz	85	54	235	22	16	7.3	6.0	.6
Lean only	2.5 oz	71	62	130	20	5	2.1	1.8	.2
Shoulder, roasted:								
Lean and fat (3 pieces, 2½ × 2½ × ¼ in)	3 oz	85	50	285	18	23	10.8	8.8	.9
Lean only	2.3 oz	64	61	130	17	6	3.6	2.3	.2
Liver, beef, fried (slice, 6½ × 2⅜ × ⅜ in)[20]	3 oz	85	56	195	22	9	2.5	3.5	.9
Pork, cured, cooked:								
Ham, light cure, lean and fat, roasted (2 pieces, 4⅛ × 2¼ × ¼ in)[22]	3 oz	85	54	245	18	19	6.8	7.9	1.7
Luncheon meat:								
Boiled ham, slice (8 per 8 oz pkg)	1 oz	28	59	65	5	5	1.7	2.0	.4
Canned, spiced or unspiced:								
Slice, approx. 3 × 2 × ½ in	1 slice	60	55	175	9	15	5.4	6.7	1.0
Pork, fresh, cooked:[18]								
Chop, loin (cut 3 per lb with bone), broiled:								
Lean and fat	2.7 oz	78	42	305	19	25	8.9	10.4	2.2
Lean only	2 oz	56	53	150	17	9	3.1	3.6	.8
Roast, oven cooked, no liquid added:								
Lean and fat (piece, 2½ × 2½ × ¾ in)	3 oz	85	46	310	21	24	8.7	10.2	2.2
Lean only	2.4 oz	68	55	175	20	10	3.5	4.1	.8
Shoulder cut, simmered:								
Lean and fat (3 pieces, 2½ × 2½ × ¼ in)	3 oz	85	46	320	20	26	9.3	10.9	2.3
Lean only	2.2 oz	63	60	135	18	6	2.2	2.6	.6
Sausages (see also Luncheon meat):								
Bologna, slice (8 per 8 oz pkg)	1 slice	28	56	85	3	8	3.0	3.4	.5
Braunschweiger, slice (6 per 6 oz pkg)	1 slice	28	53	90	4	8	2.6	3.4	.8
Brown and serve (10-11 per 8 oz pkg), browned	1 link	17	40	70	3	6	2.3	2.8	.7
Deviled ham, canned	1 tbsp	13	51	45	2	4	1.5	1.8	.4
Frankfurter (8 per 1 lb pkg), cooked (reheated)	1 frankfurter	56	57	170	7	15	5.6	6.5	1.2
Meat, potted (beef, chicken, turkey), canned	1 tbsp	13	61	30	2	2	—	—	—
Pork link (16 per 1 lb pkg), cooked	1 link	13	35	60	2	6	2.1	2.4	.5
Salami:								
Dry type, slice (12 per 4 oz pkg)	1 slice	10	30	45	2	4	1.6	1.6	.1
Cooked type, slice (8 per 8 oz pkg)	1 slice	28	51	90	5	7	3.1	3.0	.2
Vienna sausage (7 per 4 oz can)	1 sausage	16	63	40	2	3	1.2	1.4	.2
Veal, medium fat, cooked, bone removed:								
Cutlet (4⅛ × 2¼ × ½ in), braised or broiled	3 oz	85	60	185	23	9	4.0	3.4	.4
Rib (2 pieces, 4⅛ × 2¼ × ¼ in), roasted	3 oz	85	55	230	23	14	6.1	5.1	.6
Poultry and poultry products:								
Chicken, cooked:								
Breast, fried, bones removed, ½ breast (3.3 oz with bones)[23]	2.8 oz	79	58	160	26	5	1.4	1.8	1.1
Drumstick, fried, bones removed (2 oz with bones)[23]	1.3 oz	38	55	90	12	4	1.1	1.3	.9
Half broiler, broiled, bones removed (10.4 oz with bones)	6.2 oz	176	71	240	42	7	2.2	2.5	1.3

For notes, see end of table.

Nutrients in Indicated Quantity

Carbohydrate (g)	Calcium (mg)	Phosphorus (mg)	Iron (mg)	Potassium (mg)	Vitamin A Value (IU)	Thiamin (mg)	Riboflavin (mg)	Niacin (mg)	Ascorbic Acid (mg)
0	9	162	2.5	220	50	.05	.15	4.0	—
0	7	146	2.2	202	10	.05	.14	3.6	—
0	10	213	3.0	272	20	.07	.19	4.8	—
0	9	182	2.5	238	10	.05	.16	4.1	—
0	17	90	3.7	—	—	.01	.20	2.9	—
24	29	147	4.4	440	—	.02	.20	4.6	—
0	14	287	3.6	142	—	.05	.23	2.7	0
15	29	184	2.9	613	2400	.15	.17	4.7	17
39	29	149	3.8	334	1720	.30	.30	5.5	6
31	82	321	4.3	594	150	.08	.18	3.3	—
13	60	248	4.8	425	600	.28	.38	5.0	33
1	5	154	5.0	197	20	.21	1.04	6.5	1
0	8	139	1.0	200	—	.11	.19	4.1	—
0	6	121	1.1	174	—	.09	.15	3.4	—
0	9	177	1.4	241	—	.13	.23	4.7	—
0	9	169	1.4	227	—	.12	.21	4.4	—
0	9	146	1.0	206	—	.11	.20	4.0	—
0	8	140	1.0	193	—	.10	.18	3.7	—
5	9	405	7.5	323	45,390[21]	.22	3.56	14.0	23
0	8	146	2.2	199	0	.40	.15	3.1	—
0	3	47	.8	—	0	.12	.04	.7	—
1	5	65	1.3	133	0	.19	.13	1.8	—
0	9	209	2.7	216	0	.75	.22	4.5	—
0	7	181	2.2	192	0	.63	.18	3.8	—
0	9	218	2.7	233	0	.78	.22	4.8	—
0	9	211	2.6	224	0	.73	.21	4.4	—
0	9	118	2.6	158	0	.46	.21	4.1	—
0	8	111	2.3	146	0	.42	.19	3.7	—
Tr	2	36	.5	65	—	.05	.06	.7	—
1	3	69	1.7	—	1850	.05	.41	2.3	—
Tr	—	—	—	—	—	—	—	—	—
0	1	12	.3	—	0	.02	.01	.2	—
1	3	57	.8	—	—	.08	.11	1.4	—
0	—	—	—	—	—	Tr	.03	.2	—
Tr	1	21	.3	35	0	.10	.04	.5	—
Tr	1	28	.4	—	—	.04	.03	.5	—
Tr	3	57	.7	—	—	.07	.07	1.2	—
Tr	1	24	.3	—	—	.01	.02	.4	—
0	9	196	2.7	258	—	.06	.21	4.6	—
0	10	211	2.9	259	—	.11	.26	6.6	—
1	9	218	1.3	—	70	.04	.17	11.6	—
Tr	6	89	.9	—	50	.03	.15	2.7	—
0	16	355	3.0	483	160	.09	.34	15.5	—

					Nutrients in Indicated Quantity			
							Fatty Acids	
							Unsaturated	
			Water	Food Energy	Protein	Fat	Saturated (total)	Oleic	Linoleic
Foods, Approximate Measures, Units, and Weight		(g)	(%)	(cal)	(g)	(g)	(g)	(g)	(g)

Foods, Approximate Measures, Units, and Weight		(g)	Water (%)	Food Energy (cal)	Protein (g)	Fat (g)	Saturated (total) (g)	Oleic (g)	Linoleic (g)
Chicken, canned, boneless	3 oz	85	65	170	18	10	3.2	3.8	2.0
Chicken a la king, cooked (home recipe)	1 cup	245	68	470	27	34	12.7	14.3	3.3
Chicken and noodles, cooked (home recipe)	1 cup	240	71	365	22	18	5.9	7.1	3.5
Chicken chow mein:									
Canned	1 cup	250	89	95	7	Tr	—	—	—
From home recipe	1 cup	250	78	255	31	10	2.4	3.4	3.1
Chicken potpie (home recipe), baked, piece (⅓ of 9-in diameter pie)[19]	1 piece	232	57	545	23	31	11.3	10.9	5.6
Turkey, roasted, flesh without skin:									
Dark meat, piece, 2½ × 1⅝ × ¼ in	4 pieces	85	61	175	26	7	2.1	1.5	1.5
Light meat, piece, 4 × 2 × ¼ in	2 pieces	85	62	150	28	3	.9	.6	.7
Light and dark meat:									
Chopped or diced	1 cup	140	61	265	44	9	2.5	1.7	1.8
Pieces (1 slice white meat, 4 × 2 × ¼ in with 2 slices dark meat, 2½ × 1⅝ × ¼ in)	3 pieces	85	61	160	27	5	1.5	1.0	1.1
Fruits and Fruit Products									
Apples, raw, unpeeled, without cores:									
2¾-in diameter (about 3 per lb with cores)	1 apple	138	84	80	Tr	1	—	—	—
3¼-in diameter (about 2 per lb with cores)	1 apple	212	84	125	Tr	1	—	—	—
Applejuice, bottled or canned[24]	1 cup	248	88	120	Tr	Tr	—	—	—
Applesauce, canned:									
Sweetened	1 cup	255	76	230	1	Tr	—	—	—
Unsweetened	1 cup	244	89	100	Tr	Tr	—	—	—
Apricots:									
Raw, without pits (about 12 per lb with pits)	3 apricots	107	85	55	1	Tr	—	—	—
Canned in heavy syrup (halves and syrup)	1 cup	258	77	220	2	Tr	—	—	—
Dried:									
Uncooked (28 large or 37 medium halves per cup)	1 cup	130	25	340	7	1	—	—	—
Cooked, unsweetened, fruit and liquid	1 cup	250	76	215	4	1	—	—	—
Apricot nectar, canned	1 cup	251	85	145	1	Tr	—	—	—
Avocados, raw, whole, without skins and seeds:									
California, mid- and late-winter (with skin and seed, 3⅛-in diameter; wt 10 oz)	1 avocado	216	74	370	5	37	5.5	22.0	3.7
Florida, late summer and fall (with skin and seed, 3⅝-in diameter; wt 1 lb)	1 avocado	304	78	390	4	33	6.7	15.7	5.3
Banana without peel (about 2.6 per lb with peel)	1 banana	119	76	100	1	Tr	—	—	—
Banana flakes	1 tbsp	6	3	20	Tr	Tr	—	—	—
Blackberries, raw	1 cup	144	85	85	2	1	—	—	—
Blueberries, raw	1 cup	145	83	90	1	1	—	—	—
Cantaloupe; see muskmelons									
Cherries:									
Sour (tart), red, pitted, canned, water pack	1 cup	244	88	105	2	Tr	—	—	—
Sweet, raw, without pits and stems	10 cherries	68	80	45	1	Tr	—	—	—
Cranberry juice cocktail, bottled, sweetened	1 cup	253	83	165	Tr	Tr	—	—	—
Cranberry sauce, sweetened, canned, strained	1 cup	277	62	405	Tr	1	—	—	—
Dates:									
Whole, without pits	10 dates	80	23	220	2	Tr	—	—	—
Chopped	1 cup	178	23	490	4	1	—	—	—
Fruit cocktail, canned, in heavy syrup	1 cup	255	80	195	1	Tr	—	—	—
Grapefruit:									
Raw, medium, 3¾-in diameter (about 1 lb 1 oz):									
Pink or red	½ grapefruit with peel[28]	241	89	50	1	Tr	—	—	—
White	½ grapefruit with peel[28]	241	89	45	1	Tr	—	—	—
Canned, sections with syrup	1 cup	254	81	180	2	Tr	—	—	—
Grapefruit juice:									
Raw, pink, red, or white	1 cup	246	90	95	1	Tr	—	—	—
Canned, white:									
Unsweetened	1 cup	247	89	100	1	Tr	—	—	—
Sweetened	1 cup	250	86	135	1	Tr	—	—	—
Frozen, concentrate, unsweetened:									
Undiluted, 6 fl oz can	1 can	207	62	300	4	1	—	—	—
Diluted with 3 parts water by volume	1 cup	247	89	100	1	Tr	—	—	—
Dehydrated crystals, prepared with water (1 lb yields about 1 gal)	1 cup	247	90	100	1	Tr	—	—	—

For notes, see end of table.

Nutrients in Indicated Quantity

Carbohydrate (g)	Calcium (mg)	Phosphorus (mg)	Iron (mg)	Potassium (mg)	Vitamin A Value (IU)	Thiamin (mg)	Riboflavin (mg)	Niacin (mg)	Ascorbic Acid (mg)
0	18	210	1.3	117	200	.03	.11	3.7	3
12	127	358	2.5	404	1130	.10	.42	5.4	12
26	26	247	2.2	149	430	.05	.17	4.3	Tr
18	45	85	1.3	418	150	.05	.10	1.0	13
10	58	293	2.5	473	280	.08	.23	4.3	10
42	70	232	3.0	343	3090	.34	.31	5.5	5
0	—	—	2.0	338	—	.03	.20	3.6	—
0	—	—	1.0	349	—	.04	.12	9.4	—
0	11	351	2.5	514	—	.07	.25	10.8	—
0	7	213	1.5	312	—	.04	.15	6.5	—
20	10	14	.4	152	120	.04	.03	.1	6
31	15	21	.6	233	190	.06	.04	.2	8
30	15	22	1.5	250	—	.02	.05	.2	2[25]
61	10	13	1.3	166	100	.05	.03	.1	3[25]
26	10	12	1.2	190	100	.05	.02	.1	2[25]
14	18	25	.5	301	2890	.03	.04	.6	11
57	28	39	.8	604	4490	.05	.05	1.0	10
86	87	140	7.2	1273	14,170	.01	.21	4.3	16
54	55	88	4.5	795	7500	.01	.13	2.5	8
37	23	30	.5	379	2380	.03	.03	.5	36[26]
13	22	91	1.3	1303	630	.24	.43	3.5	30
27	30	128	1.8	1836	880	.33	.61	4.9	43
26	10	31	.8	440	230	.06	.07	.8	12
5	2	6	.2	92	50	.01	.01	.2	Tr
19	46	27	1.3	245	290	.04	.06	.6	30
22	22	19	1.5	117	150	.04	.09	.7	20
26	37	32	.7	317	1660	.07	.05	.5	12
12	15	13	.3	129	70	.03	.04	.3	7
42	13	8	.8	25	Tr	.03	.03	.1	81
104	17	11	.6	83	60	.03	.03	.1	6
58	47	50	2.4	518	40	.07	.08	1.8	0
130	105	112	5.3	1153	90	.16	.18	3.9	0
50	23	31	1.0	411	360	.05	.03	1.0	5
13	20	20	.5	166	540	.05	.02	.2	44
12	19	19	.5	159	10	.05	.02	.2	44
45	33	36	.8	343	30	.08	.05	.5	76
23	22	37	.5	399	([29])	.10	.05	.5	93
24	20	35	1.0	400	20	.07	.05	.5	84
32	20	35	1.0	405	30	.08	.05	.5	78
72	70	124	.8	1250	60	.29	.12	1.4	286
24	25	42	.2	420	20	.10	.04	.5	96
24	22	40	.2	412	20	.10	.05	.5	91

				Nutrients in Indicated Quantity				
							Fatty Acids		
							Saturated	Unsaturated	
Foods, Approximate Measures, Units, and Weight		(g)	Water (%)	Food Energy (cal)	Protein (g)	Fat (g)	(total) (g)	Oleic (g)	Linoleic (g)
Grapes, European type (adherent skin), raw:									
Thompson seedless	10 grapes	50	81	35	Tr	Tr	—	—	—
Tokay and Emperor, seeded types	10 grapes[30]	60	81	40	Tr	Tr	—	—	—
Grapejuice:									
Canned or bottled	1 cup	253	83	165	1	Tr	—	—	—
Frozen concentrate, sweetened:									
Undiluted, 6 fl oz can	1 can	216	53	395	1	Tr	—	—	—
Diluted with 3 parts water by volume	1 cup	250	86	135	1	Tr	—	—	—
Grape drink, canned	1 cup	250	86	135	Tr	Tr	—	—	—
Lemon, raw, size 165, without peel and seeds (about 4 per lb with peels and seeds)	1 lemon	74	90	20	1	Tr	—	—	—
Lemon juice:									
Raw	1 cup	244	91	60	1	Tr	—	—	—
Canned, or bottled, unsweetened	1 cup	244	92	55	1	Tr	—	—	—
Frozen, single strength, unsweetened, 6 fl oz can	1 can	183	92	40	1	Tr	—	—	—
Lemonade concentrate, frozen:									
Undiluted, 6 fl oz can	1 can	219	49	425	Tr	Tr	—	—	—
Diluted with 4⅓ parts water by volume	1 cup	248	89	105	Tr	Tr	—	—	—
Limeade concentrate, frozen:									
Undiluted, 6 fl oz can	1 can	218	50	410	Tr	Tr	—	—	—
Diluted with 4⅓ parts water by volume	1 cup	247	89	100	Tr	Tr	—	—	—
Limejuice:									
Raw	1 cup	246	90	65	1	Tr	—	—	—
Canned, unsweetened	1 cup	246	90	65	1	Tr	—	—	—
Muskmelons, raw, with rind, without seed cavity:									
Cantaloupe, orange-fleshed (with rind and seed cavity, 5-in diameter, 2⅓ lb)	½ melon with rind[33]	477	91	80	2	Tr	—	—	—
Honeydew (with rind and seed cavity, 6½-in diameter, 5¼ lb)	⅒ melon with rind[33]	226	91	50	1	Tr	—	—	—
Oranges, all commercial varieties, raw:									
Whole, 2⅝-in diameter, without peel and seeds (about 2½ per lb with peel and seeds)	1 orange	131	86	65	1	Tr	—	—	—
Sections without membranes	1 cup	180	86	90	2	Tr	—	—	—
Orange juice:									
Raw, all varieties	1 cup	248	88	110	2	Tr	—	—	—
Canned, unsweetened	1 cup	249	87	120	2	Tr	—	—	—
Frozen concentrate:									
Undiluted, 6 fl oz can	1 can	213	55	360	5	Tr	—	—	—
Diluted with 3 parts water by volume	1 cup	249	87	120	2	Tr	—	—	—
Dehydrated crystals, prepared with water (1 lb yields about 1 gal)	1 cup	248	88	115	1	Tr	—	—	—
Orange and grapefruit juice:									
Frozen concentrate:									
Undiluted, 6 fl oz can	1 can	210	59	330	4	1	—	—	—
Diluted with 3 parts water by volume	1 cup	248	88	110	1	Tr	—	—	—
Papayas, raw, ½-in cubes	1 cup	140	89	55	1	Tr	—	—	—
Peaches:									
Raw:									
Whole, 2½-in diameter, peeled, pitted (about 4 per lb with peels and pits)	1 peach	100	89	40	1	Tr	—	—	—
Sliced	1 cup	170	89	65	1	Tr	—	—	—
Canned, yellow-fleshed, solids and liquid (halves or slices):									
Syrup pack	1 cup	256	79	200	1	Tr	—	—	—
Water pack	1 cup	244	91	75	1	Tr	—	—	—
Dried:									
Uncooked	1 cup	160	25	420	5	1	—	—	—
Cooked, unsweetened, halves and juice	1 cup	250	77	205	3	1	—	—	—
Frozen, sliced, sweetened:									
10-oz container	1 container	284	77	250	1	Tr	—	—	—
Cup	1 cup	250	77	220	1	Tr	—	—	—
Pears:									
Raw, with skin, cored:									
Bartlett, 2½-in diameter (about 2½ per lb with cores and stems)	1 pear	164	83	100	1	1	—	—	—
Bosc, 2½-in diameter (about 3 per lb with cores and stems)	1 pear	141	83	85	1	1	—	—	—

For notes, see end of table.

			Nutrients in Indicated Quantity						

Carbohydrate (g)	Calcium (mg)	Phosphorus (mg)	Iron (mg)	Potassium (mg)	Vitamin A Value (IU)	Thiamin (mg)	Riboflavin (mg)	Niacin (mg)	Ascorbic Acid (mg)
9	6	10	.2	87	50	.03	.02	.2	2
10	7	11	.2	99	60	.03	.02	.2	2
42	28	30	.8	293	—	.10	.05	.5	Tr[25]
100	22	32	.9	255	40	.13	.22	1.5	32[31]
33	8	10	.3	85	10	.05	.08	.5	10[31]
35	8	10	.3	88	—	03[32]	03[32]	.3	([32])
6	19	12	.4	102	10	03	01	.1	39
20	17	24	.5	344	50	07	02	.2	112
19	17	24	.5	344	50	07	02	.2	102
13	13	16	.5	258	40	05	02	.2	81
112	9	13	.4	153	40	.05	06	.7	66
28	2	3	.1	40	10	.01	02	.2	17
108	11	13	.2	129	Tr	.02	.02	.2	26
27	3	3	Tr	32	Tr	Tr	Tr	Tr	6
22	22	27	.5	256	20	.05	.02	.2	79
22	22	27	.5	256	20	.05	.02	.2	52
20	38	44	1.1	682	9240	.11	.08	1.6	90
11	21	24	.6	374	60	.06	.04	.9	34
16	54	26	.5	263	260	.13	.05	.5	66
22	74	36	.7	360	360	.18	.07	.7	90
26	27	42	.5	496	500	.22	.07	1.0	124
28	25	45	1.0	496	500	.17	.05	.7	100
87	75	126	.9	1500	1620	.68	.11	2.8	360
29	25	42	.2	503	540	.23	.03	.9	120
27	25	40	.5	518	500	.20	.07	1.0	109
78	61	99	.8	1308	800	.48	.06	2.3	302
26	20	32	.2	439	270	.15	.02	.7	102
14	28	22	.4	328	2450	.06	.06	.4	78
10	9	19	.5	202	1330[34]	.02	.05	1.0	7
16	15	32	.9	343	2260[34]	.03	.09	1.7	12
51	10	31	.8	333	1100	.03	.05	1.5	8
20	10	32	.7	334	1100	.02	.07	1.5	7
109	77	187	9.6	1520	6240	.02	.30	8.5	29
54	38	93	4.8	743	3050	.01	.15	3.8	5
64	11	37	1.4	352	1850	.03	.11	2.0	116[35]
57	10	33	1.3	310	1630	.03	.10	1.8	103[35]
25	13	18	.5	213	30	.03	.07	.2	7
22	11	16	.4	83	30	.03	.06	.1	6

Foods, Approximate Measures, Units, and Weight		(g)	Water (%)	Food Energy (cal)	Protein (g)	Fat (g)	Saturated (total) (g)	Oleic (g)	Linoleic (g)
							Fatty Acids		
								Unsaturated	
D'Anjou, 3-in diameter (about 2 per lb with cores and stems)	1 pear	200	83	120	1	1	—	—	—
Canned, solids and liquid, syrup pack, heavy (halves or slices)	1 cup	255	80	195	1	1	—	—	—
Pineapple:									
Raw, diced	1 cup	155	85	80	1	Tr	—	—	—
Canned, heavy syrup pack, solids and liquid:									
Crushed, chunks, tidbits	1 cup	255	80	190	1	Tr	—	—	—
Slices and liquid:									
Large	1 slice; 2¼ tbsp liquid	105	80	80	Tr	Tr	—	—	—
Medium	1 slice; 1¼ tbsp liquid	58	80	45	Tr	Tr	—	—	—
Pineapple juice, unsweetened, canned	1 cup	250	86	140	1	Tr	—	—	—
Plums:									
Raw, without pits:									
Japanese and hybrid (2⅛-in diameter, about 6½ per lb with pits)	1 plum	66	87	30	Tr	Tr	—	—	—
Prune-type (1½-in diameter, about 15 per lb with pits)	1 plum	28	79	20	Tr	Tr	—	—	—
Canned, heavy syrup pack (Italian prunes), with pits and liquid:									
Cup	1 cup[36]	272	77	215	1	Tr	—	—	—
Portion	3 plums; 2¾ tbsp liquid[36]	140	77	110	1	Tr	—	—	—
Prunes, dried, "softenized," with pits:									
Uncooked	4 extra large or 5 large prunes[36]	49	28	110	1	Tr	—	—	—
Cooked, unsweetened, all sizes, fruit and liquid	1 cup[36]	250	66	255	2	1	—	—	—
Prune juice, canned or bottled	1 cup	256	80	195	1	Tr	—	—	—
Raisins, seedless:									
Cup, not pressed down	1 cup	145	18	420	4	Tr	—	—	—
Packet, ½ oz (1½ tbsp)	1 packet	14	18	40	Tr	Tr	—	—	—
Raspberries, red:									
Raw, capped, whole	1 cup	123	84	70	1	1	—	—	—
Frozen, sweetened, 10 oz container	1 container	284	74	280	2	1	—	—	—
Rhubarb, cooked, added sugar:									
From raw	1 cup	270	63	380	1	Tr	—	—	—
From frozen, sweetened	1 cup	270	63	385	1	1	—	—	—
Strawberries:									
Raw, whole berries, capped	1 cup	149	90	55	1	1	—	—	—
Frozen, sweetened:									
Sliced, 10 oz container	1 container	284	71	310	1	1	—	—	—
Whole, 1 lb container (about 1¾ cups)	1 container	454	76	415	2	1	—	—	—
Tangerine, raw, 2⅜-in diameter, size 176, without peel (about 4 per lb with peels and seeds)	1 tangerine	86	87	40	1	Tr	—	—	—
Tangerine juice, canned, sweetened	1 cup	249	87	125	1	Tr	—	—	—
Watermelon, raw, 4 × 8 in wedge with rind and seeds (1/16 of 32⅔ lb melon, 10 × 16 in)	1 wedge with rind and seeds	926	93	110	2	1	—	—	—
Grain Products									
Bagel, 3-in diameter:									
Egg	1 bagel	55	32	165	6	2	.5	.9	.8
Water	1 bagel	55	29	165	6	1	.2	.4	.6
Barley, pearled, light, uncooked	1 cup	200	11	700	16	2	.3	.2	.8
Biscuits, baking powder, 2-in diameter (enriched flour, vegetable shortening):									
From home recipe	1 biscuit	28	27	105	2	5	1.2	2.0	1.2
From mix	1 biscuit	28	29	90	2	3	.6	1.1	.7
Breadcrumbs (enriched)[38]:									
Dry, grated	1 cup	100	7	390	13	5	1.0	1.6	1.4
Soft; see White bread									
Breads:									
Boston brown bread, canned, slice, 3¼ × ½ in[38]	1 slice	45	45	95	2	1	.1	.2	.2
Cracked-wheat bread (¾ enriched wheat flour, ¼ cracked wheat)[38]:									
Slice (18 per loaf)	1 slice	25	35	65	2	1	.1	.2	.2
French or Vienna bread, enriched[38]									
Slice:									
French (5 × 2½ × 1 in)	1 slice	35	31	100	3	1	.2	.4	.4

For notes, see end of table.

Nutrients in Indicated Quantity

Carbohydrate (g)	Calcium (mg)	Phosphorus (mg)	Iron (mg)	Potassium (mg)	Vitamin A Value (IU)	Thiamin (mg)	Riboflavin (mg)	Niacin (mg)	Ascorbic Acid (mg)
31	16	22	.6	260	40	.04	.08	.2	8
50	13	18	.5	214	10	.03	.05	.3	3
21	26	12	.8	226	110	.14	.05	.3	26
49	28	13	.8	245	130	.20	.05	.5	18
20	12	5	.3	101	50	.08	.02	.2	7
11	6	3	.2	56	30	.05	.01	.1	4
34	38	23	.8	373	130	.13	.05	.5	80[27]
8	8	12	.3	112	160	.02	.02	.3	4
6	3	5	.1	48	80	.01	.01	.1	1
56	23	26	2.3	367	3130	.05	.05	1.0	5
29	12	13	1.2	189	1610	.03	.03	.5	3
29	22	34	1.7	298	690	.04	.07	.7	1
67	51	79	3.8	695	1590	.07	.15	1.5	2
49	36	51	1.8	602	—	.03	.03	1.0	5
112	90	146	5.1	1106	30	.16	.12	.7	1
11	9	14	.5	107	Tr	.02	.01	.1	Tr
17	27	27	1.1	207	160	.04	.11	1.1	31
70	37	48	1.7	284	200	.06	.17	1.7	60
97	211	41	1.6	548	220	.05	.14	.8	16
98	211	32	1.9	475	190	.05	.11	.5	16
13	31	31	1.5	244	90	.04	.10	.9	88
79	40	48	2.0	318	90	.06	.17	1.4	151
107	59	73	2.7	472	140	.09	.27·	2.3	249
10	34	15	.3	108	360	.05	.02	.1	27
30	44	35	.5	440	1040	.15	.05	.2	54
27	30	43	2.1	426	2510	.13	.13	.9	30
28	9	43	1.2	41	30	.14	.10	1.2	0
30	8	41	1.2	42	0	.15	.11	1.4	0
158	32	378	4.0	320	0	.24	.10	6.2	0
13	34	49	.4	33	Tr	.08	.08	.7	Tr
15	19	65	.6	32	Tr	.09	.08	.8	Tr
73	122	141	3.6	152	Tr	.35	.35	4.8	Tr
21	41	72	.9	131	0[39]	.06	.04	.7	0
13	22	32	.5	34	Tr	.08	.06	.8	Tr
19	15	30	.8	32	Tr	.14	.08	1.2	Tr

Foods, Approximate Measures, Units, and Weight		(g)	Water (%)	Food Energy (cal)	Protein (g)	Fat (g)	Saturated (total) (g)	Oleic (g)	Linoleic (g)
							Fatty Acids		
								Unsaturated	
Vienna (4¾ × 4 × ½ in)	1 slice	25	31	75	2	1	.2	.3	.3
Italian bread enriched:									
Slice, 4½ × 3¼ × ¾ in	1 slice	30	32	85	3	Tr	Tr	Tr	.1
Raisin bread, enriched[38]:									
Slice (18 per loaf)	1 slice	25	35	65	2	1	.2	.3	.2
Rye bread:									
American, light (⅔ enriched wheat flour, ⅓ rye flour):									
Slice (4¾ × 3¾ × ⁷⁄₁₆ in)	1 slice	25	36	60	2	Tr	Tr	Tr	.1
Pumpernickel (⅔ rye flour, ⅓ enriched wheat flour):									
Slice (5 × 4 × ⅜ in)	1 slice	32	34	80	3	Tr	.1	Tr	.2
White bread, enriched[38]:									
Soft-crumb type[38]:									
Slice (18 per loaf)	1 slice	25	36	70	2	1	.2	.3	.3
Slice, toasted	1 slice	22	25	70	2	1	.2	.3	.3
Slice (22 per loaf)	1 slice	20	36	55	2	1	.2	.2	.2
Slice, toasted	1 slice	17	25	55	2	1	.2	.2	.2
Slice (24 per loaf)	1 slice	28	36	75	2	1	.2	.3	.3
Slice, toasted	1 slice	24	25	75	2	1	.2	.3	.3
Slice (28 per loaf)	1 slice	24	36	65	2	1	.2	.3	.2
Slice, toasted	1 slice	21	25	65	2	1	.2	.3	.2
Cubes	1 cup	30	36	80	3	1	.2	.3	.3
Crumbs	1 cup	45	36	120	4	1	.3	.5	.5
Firm-crumb type[38]:									
Slice (20 per loaf)	1 slice	23	35	65	2	1	.2	.3	.3
Slice, toasted	1 slice	20	24	65	2	1	.2	.3	.3
Slice (34 per loaf)	1 slice	27	35	75	2	1	.2	.3	.3
Slice, toasted	1 slice	23	24	75	2	1	.2	.3	.3
Whole-wheat bread:									
Soft-crumb type:									
Slice (16 per loaf)	1 slice	28	36	65	3	1	.1	.2	.2
Slice, toasted	1 slice	24	24	65	3	1	.1	.2	.2
Firm-crumb type:									
Slice (18 per loaf)	1 slice	25	36	60	3	1	.1	.2	.3
Slice, toasted	1 slice	21	24	60	3	1	.1	.2	.3
Breakfast cereals:									
Hot type, cooked:									
Corn (hominy) grits, degermed:									
Enriched	1 cup	245	87	125	3	Tr	Tr	Tr	.1
Unenriched	1 cup	245	87	125	3	Tr	Tr	Tr	.1
Farina, quick-cooking, enriched	1 cup	245	89	105	3	Tr	Tr	Tr	.1
Oatmeal or rolled oats	1 cup	240	87	130	5	2	.4	.8	.9
Wheat, rolled	1 cup	240	80	180	5	1	—	—	—
Wheat, whole-meal	1 cup	245	88	110	4	1	—	—	—
Ready-to-eat:									
Bran flakes (40% bran), added sugar, salt, iron, vitamins	1 cup	35	3	105	4	1	—	—	—
Bran flakes with raisins, added sugar, salt, iron, vitamins	1 cup	50	7	145	4	1	—	—	—
Corn flakes:									
Plain, added sugar, salt, iron, vitamins	1 cup	25	4	95	2	Tr	—	—	—
Sugar-coated, added salt, iron, vitamins	1 cup	40	2	155	2	Tr	—	—	—
Corn, oat flour, puffed, added sugar, salt, iron, vitamins	1 cup	20	4	80	2	1	—	—	—
Corn, shredded, added sugar, salt, iron, thiamin, niacin	1 cup	25	3	95	2	Tr	—	—	—
Oats, puffed, added sugar, salt, minerals, vitamins	1 cup	25	3	100	3	1	—	—	—
Rice, puffed:									
Plain, added iron, thiamin, niacin	1 cup	15	4	60	1	Tr	—	—	—
Presweetened, added salt, iron, vitamins	1 cup	28	3	115	1	0	—	—	—
Wheat flakes, added sugar, salt, iron, vitamins	1 cup	30	4	105	3	Tr	—	—	—
Wheat, puffed:									
Plain, added iron, thiamin, niacin	1 cup	15	3	55	2	Tr	—	—	—
Presweetened, added salt, iron, vitamins	1 cup	38	3	140	3	Tr	—	—	—

Nutrients in Indicated Quantity

For notes, see end of table.

Nutrients in Indicated Quantity

Carbohydrate (g)	Calcium (mg)	Phosphorus (mg)	Iron (mg)	Potassium (mg)	Vitamin A Value (IU)	Thiamin (mg)	Riboflavin (mg)	Niacin (mg)	Ascorbic Acid (mg)
14	11	21	.6	23	Tr	.10	.06	.8	Tr
17	5	23	.7	22	0	.12	.07	1.0	0
13	18	22	.6	58	Tr	.09	.06	.6	Tr
13	19	37	.5	36	0	.07	.05	.7	0
17	27	73	.8	145	0	.09	.07	.6	0
13	21	24	.6	26	Tr	.10	.06	.8	Tr
13	21	24	.6	26	Tr	.08	.06	.8	Tr
10	17	19	.5	21	Tr	.08	.05	.7	Tr
10	17	19	.5	21	Tr	.06	.05	.7	Tr
14	24	27	.7	29	Tr	.11	.07	.9	Tr
14	24	27	.7	29	Tr	.09	.07	.9	Tr
12	20	23	.6	25	Tr	.10	.06	.8	Tr
12	20	23	.6	25	Tr	.08	.06	.8	Tr
15	25	29	.8	32	Tr	.12	.07	1.0	Tr
23	38	44	1.1	47	Tr	.18	.11	1.5	Tr
12	22	23	.6	28	Tr	.09	.06	.8	Tr
12	22	23	.6	28	Tr	.07	.06	.8	Tr
14	26	28	.7	33	Tr	.11	.06	.9	Tr
14	26	28	.7	33	Tr	.09	.06	.9	Tr
14	24	71	.8	72	Tr	.09	.03	.8	Tr
14	24	71	.8	72	Tr	.07	.03	.8	Tr
12	25	57	.8	68	Tr	.06	.03	.7	Tr
12	25	27	.8	68	Tr	.05	.03	.7	Tr
27	2	25	.7	27	Tr[40]	.10	.07	1.0	0
27	2	25	.2	27	Tr[40]	.05	.02	.5	0
22	147	113[41]	([42])	25	0	.12	.07	1.0	0
23	22	137	1.4	146	0	.19	.05	.2	0
41	19	182	1.7	202	0	.17	.07	2.2	0
23	17	127	1.2	118	0	.15	.05	1.5	0
28	19	125	5.6	137	1540	.46	.52	6.2	0
40	28	146	7.9	154	2200[43]	([44])	([44])	([44])	0
21	([44])	9	([44])	30	([44])	([44])	([44])	([44])	13[45]
37	1	10	([44])	27	1760	.53	.60	7.1	21[45]
16	4	18	5.7	—	880	.26	.30	3.5	11
22	1	10	.6	—	0	.33	.05	4.4	13
19	44	102	4.0	—	1100	.33	.38	4.4	13
13	3	14	.3	15	0	.07	.01	.7	0
26	3	14	([44])	43	1240[45]	([44])	([44])	([44])	15[45]
24	12	83	4.8	81	1320	.40	.45	5.3	16
12	4	48	.6	51	0	.08	.03	1.2	0
33	7	52	([44])	63	1680	.50	.57	6.7	20[45]

| | | | | | | Fatty Acids | | |
| | | | | | | Saturated | Unsaturated | |
Foods, Approximate Measures, Units, and Weight		(g)	Water (%)	Food Energy (cal)	Protein (g)	Fat (g)	(total) (g)	Oleic (g)	Linoleic (g)
Wheat, shredded, plain	1 oblong biscuit or ½ cup spoon-size biscuits	25	7	90	2	1	—	—	—
Wheat germ, without salt and sugar, toasted	1 tbsp	6	4	25	2	1	—	—	—
Buckwheat flour, light, sifted	1 cup	98	12	340	6	1	.2	.4	.4
Bulgur, canned, seasoned	1 cup	135	56	245	8	4	—	—	—
Cake icings; see Sugars and sweets									
Cakes made from cake mixes with enriched flour[46]:									
Angelfood:									
Piece, 1/12 of cake	1 piece	53	34	135	3	Tr	—	—	—
Coffeecake:									
Piece, 1/6 of cake	1 piece	72	30	230	5	7	2.0	2.7	1.5
Cupcakes, made with egg, milk, 2½-in diameter:									
Without icing	1 cupcake	25	26	90	1	3	.8	1.2	.7
With chocolate icing	1 cupcake	36	22	130	2	5	2.0	1.6	.6
Devil's food with chocolate icing:									
Piece, 1/16 of cake	1 piece	69	24	235	3	8	3.1	2.8	1.1
Cupcake, 2½-in diameter	1 cupcake	35	24	120	2	4	1.6	1.4	.5
Gingerbread:									
Piece, 1/9 of cake	1 piece	63	37	175	2	4	1.1	1.8	1.1
White, 2 layer with chocolate icing:									
Piece, 1/16 of cake	1 piece	71	21	250	3	8	2.0	2.9	1.2
Yellow, 2 layer with chocolate icing:									
Piece, 1/16 of cake	1 piece	69	26	235	3	8	3.0	3.0	1.3
Cakes made from home recipes using enriched flour[47]:									
Boston cream pie with custard filling:									
Whole cake (8-in diameter)	1 cake	825	35	2490	41	78	23.0	30.1	15.2
Piece, 1/12 of cake	1 piece	69	35	210	3	6	1.9	2.5	1.3
Fruitcake, dark:									
Slice, 1/30 of loaf	1 slice	15	18	55	1	2	.5	1.1	.5
Plain, sheet cake:									
Without icing:									
Whole cake (9-in sq)	1 cake	777	25	2830	35	108	29.5	44.4	23.9
Piece, 1/9 of cake	1 piece	86	25	315	4	12	3.3	4.9	2.6
With uncooked white icing:									
Piece, 1/9 of cake	1 piece	121	21	445	4	14	4.7	5.5	2.7
Pound[49]:									
Loaf, 8½ × 3½ × 3¼ in	1 loaf	565	16	2725	31	170	42.9	73.1	39.6
Slice, 1/17 of loaf	1 slice	33	16	160	2	10	2.5	4.3	2.3
Spongecake:									
Whole cake (9¾-in diameter tube cake)	1 cake	790	32	2345	60	45	13.1	15.8	5.7
Piece, 1/12 of cake	1 piece	66	32	195	5	4	1.1	1.3	.5
Cookies made with enriched flour[50,51]:									
Brownies with nuts:									
Home-prepared, 1¾ × 1¾ × ⅞ in:									
From home recipe	1 brownie	20	10	95	1	6	1.5	3.0	1.2
From commercial recipe	1 brownie	20	11	85	1	4	.9	1.4	1.3
Frozen, with chocolate icing, 1½ × 1¾ × ⅞ in[52]	1 brownie	25	13	105	1	5	2.0	2.2	.7
Chocolate chip:									
Commercial, 2¼-in diameter, ⅜ in thick	4 cookies	42	3	200	2	9	2.8	2.9	2.2
From home recipe, 2 ⅓-in diameter	4 cookies	40	3	205	2	12	3.5	4.5	2.9
Fig bars, square (1⅝ × 1⅝ × ⅜ in) or rectangular (1½ × 1¾ × ½ in)	4 cookies	56	14	200	2	3	.8	1.2	.7
Gingersnaps, 2-in diameter, ¼ in thick	4 cookies	28	3	90	2	2	.7	1.0	.6
Macaroons, 2¾-in diameter, ¼ in thick	2 cookies	38	4	180	2	9	—	—	—
Oatmeal with raisins, 2⅝-in diameter, ¼ in thick	4 cookies	52	3	235	3	8	2.0	3.3	2.0
Plain, prepared from commercial chilled dough, 2½-in diameter, ¼ in thick	4 cookies	48	5	240	2	12	3.0	5.2	2.9
Sandwich type (chocolate or vanilla), 1¾-in diameter, ⅜ in thick	4 cookies	40	2	200	2	9	2.2	3.9	2.2
Vanilla wafers, 1¾-in diameter, ¼ in thick	10 cookies	40	3	185	2	6	—	—	—

For notes, see end of table.

Nutrients in Indicated Quantity

Carbohydrate (g)	Calcium (mg)	Phosphorus (mg)	Iron (mg)	Potassium (mg)	Vitamin A Value (IU)	Thiamin (mg)	Riboflavin (mg)	Niacin (mg)	Ascorbic Acid (mg)
20	11	97	.9	87	0	.06	.03	1.1	0
3	3	70	.5	57	10	.11	.05	.3	1
78	11	86	1.0	314	0	.08	.04	.4	0
44	27	263	1.9	151	0	.08	.05	4.1	0
32	50	63	.2	32	0	.03	.08	.3	0
38	44	125	1.2	78	120	.14	.15	1.3	Tr
14	40	59	.3	21	40	.05	.05	.4	Tr
21	47	71	.4	42	60	.05	.06	.4	Tr
40	41	72	1.0	90	100	.07	.10	.6	Tr
20	21	37	.5	46	50	.03	.05	.3	Tr
32	57	63	.9	173	Tr	.09	.11	.8	Tr
45	70	127	.7	82	40	.09	.11	.8	Tr
40	63	126	.8	75	100	.08	.10	.7	Tr
412	553	833	8.2	734[48]	1730	1.04	1.27	9.6	2
34	46	70	.7	61[48]	140	.09	.11	.8	Tr
9	11	17	.4	74	20	.02	.02	.2	Tr
434	497	793	8.5	614[48]	1320	1.21	1.40	10.2	2
48	55	88	.9	68[48]	150	.13	.15	1.1	Tr
77	61	91	.8	74	240	.14	.16	1.1	Tr
273	107	418	7.9	345	1410	.90	.99	7.3	0
16	6	24	.5	20	80	.05	.06	.4	0
427	237	885	13.4	687	3560	1.10	1.64	7.4	0
36	20	74	1.1	57	300	.09	.14	.6	Tr
10	8	30	.4	38	40	.04	.03	.2	Tr
13	9	27	.4	34	20	.03	.02	.2	Tr
15	10	31	.4	44	50	.03	.03	.2	Tr
29	16	48	1.0	56	50	.10	.17	.9	Tr
24	14	40	.8	47	40	.06	.06	.5	Tr
42	44	34	1.0	111	60	.04	.14	.9	Tr
22	20	13	.7	129	20	.08	.06	.7	0
25	10	32	.3	176	0	.02	.06	.2	0
38	11	53	1.4	192	30	.15	.10	1.0	Tr
31	17	35	.6	23	30	.10	.08	.9	0
28	10	96	.7	15	0	.06	.10	.7	0
30	16	25	.6	29	50	.10	.09	.8	0

Foods, Approximate Measures, Units, and Weight		(g)	Water (%)	Food Energy (cal)	Protein (g)	Fat (g)	Saturated (total) (g)	Oleic (g)	Linoleic (g)
							Fatty Acids		
								Unsaturated	
Cornmeal									
Whole-ground, unbolted, dry form	1 cup	122	12	435	11	5	.5	1.0	2.5
Bolted (nearly whole-grain), dry form	1 cup	122	12	440	11	4	.5	.9	2.1
Degermed, enriched:									
Dry form	1 cup	138	12	500	11	2	.2	.4	.9
Cooked	1 cup	240	88	120	3	Tr	Tr	.1	.2
Degermed, unenriched:									
Dry form	1 cup	138	12	500	11	2	.2	.4	.9
Cooked	1 cup	240	88	120	3	Tr	Tr	.1	.2
Crackers[38]:									
Graham, plain, 2½-in square	2 crackers	14	6	55	1	1	.3	.5	.3
Rye wafers, whole-grain, 1⅞ × 3½ in	2 wafers	13	6	45	2	Tr	—	—	—
Saltines, made with enriched flour	4 crackers or 1 packet	11	4	50	1	1	.3	.5	.4
Danish pastry (enriched flour), plain without fruit or nuts[54]:									
Round piece, about 4¼-in diameter × 1 in	1 pastry	65	22	275	5	15	4.7	6.1	3.2
Ounce	1 oz	28	22	120	2	7	2.0	2.7	1.4
Doughnuts, made with enriched flour[38]:									
Cake type, plain, 2½-in diameter, 1 in high	1 doughnut	25	24	100	1	5	1.2	2.0	1.1
Yeast-leavened, glazed, 3¾-in diameter, 1¼ in high	1 doughnut	50	26	205	3	11	3.3	5.8	3.3
Macaroni, enriched, cooked (cut lengths, elbows, shells):									
Firm stage (hot)	1 cup	130	64	190	7	1	—	—	—
Tender stage:									
Cold macaroni	1 cup	105	73	115	4	Tr	—	—	—
Hot macaroni	1 cup	140	73	155	5	1	—	—	—
Macaroni (enriched) and cheese[55]:									
Canned	1 cup	240	80	230	9	10	4.2	3.1	1.4
From home recipe (served hot)[56]	1 cup	200	58	430	17	22	8.9	8.8	2.9
Muffins made with enriched flour[38]:									
From home recipe:									
Blueberry, 2⅜-in diameter, 1½ in high	1 muffin	40	39	110	3	4	1.1	1.4	.7
Bran	1 muffin	40	35	105	3	4	1.2	1.4	.8
Corn (enriched degermed cornmeal and flour), 2⅜-in diameter, 1½ in high	1 muffin	40	33	125	3	4	1.2	1.6	.9
Plain, 3-in diameter, 1½ in high	1 muffin	40	38	120	3	4	1.0	1.7	1.0
From mix, egg, milk:									
Corn, 2⅜-in diameter, 1½ in high[58]	1 muffin	40	30	130	3	4	1.2	1.7	.9
Noodles (egg noodles), enriched, cooked	1 cup	160	71	200	7	2	—	—	—
Noodles, chow mein, canned	1 cup	45	1	220	6	11	—	—	—
Pancakes (4-in diameter)[38]:									
Buckwheat, made from mix (with buckwheat and enriched flour), egg and milk added	1 cake	27	58	55	2	2	.8	.9	.4
Plain:									
Made from home recipe using enriched flour	1 cake	27	50	60	2	2	.5	.8	.5
Made from mix with enriched flour, egg and milk added	1 cake	27	51	60	2	2	.7	.7	.3
Pies, piecrust made with enriched flour, vegetable shortening (9-in diameter):									
Apple:									
Sector, ⅐ of pie	1 sector	135	48	345	3	15	3.9	6.4	3.6
Banana cream:									
Sector, ⅐ of pie	1 sector	130	54	285	6	12	3.8	4.7	2.3
Blueberry:									
Sector, ⅐ of pie	1 sector	135	51	325	3	15	3.5	6.2	3.6
Cherry:									
Sector, ⅐ of pie	1 sector	135	47	350	4	15	4.0	6.4	3.6
Custard:									
Sector, ⅐ of pie	1 sector	130	58	285	8	14	4.8	5.5	2.5
Lemon meringue:									
Sector, ⅐ of pie	1 sector	120	47	305	4	12	3.7	4.8	2.3
Mince:									
Sector, ⅐ of pie	1 sector	135	43	365	3	16	4.0	6.6	3.6
Peach:									
Sector, ⅐ of pie	1 sector	135	48	345	3	14	3.5	6.2	3.6
Pecan:									
Sector, ⅐ of pie	1 sector	118	20	495	6	27	4.0	14.4	6.3
Pumpkin:									
Sector, ⅐ of pie	1 sector	130	59	275	5	15	5.4	5.4	2.4

For notes, see end of table.

Nutrients in Indicated Quantity

Carbohydrate (g)	Calcium (mg)	Phosphorus (mg)	Iron (mg)	Potassium (mg)	Vitamin A Value (IU)	Thiamin (mg)	Riboflavin (mg)	Niacin (mg)	Ascorbic Acid (mg)
90	24	312	2.9	346	620[53]	.46	.13	2.4	0
91	21	272	2.2	303	590[53]	.37	.10	2.3	0
108	8	137	4.0	166	610[53]	.61	.36	4.8	0
26	2	34	1.0	38	140[53]	.14	.10	1.2	0
108	8	137	1.5	166	610[53]	.19	.07	1.4	0
26	2	34	.5	38	140[53]	.05	.02	.2	0
10	6	21	.5	55	0	.02	.08	.5	0
10	7	50	.5	78	0	.04	.03	.2	0
8	2	10	.5	13	0	.05	.05	.4	0
30	33	71	1.2	73	200	.18	.19	1.7	Tr
13	14	31	.5	32	90	.08	.08	.7	Tr
13	10	48	.4	23	20	.05	.05	.4	Tr
22	16	33	.6	34	25	.10	.10	.8	0
39	14	85	1.4	103	0	.23	.13	1.8	0
24	8	53	.9	64	0	.15	.08	1.2	0
32	11	70	1.3	85	0	.20	.11	1.5	0
26	199	182	1.0	139	260	.12	.24	1.0	Tr
40	362	322	1.8	240	860	.20	.40	1.8	Tr
17	34	53	.6	46	90	.09	.10	.7	Tr
17	57	162	1.5	172	90	.07	.10	1.7	Tr
19	42	68	.7	54	120[57]	.10	.10	.7	Tr
17	42	60	.6	50	40	.09	.12	.9	Tr
20	96	152	.6	44	100[57]	.08	.09	.7	Tr
37	16	94	1.4	70	110	.22	.13	1.9	0
26	—	—	—	—	—	—	—	—	—
6	59	91	.4	66	60	.04	.05	.2	Tr
9	27	38	.4	33	30	.06	.07	.5	Tr
9	58	70	.3	42	70	.04	.06	.2	Tr
51	11	30	.9	108	40	.15	.11	1.3	2
40	86	107	1.0	264	330	.11	.22	1.0	1
47	15	31	1.4	88	40	.15	.11	1.4	4
52	19	34	.9	142	590	.16	.12	1.4	Tr
30	125	147	1.2	178	300	.11	.27	.8	0
45	17	59	1.0	60	200	.09	.12	.7	4
56	38	51	1.9	240	Tr	.14	.12	1.4	1
52	14	39	1.2	201	990	.15	.14	2.0	4
61	55	122	3.7	145	190	.26	.14	1.0	Tr
32	66	90	1.0	208	3210	.11	.18	1.0	Tr

Foods, Approximate Measures, Units, and Weight		(g)	Water (%)	Food Energy (cal)	Protein (g)	Fat (g)	Saturated (total) (g)	Oleic (g)	Linoleic (g)
								Unsaturated	
Piecrust (home recipe) made with enriched flour and vegetable shortening, baked	1 pie shell, 9-in diameter	180	15	900	11	60	14.8	26.1	14.9
Pizza (cheese) baked, 4¾-in sector; ⅛ of 12-in diameter pie[19]	1 sector	60	45	145	6	4	1.7	1.5	0.6
Popcorn, popped:									
Plain, large kernel	1 cup	6	4	25	1	Tr	Tr	.1	.2
With oil (coconut) and salt added, large kernel	1 cup	9	3	40	1	2	1.5	.2	.2
Sugar coated	1 cup	35	4	135	2	1	.5	.2	.4
Pretzels, made with enriched flour:									
Dutch, twisted, 2¾ × 2⅝ in	1 pretzel	16	5	60	2	1	—	—	—
Thin, twisted, 3¼ × 2¼ × ¼ in	10 pretzels	60	5	235	6	3	—	—	—
Stick, 2¼ in long	10 pretzels	3	5	10	Tr	Tr	—	—	—
Rice, white, enriched:									
Instant, ready-to-serve, hot	1 cup	165	73	180	4	Tr	Tr	Tr	Tr
Long grain:									
Raw	1 cup	185	12	670	12	1	.2	.2	.2
Cooked, served hot	1 cup	205	73	225	4	Tr	.1	.1	.1
Parboiled:									
Raw	1 cup	185	10	685	14	1	.2	.1	.2
Cooked, served hot	1 cup	175	73	185	4	Tr	.1	.1	.1
Rolls, enriched:									
Commercial:									
Brown-and-serve (12 per 12-oz pkg), browned	1 roll	26	27	85	2	2	.4	.7	.5
Cloverleaf or pan, 2½-in diameter, 2 in high	1 roll	28	31	85	2	2	.4	.6	.4
Frankfurter and hamburger (8 per 11½-oz pkg)	1 roll	40	31	120	3	2	.5	.8	.6
Hard, 3¾-in diameter, 2 in high	1 roll	50	25	155	5	2	.4	.6	.5
Hoagie or submarine, 11½ × 3 × 2½ in	1 roll	135	31	390	12	4	.9	1.4	1.4
From home recipe:									
Cloverleaf, 2½-in diameter, 2 in high	1 roll	35	26	120	3	3	.8	1.1	.7
Spaghetti, enriched, cooked:									
Firm stage, "al dente," served hot	1 cup	130	64	190	7	1	—	—	—
Tender stage, served hot	1 cup	140	73	155	5	1	—	—	—
Spaghetti (enriched) in tomato sauce with cheese:									
From home recipe	1 cup	250	77	260	9	9	2.0	5.4	.7
Canned	1 cup	250	80	190	6	2	.5	.3	.4
Spaghetti (enriched) with meat balls and tomato sauce:									
From home recipe	1 cup	248	70	330	19	12	3.3	6.3	.9
Canned	1 cup	250	78	260	12	10	2.2	3.3	3.9
Toaster pastries	1 pastry	50	12	200	3	6	—	—	—
Waffles, made with enriched flour, 7-in diameter[38]:									
From home recipe	1 waffle	75	41	210	7	7	2.3	2.8	1.4
From mix, egg and milk added	1 waffle	75	42	205	7	8	2.8	2.9	1.2
Wheat flours:									
All-purpose or family flour, enriched:									
Sifted, spooned	1 cup	115	12	420	12	1	.2	.1	0.5
Unsifted, spooned	1 cup	125	12	455	13	1	.2	.1	.5
Cake or pastry flour, enriched, sifted, spooned	1 cup	96	12	350	7	1	.1	.1	.3
Self-rising, enriched, unsifted, spooned	1 cup	125	12	440	12	1	.2	.1	.5
Whole-wheat, from hard wheats, stirred	1 cup	120	12	400	16	2	.4	.2	1.0
Legumes (Dry), Nuts, Seeds; Related Products									
Almonds, shelled:									
Chopped (about 130 almonds)	1 cup	130	5	775	24	70	5.6	47.7	12.8
Slivered, not pressed down (about 115 almonds)	1 cup	115	5	690	21	62	5.0	42.2	11.3
Beans, dry:									
Common varieties as Great Northern, navy, and others:									
Cooked, drained:									
Great Northern	1 cup	180	69	210	14	1	—	—	—
Pea (navy)	1 cup	190	69	225	15	1	—	—	—
Canned, solids and liquid:									
White with:									
Frankfurters (sliced)	1 cup	255	71	365	19	18	—	—	—
Pork and tomato sauce	1 cup	255	71	310	16	7	2.4	2.8	.6
Pork and sweet sauce	1 cup	255	66	385	16	12	4.3	5.0	1.1
Red kidney	1 cup	255	76	230	15	1	—	—	—

For notes, see end of table.

Nutrients in Indicated Quantity

Carbohydrate (g)	Calcium (mg)	Phosphorus (mg)	Iron (mg)	Potassium (mg)	Vitamin A Value (IU)	Thiamin (mg)	Riboflavin (mg)	Niacin (mg)	Ascorbic Acid (mg)
79	25	90	3.1	89	0	.47	.40	5.0	0
22	86	89	1.1	67	230	.16	.18	1.6	4
5	1	17	.2	—	—	—	.01	.1	0
5	1	19	.2	—	—	—	.01	.2	0
30	2	47	.5	—	—	—	.02	.4	0
12	4	21	.2	21	0	.05	.04	.7	0
46	13	79	.9	78	0	.20	.15	2.5	0
2	1	4	Tr	4	0	.01	.01	.1	0
40	5	31	1.3	—	0	.21	([59])	1.7	0
149	44	174	5.4	170	0	.81	.06	6.5	c
50	21	57	1.8	57	0	.23	.02	2.1	0
150	111	370	5.4	278	0	.81	.07	6.5	0
41	33	100	1.4	75	0	.19	.02	2.1	0
14	20	23	.5	25	Tr	.10	.06	.9	Tr
15	21	24	.5	27	Tr	.11	.07	.9	Tr
21	30	34	.8	38	Tr	.16	.10	1.3	Tr
30	24	46	1.2	49	Tr	.20	.12	1.7	Tr
75	58	115	3.0	122	Tr	.54	.32	4.5	Tr
20	16	36	.7	41	30	.12	.12	1.2	Tr
39	14	85	1.4	103	0	.23	.13	1.8	0
32	11	70	1.3	85	0	.20	.11	1.5	0
37	80	135	2.3	408	1080	.25	.18	2.3	13
39	40	88	2.8	303	930	.35	.28	4.5	10
39	124	236	3.7	665	1590	.25	.30	4.0	22
29	53	113	3.3	245	1000	.15	.18	2.3	5
36	54[60]	67[60]	1.9	74[60]	500	.16	.17	2.1	([60])
28	85	130	1.3	109	250	.17	.23	1.4	Tr
27	179	257	1.0	146	170	.14	.22	.9	Tr
88	18	100	3.3	109	0	0.74	0.46	6.1	0
95	20	109	3.6	119	0	.80	.50	6.6	0
76	16	70	2.8	91	0	.61	.38	5.1	0
93	331	583	3.6	—	0	.80	.50	6.6	0
85	49	446	4.0	444	0	.66	.14	5.2	0
25	304	655	6.1	1005	0	.31	1.20	4.6	Tr
22	269	580	5.4	889	0	.28	1.06	4.0	Tr
38	90	266	4.9	749	0	.25	.13	1.3	0
40	95	281	5.1	790	0	.27	.13	1.3	0
32	94	303	4.8	668	330	.18	.15	3.3	Tr
48	138	235	4.6	536	330	.20	.08	1.5	5
54	161	291	5.9	—	—	.15	.10	1.3	—
42	74	278	4.6	673	10	.13	.10	1.5	—

Foods, Approximate Measures, Units, and Weight		(g)	Water (%)	Food Energy (cal)	Protein (g)	Fat (g)	Saturated (total) (g)	Oleic (g)	Linoleic (g)
								Fatty Acids	
								Unsaturated	
Lima, cooked, drained	1 cup	190	64	260	16	1	—	—	—
Blackeye peas, dry, cooked (with residual cooking liquid)	1 cup	250	80	190	13	1	—	—	—
Brazil nuts, shelled (6-8 large kernels)	1 oz	28	5	185	4	19	4.8	6.2	7.1
Cashew nuts, roasted in oil	1 cup	140	5	785	24	64	12.9	36.8	10.2
Coconut meat, fresh:									
Piece, about 2 × 2 × ½ in	1 piece	45	51	155	2	16	14.0	.9	.3
Shredded or grated, not pressed down	1 cup	80	51	275	3	28	24.8	1.6	.5
Filberts (hazelnuts), chopped (about 60 kernels)	1 cup	115	6	730	14	72	5.1	55.2	7.3
Lentils, whole, cooked	1 cup	200	72	210	16	Tr	—	—	—
Peanuts, roasted in oil, salted (whole, halves, chopped)	1 cup	144	2	840	37	72	13.7	33.0	20.7
Peanut butter	1 tbsp	16	2	95	4	8	1.5	3.7	2.3
Peas, split, dry, cooked	1 cup	200	70	230	16	1	—	—	—
Pecans, chopped or pieces (about 120 large halves)	1 cup	118	3	810	11	84	7.2	50.5	20.0
Pumpkin and squash kernels, dry, hulled	1 cup	140	4	775	41	65	11.8	23.5	27.5
Sunflower seeds, dry, hulled	1 cup	145	5	810	35	69	8.2	13.7	43.2
Walnuts:									
Black:									
Chopped or broken kernels	1 cup	125	3	785	26	74	6.3	13.3	45.7
Ground (finely)	1 cup	80	3	500	16	47	4.0	8.5	29.2
Persian or English, chopped (about 60 halves)	1 cup	120	4	780	18	77	8.4	11.8	42.2
Sugars and Sweets									
Cake icings:									
Boiled, white:									
Plain	1 cup	94	18	295	1	0	0	0	—
With coconut	1 cup	166	15	605	3	13	11.0	.9	Tr
Uncooked:									
Chocolate made with milk and butter	1 cup	275	14	1035	9	38	23.4	11.7	1.0
Creamy fudge from mix and water	1 cup	245	15	830	7	16	5.1	6.7	3.1
White	1 cup	319	11	1200	2	21	12.7	5.1	.5
Candy:									
Caramels, plain or chocolate	1 oz	28	8	115	1	3	1.6	1.1	.1
Chocolate:									
Milk, plain	1 oz	28	1	145	2	9	5.5	3.0	.3
Semisweet, small pieces (60 per oz)	1 cup or 6-oz pkg	170	1	860	7	61	36.2	19.8	1.7
Chocolate-coated peanuts	1 oz	28	1	160	5	12	4.0	4.7	2.1
Fondant, uncoated (mints, candy corn, other)	1 oz	28	8	105	Tr	1	.1	.3	.1
Fudge, chocolate, plain	1 oz	28	8	115	1	3	1.3	1.4	.6
Gum drops	1 oz	28	12	100	Tr	Tr	—	—	—
Hard	1 oz	28	1	110	0	Tr	—	—	—
Marshmallows	1 oz	28	17	90	1	Tr	—	—	—
Chocolate-flavored beverage powders (about 4 heaping tsp per oz):									
With nonfat dry milk	1 oz	28	2	100	5	1	.5	.3	Tr
Without milk	1 oz	28	1	100	1	1	.4	.2	Tr
Honey, strained or extracted	1 tbsp	21	17	65	Tr	0	0	0	0
Jams and preserves	1 tbsp	20	29	55	Tr	Tr	—	—	—
	1 packet	14	29	40	Tr	Tr	—	—	—
Jellies	1 tbsp	18	29	50	Tr	Tr	—	—	—
	1 packet	14	29	40	Tr	Tr	—	—	—
Syrups:									
Chocolate-flavored syrup or topping:									
Thin type	1 fl oz or 2 tbsp	38	32	90	1	1	.5	.3	Tr
Fudge type	1 fl oz or 2 tbsp	38	25	125	2	5	3.1	1.6	.1
Molasses, cane:									
Light (first extraction)	1 tbsp	20	24	50	—	—	—	—	—
Blackstrap (third extraction)	1 tbsp	20	24	45	—	—	—	—	—
Sorghum	1 tbsp	21	23	55	—	—	—	—	—
Table blends, chiefly corn, light and dark	1 tbsp	21	24	60	0	0	0	0	0
Sugars:									
Brown, pressed down	1 cup	220	2	820	0	0	0	0	0
White:									
Granulated	1 cup	200	1	770	0	0	0	0	0
	1 tbsp	12	1	45	0	0	0	0	0
	1 packet	6	1	23	0	0	0	0	0
Powdered, sifted, spooned into cup	1 cup	100	1	385	0	0	0	0	0

For notes, see end of table.

Nutrients in Indicated Quantity

Carbohydrate (g)	Calcium (mg)	Phosphorus (mg)	Iron (mg)	Potassium (mg)	Vitamin A Value (IU)	Thiamin (mg)	Riboflavin (mg)	Niacin (mg)	Ascorbic Acid (mg)
49	55	293	5.9	1163	—	.25	.11	1.3	—
35	43	238	3.3	573	30	.40	.10	1.0	—
3	53	196	1.0	203	Tr	.27	.03	.5	—
41	53	522	5.3	650	140	.60	.35	2.5	—
4	6	43	.8	115	0	.02	.01	.2	1
8	10	76	1.4	205	0	.04	.02	.4	2
19	240	388	3.9	810	—	.53	—	1.0	Tr
39	50	238	4.2	498	40	.14	.12	1.2	0
27	107	577	3.0	971	—	.46	.19	24.8	0
3	9	61	.3	100	—	.02	.02	2.4	0
42	22	178	3.4	592	80	.30	.18	1.8	—
17	86	341	2.8	712	150	1.01	.15	1.1	2
21	71	1602	15.7	1386	100	.34	.27	3.4	—
29	174	1214	10.3	1334	70	2.84	.33	7.8	—
19	Tr	713	7.5	575	380	.28	.14	.9	—
12	Tr	456	4.8	368	240	.18	.09	.6	—
19	119	456	3.7	540	40	.40	.16	1.1	2
75	2	2	Tr	17	0	Tr	0.03	Tr	0
124	10	50	.8	277	0	.02	.07	.3	0
185	165	305	3.3	536	580	.06	.28	.6	1
183	96	218	2.7	238	Tr	.05	.20	.7	Tr
260	48	38	Tr	57	860	Tr	.06	Tr	Tr
22	42	35	.4	54	Tr	.01	.05	.1	Tr
16	65	65	.3	109	80	.02	.10	.1	Tr
97	51	255	4.4	553	30	.02	.14	.9	0
11	33	84	.4	143	Tr	.10	.05	2.1	Tr
25	4	2	.3	1	0	Tr	Tr	Tr	0
21	22	24	.3	42	Tr	.01	.03	.1	Tr
25	2	Tr	.1	1	0	0	Tr	Tr	0
28	6	2	.5	1	0	0	0	0	0
23	5	2	.5	2	0	0	Tr	Tr	0
20	167	155	.5	227	10	.04	.21	.2	1
25	9	48	.6	142	—	.01	.03	.1	0
17	1	1	.1	11	0	Tr	.01	.1	Tr
14	4	2	.2	18	Tr	Tr	.01	Tr	Tr
10	3	1	.1	12	Tr	Tr	Tr	Tr	Tr
13	4	1	.3	14	Tr	Tr	.01	Tr	1
10	3	1	.2	11	Tr	Tr	Tr	Tr	1
24	6	35	.6	106	Tr	.01	.03	.2	0
20	48	60	.5	107	60	.02	.08	.2	Tr
13	33	9	.9	183	—	.01	.01	Tr	—
11	137	17	3.2	585	—	.02	.04	.4	—
14	35	5	2.6	—	—	—	.02	Tr	—
15	9	3	.8	1	0	0	0	0	0
212	187	42	7.5	757	0	.02	.7	.4	0
199	0	0	.2	6	0	0	0	0	0
12	0	0	Tr	Tr	0	0	0	0	0
6	0	0	Tr	Tr	0	0	0	0	0
100	0	0	.1	3	0	0	0	0	0

						Fatty Acids		
						Saturated	Unsaturated	
Foods, Approximate Measures, Units, and Weight	(g)	Water (%)	Food Energy (cal)	Protein (g)	Fat (g)	(total) (g)	Oleic (g)	Linoleic (g)
Vegetable and Vegetable Products								
Asparagus, green:								
Cooked, drained:								
Cuts and tips, 1½- to 2-in lengths:								
From raw	1 cup	145	94	30	3	Tr	—	—	—
From frozen	1 cup	180	93	40	6	Tr	—	—	—
Spears, ½-in diameter at base:								
From raw	4 spears	60	94	10	1	Tr	—	—	—
From frozen	4 spears	60	92	15	2	Tr	—	—	—
Canned, spears, ½-in diameter at base	4 spears	80	93	15	2	Tr	—	—	—
Beans:								
Lima, immature seeds, frozen, cooked, drained:								
Thick-seeded types (Fordhooks)	1 cup	170	74	170	10	Tr	—	—	—
Thin-seeded types (baby limas)	1 cup	180	69	210	13	Tr	—	—	—
Snap:								
Green:								
Cooked, drained:								
From raw (cuts and French style)	1 cup	125	92	30	2	Tr	—	—	—
From frozen:								
Cuts	1 cup	135	92	35	2	Tr	—	—	—
French style	1 cup	130	92	35	2	Tr	—	—	—
Canned, drained solids (cuts)	1 cup	135	92	30	2	Tr	—	—	—
Yellow or wax:								
Cooked, drained:								
From raw (cuts and French style)	1 cup	125	93	30	2	Tr	—	—	—
From frozen (cuts)	1 cup	135	92	35	2	Tr	—	—	—
Canned, drained solids (cuts)	1 cup	135	92	30	2	Tr	—	—	—
Beans, mature. See Beans, dry and Blackeye peas, dry.								
Bean sprouts (mung):								
Raw	1 cup	105	89	35	4	Tr	—	—	—
Cooked, drained	1 cup	125	91	35	4	Tr	—	—	—
Beets:								
Cooked, drained, peeled:								
Whole beets, 2-in diameter	2 beets	100	91	30	1	Tr	—	—	—
Diced or sliced	1 cup	170	91	55	2	Tr	—	—	—
Canned, drained solids:								
Whole beets, small	1 cup	160	89	60	2	Tr	—	—	—
Diced or sliced	1 cup	170	89	65	2	Tr	—	—	—
Beet greens, leaves and stems, cooked, drained	1 cup	145	94	25	2	Tr	—	—	—
Blackeye peas, immature seeds, cooked and drained:								
From raw	1 cup	165	72	180	13	1	—	—	—
From frozen	1 cup	170	66	220	15	1	—	—	—
Broccoli, cooked, drained:								
From raw:								
Stalk, medium size	1 stalk	180	91	45	6	1	—	—	—
Stalks cut into ½-in pieces	1 cup	155	91	40	5	Tr	—	—	—
From frozen:								
Stalk, 4½ to 5 in long	1 stalk	30	91	10	1	Tr	—	—	—
Chopped	1 cup	185	92	50	5	1	—	—	—
Brussels sprouts, cooked, drained:								
From raw, 7-8 sprouts (1¼- to 1½-in diameter)	1 cup	155	88	55	7	1	—	—	—
From frozen	1 cup	155	89	50	5	Tr	—	—	—
Cabbage:								
Common varieties:								
Raw:								
Coarsely shredded or sliced	1 cup	70	92	15	1	Tr	—	—	—
Finely shredded or chopped	1 cup	90	92	20	1	Tr	—	—	—
Cooked, drained	1 cup	145	94	30	2	Tr	—	—	—
Red, raw, coarsely shredded or sliced	1 cup	70	90	20	1	Tr	—	—	—
Savoy, raw, coarsely shredded or sliced	1 cup	70	92	15	2	Tr	—	—	—
Cabbage, celery (also called pe-tsai or wongbok), raw, 1-in pieces	1 cup	75	95	10	1	Tr	—	—	—
Cabbage, white mustard (also called bokchoy or pakchoy), cooked, drained	1 cup	170	95	25	2	Tr	—	—	—
Carrots:								
Raw, without crowns and tips, scraped:								
Whole, 7½ × 1⅛ in, or strips, 2½ to 3 in long	1 carrot or 18 strips	72	88	30	1	Tr	—	—	—

For notes, see end of table.

					Nutrients in Indicated Quantity				
Carbohydrate (g)	Calcium (mg)	Phosphorus (mg)	Iron (mg)	Potassium (mg)	Vitamin A Value (IU)	Thiamin (mg)	Riboflavin (mg)	Niacin (mg)	Ascorbic Acid (mg)
5	30	73	.9	265	1310	.23	.26	2.0	38
6	40	115	2.2	396	1530	.25	.23	1.8	41
2	13	30	.4	110	540	.10	.11	.8	16
2	13	40	.7	143	470	.10	.08	.7	16
3	15	42	1.5	133	640	.05	.08	.6	12
32	34	153	2.9	724	390	.12	.09	1.7	29
40	63	227	4.7	709	400	.16	.09	2.2	22
7	63	45	.8	189	680	.09	.11	.6	15
8	54	43	.9	205	780	.09	.12	.5	7
8	49	39	1.2	177	690	.08	.10	.4	9
7	61	34	2.0	128	630	.04	.07	.4	5
6	63	46	.8	189	290	.09	.11	.6	16
8	47	42	.9	221	140	.09	.11	.5	8
7	61	34	2.0	128	140	.04	.07	.4	7
7	20	67	1.4	234	20	.14	.14	.8	20
7	21	60	1.1	195	30	.11	.13	.9	8
7	14	23	.5	208	20	.03	.04	.3	6
12	24	39	.9	354	30	.05	.07	.5	10
14	30	29	1.1	267	30	.02	.05	.2	5
15	32	31	1.2	284	30	.02	.05	.2	5
5	144	36	2.8	481	7400	.10	.22	.4	22
30	40	241	3.5	625	580	.50	.18	2.3	28
40	43	286	4.8	573	290	.68	.19	2.4	15
8	158	112	1.4	481	4500	.16	.36	1.4	162
7	136	96	1.2	414	3880	.14	.31	1.2	140
1	12	17	.2	66	570	.02	.03	.2	22
9	100	104	1.3	392	4810	.11	.22	.9	105
10	50	112	1.7	423	810	.12	.22	1.2	135
10	33	95	1.2	457	880	.12	.16	.9	126
4	34	20	.3	163	90	.04	.04	.2	33
5	44	26	.4	210	120	.05	.05	.3	42
6	64	29	.4	236	190	.06	.06	.4	48
5	29	25	.6	188	30	.06	.04	.3	43
3	47	38	.6	188	140	.04	.06	.2	39
2	32	30	.5	190	110	.04	.03	.5	19
4	252	56	1.0	364	5270	.07	.14	1.2	26
7	27	26	.5	246	7930	.04	.04	.4	6

| | | | | | | | | Fatty Acids | | |
| | | | | | | | | Saturated | Unsaturated | |
Foods, Approximate Measures, Units, and Weight		(g)	Water (%)	Food Energy (cal)	Protein (g)	Fat (g)		(total) (g)	Oleic (g)	Linoleic (g)
Grated	1 cup	110	88	45	1	Tr		—	—	—
Cooked (crosswise cuts), drained	1 cup	155	91	50	1	Tr		—	—	—
Canned:										
Sliced, drained solids	1 cup	155	91	45	1	Tr		—	—	—
Strained or junior (baby food)	1 oz (1¾ to 2 tbsp)	28	92	10	Tr	Tr		—	—	—
Cauliflower:										
Raw, chopped	1 cup	115	91	31	3	Tr		—	—	—
Cooked, drained:										
From raw (flower buds)	1 cup	125	93	30	3	Tr		—	—	—
From frozen (flowerets)	1 cup	180	94	30	3	Tr		—	—	—
Celery, Pascal type, raw:										
Stalk, large outer, 8 × 1½ in, at root end	1 stalk	40	94	5	Tr	Tr		—	—	—
Pieces, diced	1 cup	120	94	20	1	Tr		—	—	—
Collards, cooked, drained:										
From raw (leaves without stems)	1 cup	190	90	65	7	1		—	—	—
From frozen (chopped)	1 cup	170	90	50	5	1		—	—	—
Corn, sweet:										
Cooked, drained:										
From raw, ear 5 × 1¾ in	1 ear[61]	140	74	70	2	1		—	—	—
From frozen:										
Ear, 5 in long	1 ear[61]	229	73	120	4	1		—	—	—
Kernels	1 cup	165	77	130	5	1		—	—	—
Canned:										
Cream style	1 cup	256	76	210	5	2		—	—	—
Whole kernel:										
Vacuum pack	1 cup	210	76	175	5	1		—	—	—
Wet pack, drained solids	1 cup	165	76	140	4	1		—	—	—
Cowpeas; see Blackeye peas										
Cucumber slices, ⅛ in thick (large, 2⅛-in diameter; small, 1¾-in diameter):										
With peel	6 large or 8 small slices	28	95	5	Tr	Tr		—	—	—
Without peel	6½ large or 9 small pieces	28	96	5	Tr	Tr		—	—	—
Dandelion greens, cooked, drained	1 cup	105	90	35	2	1		—	—	—
Endive, curly (including escarole), raw, small pieces	1 cup	50	93	10	1	Tr		—	—	—
Kale, cooked, drained:										
From raw (leaves without stems and midribs)	1 cup	110	88	45	5	1		—	—	—
From frozen (leaf style)	1 cup	130	91	40	4	1		—	—	—
Lettuce, raw:										
Butterhead, as Boston types:										
Head, 5-in diameter	1 head[63]	220	95	25	2	Tr		—	—	—
Leaves	1 outer or 2 inner or 3 heart leaves	15	95	Tr	Tr	Tr		—	—	—
Crisphead, as Iceberg:										
Head, 6-in diameter	1 head[64]	567	96	70	5	1		—	—	—
Wedge, ¼ of head	1 wedge	135	96	20	1	Tr		—	—	—
Pieces, chopped or shredded	1 cup	55	96	5	Tr	Tr		—	—	—
Looseleaf (bunching varieties including romaine or cos), chopped or shredded pieces	1 cup	55	94	10	1	Tr		—	—	—
Mushrooms, raw, sliced or chopped	1 cup	70	90	20	2	Tr		—	—	—
Mustard greens, without stems and midribs, cooked, drained	1 cup	140	93	30	3	1		—	—	—
Okra pods, 3 × ⅝ in, cooked	10 pods	106	91	30	2	Tr		—	—	—
Onions:										
Mature:										
Raw:										
Chopped	1 cup	170	89	65	3	Tr		—	—	—
Sliced	1 cup	115	89	45	2	Tr		—	—	—
Cooked (whole or sliced), drained	1 cup	210	92	60	3	Tr		—	—	—
Young green, bulb (⅜-in diameter) and white portion of top	6 onions	30	88	15	Tr	Tr		—	—	—
Parsley, raw, chopped	1 tbsp	4	85	Tr	Tr	Tr		—	—	—
Parsnips, cooked (diced or 2-in lengths)	1 cup	155	82	100	2	1		—	—	—
Peas, green:										
Canned:										
Whole, drained solids	1 cup	170	77	150	8	1		—	—	—
Strained (baby food)	1 oz (1¾ to 2 tbsp)	28	86	15	1	Tr		—	—	—
Frozen, cooked, drained	1 cup	160	82	110	8	Tr		—	—	—

For notes, see end of table.

Nutrients in Indicated Quantity

Carbohydrate (g)	Calcium (mg)	Phosphorus (mg)	Iron (mg)	Potassium (mg)	Vitamin A Value (IU)	Thiamin (mg)	Riboflavin (mg)	Niacin (mg)	Ascorbic Acid (mg)
11	41	40	.8	375	12,100	.07	.06	.7	9
11	51	48	.9	344	16,280	.08	.08	.8	9
10	47	34	1.1	186	23,250	.03	.05	.6	3
2	7	6	.1	51	3690	.01	.01	.1	1
6	29	64	1.3	339	70	.13	.12	.8	90
5	26	53	.9	258	80	.11	.10	.8	69
6	31	68	.9	373	50	.07	.09	.7	74
2	16	11	.1	136	110	01	.01	.1	4
5	47	34	.4	409	320	.04	.04	.4	11
10	357	99	1.5	498	14,820	.21	.38	2.3	144
10	299	87	1.7	401	11,560	.10	.24	1.0	56
16	2	69	.5	151	310[62]	.09	.08	1.1	7
27	4	121	1.0	291	440[62]	.18	.10	2.1	9
31	5	120	1.3	304	580[62]	.15	.10	2.5	8
51	8	143	1.5	248	840[62]	.08	.13	2.6	13
43	6	153	1.1	204	740[62]	.06	.13	2.3	11
33	8	81	.8	160	580[62]	.05	.08	1.5	7
1	7	8	.3	45	70	.01	.01	.1	3
1	5	5	.1	45	Tr	.01	.01	.1	3
7	147	44	1.9	244	12,290	.14	.17	—	19
2	41	27	.9	147	1650	.04	.07	.3	5
7	206	64	1.8	243	9130	.11	.20	1.8	102
7	157	62	1.3	251	10,660	.08	.20	.9	49
4	57	42	3.3	430	1580	.10	.10	.5	13
Tr	5	4	.3	40	150	.01	.01	Tr	1
16	108	118	2.7	943	1780	.32	.32	1.6	32
4	27	30	.7	236	450	.08	.08	.4	8
2	11	12	.3	96	180	.03	.03	.2	3
2	37	14	.8	145	1050	.03	.04	.2	10
3	4	81	.6	290	Tr	.07	.32	2.9	2
6	193	45	2.5	308	8120	.11	.20	.8	67
6	98	43	.5	184	520	.14	.19	1.0	21
15	46	61	.9	267	Tr[65]	.05	.07	.3	17
10	31	41	.6	181	Tr[65]	.03	.05	.2	12
14	50	61	8	231	Tr[65]	.06	.06	.4	15
3	12	12	.2	69	Tr[65]	.02	.01	.1	8
Tr	7	2	.2	25	300	Tr	.01	Tr	6
23	70	96	.9	587	50	.11	.12	.2	16
29	44	129	3.2	163	1170	.15	.10	1.4	14
3	3	18	.3	28	140	.02	.03	.3	3
19	30	138	3.0	216	960	.43	.14	2.7	21

| | | | | | | Fatty Acids | | |
| | | | | | | | Unsaturated | |
Foods, Approximate Measures, Units, and Weight		(g)	Water (%)	Food Energy (cal)	Protein (g)	Fat (g)	Saturated (total) (g)	Oleic (g)	Linoleic (g)
Peppers, hot, red, without seeds, dried (ground chili powder, added seasonings)	1 tsp	2	9	5	Tr	Tr	—	—	—
Peppers, sweet (about 5 per lb, whole), stem and seeds removed:									
Raw	1 pod	74	93	15	1	Tr	—	—	—
Cooked, boiled, drained	1 pod	73	95	15	1	Tr	—	—	—
Potatoes, cooked:									
Baked, peeled after baking (about 2 per lb, raw)	1 potato	156	75	145	4	Tr	—	—	—
Boiled (about 3 per lb, raw):									
Peeled after boiling	1 potato	137	80	105	3	Tr	—	—	—
Peeled before boiling	1 potato	135	83	90	3	Tr	—	—	—
French-fried, strip, 2 to 3½ in long:									
Prepared from raw	10 strips	50	45	135	2	7	1.7	1.2	3.3
Frozen, oven heated	10 strips	50	53	110	2	4	1.1	.8	2.1
Hashed brown, prepared from frozen	1 cup	155	56	345	3	18	4.6	3.2	9.0
Mashed, prepared from:									
Raw:									
Milk added	1 cup	210	83	135	4	2	.7	.4	Tr
Milk and butter added	1 cup	210	80	195	4	9	5.6	2.3	0.2
Dehydrated flakes (without milk), water, milk, butter, and salt added	1 cup	210	79	195	4	7	3.6	2.1	.2
Potato chips, 1¾ × 2½-in oval cross section	10 chips	20	2	115	1	8	2.1	1.4	4.0
Potato salad, made with cooked salad dressing	1 cup	250	76	250	7	7	2.0	2.7	1.3
Pumpkin, canned	1 cup	245	90	80	2	1	—	—	—
Radishes, raw (prepackaged) stem ends, rootlets cut off	4 radishes	18	95	5	Tr	Tr	—	—	—
Sauerkraut, canned, solids and liquid	1 cup	235	93	40	2	Tr	—	—	—
Southern peas; see Blackeye peas									
Spinach:									
Raw, chopped	1 cup	55	91	15	2	Tr	—	—	—
Cooked, drained:									
From raw	1 cup	180	92	40	5	1	—	—	—
From frozen:									
Chopped	1 cup	205	92	45	6	1	—	—	—
Leaf	1 cup	190	92	45	6	1	—	—	—
Canned, drained solids	1 cup	205	91	50	6	1	—	—	—
Squash, cooked:									
Summer (all varieties), diced, drained	1 cup	210	96	30	2	Tr	—	—	—
Winter (all varieties), baked, mashed	1 cup	205	81	130	4	1	—	—	—
Sweet potatoes:									
Cooked (raw, 5 × 2 in; about 2½ per lb):									
Baked in skin, peeled	1 potato	114	64	160	2	1	—	—	—
Broiled in skin, peeled	1 potato	151	71	170	3	1	—	—	—
Candied, 2½ × 2-in piece	1 piece	105	60	175	1	3	2.0	.8	.1
Canned:									
Solid pack (mashed)	1 cup	255	72	275	5	1	—	—	—
Vacuum pack, piece 2¾ × 1 in	1 piece	40	72	45	1	Tr	—	—	—
Tomatoes:									
Raw, 2⅗-in diameter (3 per 12 oz pkg)	1 tomato[66]	135	94	25	1	Tr	—	—	—
Canned, solids and liquid	1 cup	241	94	50	2	Tr	—	—	—
Tomato catsup	1 cup	273	69	290	5	1	—	—	—
	1 tbsp	15	69	15	Tr	Tr	—	—	—
Tomato juice, canned:									
Cup	1 cup	243	94	45	2	Tr	—	—	—
Glass (6 fl oz)	1 glass	182	94	35	2	Tr	—	—	—
Turnips, cooked, diced	1 cup	155	35	35	1	Tr	—	—	—
Turnip greens, cooked, drained:									
From raw (leaves and stems)	1 cup	145	94	30	3	Tr	—	—	—
From frozen (chopped)	1 cup	165	93	40	4	Tr	—	—	—
Vegetables, mixed, frozen, cooked	1 cup	182	83	115	6	1	—	—	—
Miscellaneous Items									
Baking powders for home use:									
Sodium aluminum sulfate:									
With monocalcium phosphate monohydrate	1 tsp	3.0	2	5	Tr	Tr	0	0	0
With monocalcium phosphate monohydrate, calcium sulfate	1 tsp	2.9	1	5	Tr	Tr	0	0	0
Straight phosphate	1 tsp	3.8	2	5	Tr	Tr	0	0	0
Low sodium	1 tsp	4.3	2	5	Tr	Tr	0	0	0
Barbecue sauce	1 cup	250	81	230	4	17	2.2	4.3	10.0

For notes, see end of table.

Nutrients in Indicated Quantity

Carbohydrate (g)	Calcium (mg)	Phosphorus (mg)	Iron (mg)	Potassium (mg)	Vitamin A Value (IU)	Thiamin (mg)	Riboflavin (mg)	Niacin (mg)	Ascorbic Acid (mg)
1	5	4	.3	20	1300	Tr	.02	.2	Tr
4	7	16	.5	157	310	.06	.06	.4	94
3	7	12	.4	109	310	.05	.05	.4	70
33	14	101	1.1	782	Tr	.15	.07	2.7	31
23	10	72	.8	556	Tr	.12	.05	2.0	22
20	8	57	.7	385	Tr	.12	.05	1.6	22
18	8	56	.7	427	Tr	.07	.04	1.6	11
17	5	43	.9	326	Tr	.07	.01	1.3	11
45	28	78	1.9	439	Tr	.11	.03	1.6	12
27	50	103	.8	548	40	.17	.11	2.1	21
26	50	101	.8	525	360	.17	.11	2.1	19
30	65	99	.6	601	270	.08	.08	1.9	11
10	8	28	.4	226	Tr	.04	.01	1.0	3
41	80	160	1.5	798	350	.20	.18	2.8	28
19	61	64	1.0	588	15,680	.07	.12	1.5	12
1	5	6	.2	58	Tr	.01	.01	.1	5
9	85	42	1.2	329	120	.07	.09	.5	33
2	51	28	1.7	259	4460	.06	.11	.3	28
6	167	68	4.0	583	14,580	.13	.25	.9	50
8	232	90	4.3	683	16,200	.14	.31	.8	39
7	200	84	4.8	688	15,390	.15	.27	1.0	53
7	242	53	5.3	513	16,400	.04	.25	.6	29
7	53	53	.8	296	820	.11	.17	1.7	21
32	57	98	1.6	945	8610	.10	.27	1.4	27
37	46	66	1.0	342	9230	.10	.08	.8	25
40	48	71	1.1	367	11,940	.14	.09	.9	26
36	39	45	.9	200	6620	.06	.04	.4	11
63	64	105	2.0	510	19,890	.13	.10	1.5	36
10	10	16	.3	80	3120	.02	.02	.2	6
6	16	33	.6	300	1110	.07	.05	.9	28[67]
10	14[68]	46	1.2	523	2170	.12	.07	1.7	41
69	60	137	2.2	991	3820	.25	.19	4.4	41
4	3	8	.1	54	210	.01	.01	.2	2
10	17	44	2.2	552	1940	.12	.07	1.9	39
8	13	33	1.6	413	1460	.09	.05	1.5	29
8	54	34	.6	291	Tr	.06	.08	.5	34
5	252	49	1.5	—	8270	.15	.33	.7	68
6	195	64	2.6	246	11,390	.08	.15	.7	31
24	46	115	2.4	348	9010	.22	.13	2.0	15
1	58	87	—	5	0	0	0	0	0
1	183	45	—	—	0	0	0	0	0
	239	359	—	6	0	0	0	0	0
2	207	314	—	471	0	0	0	0	0
20	53	50	2.0	435	900	.03	.03	.8	13

| | | | | | | Fatty Acids | | |
| | | | | | | | Unsaturated | |
Foods, Approximate Measures, Units, and Weight		(g)	Water (%)	Food Energy (cal)	Protein (g)	Fat (g)	Saturated (total) (g)	Oleic (g)	Linoleic (g)
Beverages, alcoholic:									
Beer	12 fl oz	360	92	150	1	0	0	0	0
Gin, rum, vodka, whisky:									
80 proof	1½ fl oz jigger	42	67	95	—	—	0	0	0
86 proof	1½ fl oz jigger	42	64	105	—	—	0	0	0
90 proof	1½ fl oz jigger	42	62	110	—	—	0	0	0
Wines:									
Dessert	3½ fl oz glass	103	77	140	Tr	0	0	0	0
Table	3½ fl oz glass	102	86	85	Tr	0	0	0	0
Beverages, carbonated, sweetened, nonalcoholic:									
Carbonated water	12 fl oz	366	92	115	0	0	0	0	0
Cola type	12 fl oz	369	90	145	0	0	0	0	0
Fruit-flavored sodas and Tom Collins mixer	12 fl oz	372	88	170	0	0	0	0	0
Ginger ale	12 fl oz	366	92	115	0	0	0	0	0
Root beer	12 fl oz	370	90	150	0	0	0	0	0
Chili powder; see Peppers, hot, red									
Chocolate:									
Bitter or baking	1 oz	28	2	145	3	15	8.9	4.9	.4
Semisweet; see Candy, chocolate									
Gelatin, dry	1 7 g envelope	7	13	25	6	Tr	0	0	0
Gelatin dessert prepared with gelatin dessert powder and water	1 cup	240	84	140	4	0	0	0	0
Mustard, prepared, yellow	1 tsp or individual serving pouch or cup	5	80	5	Tr	Tr	—	—	—
Olives, pickled, canned:									
Green	4 medium or 3 extra large or 2 giant[69]	16	78	15	Tr	2	.2	1.2	.1
Ripe, Mission	3 small or 2 large[69]	10	73	15	Tr	2	.2	1.2	.1
Pickles, cucumber:									
Dill, medium, whole, 3¾ in long, 1¼-in diameter	1 pickle	65	93	5	Tr	Tr	—	—	—
Fresh-pack, slices 1½-in diameter, ¼ in thick	2 slices	15	79	10	Tr	Tr	—	—	—
Sweet gherkin, small, whole, about 2½ in long, ¾-in diameter	1 pickle	15	61	20	Tr	Tr	—	—	—
Relish, finely chopped, sweet	1 tbsp	15	63	20	Tr	Tr	—	—	—
Popsicle, 3 fl oz size	1 popsicle	95	80	70	0	0	0	0	0
Soups:									
Canned, condensed:									
Prepared with equal volume of milk:									
Cream of chicken	1 cup	245	85	180	7	10	4.2	3.6	1.3
Cream of mushroom	1 cup	245	83	215	7	14	5.4	2.9	4.6
Tomato	1 cup	250	84	175	7	7	3.4	1.7	1.0
Prepared with equal volume of water:									
Bean with pork	1 cup	250	84	170	8	6	1.2	1.8	2.4
Beef broth, bouillon, consomme	1 cup	240	96	30	5	0	0	0	0
Beef noodle	1 cup	240	93	65	4	3	.6	.7	.8
Clam chowder, Manhattan type (with tomatoes, without milk)	1 cup	245	92	80	2	3	.5	.4	1.3
Cream of chicken	1 cup	240	92	95	3	6	1.6	2.3	1.1
Cream of mushroom	1 cup	240	90	135	2	10	2.6	1.7	4.5
Minestrone	1 cup	245	90	105	5	3	.7	.9	1.3
Split pea	1 cup	245	85	145	9	3	1.1	1.2	.4
Tomato	1 cup	245	91	90	2	3	.5	.5	1.0
Vegetable beef	1 cup	245	92	80	5	2	—	—	—
Vegetarian	1 cup	245	92	80	2	2	—	—	—
Dehydrated:									
Bouillon cube, ½ in	1 cube	4	4	5	1	Tr	—	—	—
Mixes:									
Unprepared:									
Onion	1½ oz pkg	43	3	150	6	5	1.1	2.3	1.0
Prepared with water:									
Chicken noodle	1 cup	240	95	55	2	1	—	—	—
Onion	1 cup	240	96	35	1	1	—	—	—
Tomato vegetable with noodles	1 cup	240	93	65	1	1	—	—	—
Vinegar, cider	1 tbsp	15	94	Tr	Tr	0	0	0	0
White sauce, medium, with enriched flour	1 cup	250	73	405	10	31	19.3	7.8	.8
Yeast:									
Baker's dry, active	1 pkg	7	5	20	3	Tr	—	—	—
Brewer's, dry	1 tbsp	8	5	25	3	Tr	—	—	—

For notes, see end of table.

Nutrients in Indicated Quantity

Carbohydrate (g)	Calcium (mg)	Phosphorus (mg)	Iron (mg)	Potassium (mg)	Vitamin A Value (IU)	Thiamin (mg)	Riboflavin (mg)	Niacin (mg)	Ascorbic Acid (mg)
14	18	108	Tr	90	—	.01	.11	2.2	—
Tr	—	—	—	1	—	—	—	—	—
Tr	—	—	—	1	—	—	—	—	—
Tr	—	—	—	1	—	—	—	—	—
8	8	—	—	77	—	.01	.02	.2	—
4	9	10	.4	94	—	Tr	.01	.1	—
29	—	—	—	—	0	0	0	0	0
37	—	—	—	—	0	0	0	0	0
45	—	—	—	—	0	0	0	0	0
29	—	—	—	0	0	0	0	0	0
39	—	—	—	0	0	0	0	0	0
8	22	109	1.9	235	20	.01	.07	.4	0
0	—	—	—	—	—	—	—	—	—
34	—	—	—	—	—	—	—	—	—
Tr	4	4	.1	7	—	—	—	—	—
Tr	8	2	.2	7	40	—	—	—	—
Tr	9	1	.1	2	10	Tr	Tr	—	—
1	17	14	.7	130	70	Tr	.01	Tr	4
3	5	4	.3	—	20	Tr	Tr	Tr	1
5	2	2	.2	—	10	Tr	Tr	Tr	1
5	3	2	.1	—	—	—	—	—	—
18	0	—	Tr	—	0	0	0	0	0
15	172	152	0.5	260	610	0.05	0.27	0.7	2
16	191	169	.5	279	250	.05	.34	.7	1
23	168	155	.8	418	1200	.10	.25	1.3	15
22	63	128	2.3	395	650	.13	.08	1.0	3
3	Tr	31	.5	130	Tr	Tr	.02	1.2	—
7	7	48	1.0	77	50	.05	.07	1.0	Tr
12	34	47	1.0	184	880	.02	.02	1.0	—
8	24	34	.5	79	410	.02	.05	.5	Tr
10	41	50	.5	98	70	.02	.12	.7	Tr
14	37	59	1.0	314	2350	.07	.05	1.0	—
21	29	149	1.5	270	440	.25	.15	1.5	1
16	15	34	.7	230	1000	.05	.05	1.2	12
10	12	49	.7	162	2700	.05	.05	1.0	—
13	20	39	1.0	172	2940	.05	.05	1.0	—
Tr	—	—	—	4	—	—	—	—	—
23	42	49	.6	238	30	.05	.03	.3	6
8	7	19	.2	19	50	.07	.05	.5	Tr
6	10	12	.2	58	Tr	Tr	Tr	Tr	2
12	7	19	.2	29	480	.05	.02	.5	5
1	1	1	.1	15	—	—	—	—	—
22	288	233	.5	348	1150	.12	.43	.7	2
3	3	90	1.1	140	Tr	.16	.38	2.6	Tr
3	17[70]	140	1.4	152	Tr	1.25	.34	3.0	Tr

Footnotes

[1] Vitamin A value is largely from beta-carotene used for coloring. Riboflavin value for powdered sweet creamers applies to products with added riboflavin.

[2] Applies to product without added vitamin A. With added vitamin A, value is 500 IU.

[3] Applies to product without added vitamin A added.

[4] Applies to product with added vitamin A. Without added vitamin A, value is 20 IU.

[5] Yields 1 qt of fluid milk when reconstituted according to package directions.

[6] Applies to product with added vitamin A.

[7] Weight applies to product with label claim of 1⅓ cups equal 3.2 oz.

[8] Applies to products made from thick shake mixes and that do not contain added ice cream. Products made from milk shake mixes are higher in fat and usually contain added ice cream.

[9] Content of fat, vitamin A, and carbohydrate varies. Consult the label when precise values are needed for special diets.

[10] Applies to product made with milk containing no added vitamin A.

[11] Based on year-round average.

[12] Based on average vitamin A content of fortified margarine. Federal specifications for fortified margarine require a minimum of 15,000 IU of vitamin A per pound.

[13] Fatty acid values apply to product made with regular-type margarine.

[14] Dipped in egg, milk or water, and breadcrumbs; fried in vegetable shortening.

[15] If bones are discarded, value for calcium will be greatly reduced.

[16] Dipped in egg, breadcrumbs, and flour or batter.

[17] Prepared with tuna, celery, salad dressing (mayonnaise type), pickle, onion, and egg.

[18] Outer layer of fat on the cut was removed to within approximately ½ in of the lean. Deposits of fat within the cut were not removed.

[19] Crust made with vegetable shortening and enriched flour.

[20] Regular-type margarine used.

[21] Value varies widely.

[22] About one fourth of the outer layer of fat on the cut was removed. Deposits of fat within the cut were not removed.

[23] Vegetable shortening used.

[24] Also applies to pasteurized apple cider.

[25] Applies to product without added ascorbic acid. For value of product with added ascorbic acid, refer to label.

[26] Based on product with label claim of 45% of U.S. RDA in 6 fl oz.

[27] Based on product with label claim of 100% of U.S. RDA in 6 fl oz.

[28] Weight includes peel and membranes between sections. Without these parts, the weight of the edible portion is 123 g for ½ pink or red grapefruit and 118 g for ½ white grapefruit.

[29] For white-fleshed varieties, value is about 20 IU per cup; for red-fleshed varieties, 1080 IU.

[30] Weight includes seeds. Without seeds, weight of the edible portion is 57 g.

[31] Applies to product without added ascorbic acid. With added ascorbic acid, based on claim that 6 fl oz of reconstituted juice contains 45% or 50% of the U.S. RDA, value in milligrams is 108 or 120 for a 6 fl oz can (undiluted, frozen concentrate grape juice), 36 or 40 for 1 cup of diluted juice (diluted frozen concentrate grape juice).

[32] For products with added thiamin and riboflavin but without added ascorbic acid, values in milligrams would be .60 for thiamin, .80 for riboflavin, and Tr for ascorbic acid. For products with only ascorbic acid added, value varies with the brand. Consult the label.

[33] Weight includes rind. Without rind, the weight of the edible portion is 272 g for cantaloup and 149 g for honeydew melon.

[34] Represents yellow-fleshed varieties. For white-fleshed varieties, value is 50 IU for 1 peach, 90 IU for 1 cup of slices.

[35] Value represents products with added ascorbic acid. For products without added ascorbic acid, value in milligrams is 116 for a 10 oz container, 103 for 1 cup.

[36]Weight includes pits. After removal of the pits, the weight of the edible portion is 258 g for 1 cup plums in heavy syrup, 133 g for 3 plums in heavy syrup, 43 g for 4 dried prunes, and 213 g for 1 cup cooked, unsweetened prunes.

[37]Weight includes rind and seeds. Without rind and seeds, weight of the edible portion is 426 g.

[38]Made with vegetable shortening.

[39]Applies to product made with white cornmeal. With yellow cornmeal, value is 30 IU.

[40]Applies to white varieties. For yellow varieties, value is 150 IU.

[41]Applies to products that do not contain disodium phosphate. If disodium phosphate is an ingredient, value is 162 mg.

[42]Value may range from less than 1 mg to about 8 mg, depending on the brand. Consult the label.

[43]Applies to product with added nutrient. Without added nutrient, value is trace.

[44]Value varies with the brand. Consult the label.

[45]Applies to product with added nutrient. Without added nutrient, value is trace.

[46]Excepting angelfood cake, cakes were made from mixes containing vegetable shortening; icings, with butter.

[47]Excepting spongecake, vegetable shortening used for cake portion; butter, for icing. If butter or margarine used for cake portion, vitamin A values would be higher.

[48]Applies to product made with a sodium aluminum-sulfate type of baking power. With a low-sodium type of baking powder containing potassium, value would be about twice the amount shown.

[49]Equal weights of flour, sugar, eggs, and vegetable shortening.

[50]Products are commercial unless otherwise specified.

[51]Made with enriched flour and vegetable shortening except for macaroons, which do not contain flour or shortening.

[52]Icing made with butter.

[53]Applies to yellow varieties; white varieties contain only a trace.

[54]Contains vegetable shortening and butter.

[55]Made with corn oil.

[56]Made with regular margarine.

[57]Applies to product made with yellow cornmeal.

[58]Made with enriched degermed cornmeal and enriched flour.

[59]Product may or may not be enriched with riboflavin. Consult the label.

[60]Value varies with the brand. Consult the label.

[61]Weight includes cob. Without cob, weight is 77 g for 1 ear cooked, drained sweet corn, 126 g for 1 frozen 5-in ear.

[62]Based on yellow varieties. For white varieties, value is trace.

[63]Weight includes refuse of outer leaves and core. Without these parts, weight is 163 g.

[64]Weight includes core. Without core, weight is 539 g.

[65]Value based on white-fleshed varieties. For yellow-fleshed varieties, value in IU is 70 for 1 cup chopped raw onions, 50 for 1 cup sliced raw onions, and 80 for 1 cup cooked onions.

[66]Weight inclues cores and stem ends. Without these parts, weight is 123 g.

[67]Based on year-round average. For tomatoes marketed from November through May, value is about 12 mg; from June through October, 32 mg.

[68]Applies to product without calcium salts added. Value for products with calcium salts added may be as much as 63 mg for whole tomatoes, 241 mg for cut forms.

[69]Weight includes pits. Without pits, weight is 13 g for 4 medium (or 3 extra large or 2 giant) green pickled olives, 9 g for 3 small (or 2 large) ripe pickled olives.

[70]Value may vary from 6 to 60 mg.

APPENDIX B
Cholesterol content of foods

Item	Amount of cholesterol in 100 g edible portion[1] (mg)	Amount of cholesterol in Edible portion of 450 g (1 lb) as purchased (mg)	Refuse from item as purchased (%)
Beef, raw			
With bone[2]	70	270	15
Without bone[2]	70	320	0
Brains, raw	>2000	>9000	0
Butter	250	1135	0
Cavier or fish roe	>300	>1300	0
Cheese			
Cheddar	100	455	0
Cottage, creamed	15	70	0
Cream	120	545	0
Other (25%-30% fat)	85	385	0
Cheese spread	65	295	0
Chicken, flesh only, raw	60	—	0
Crab			
In shell[2]	125	270	52
Meat only[2]	125	565	0
Egg, whole	550	2200	12
Egg white	0	0	0
Egg yolk			
Fresh	1500	6800	0
Frozen	1280	5800	0
Dried	2950	13,380	0
Fish			
Steak[2]	70	265	16
Fillet[2]	70	320	0
Heart, raw	150	680	0
Ice cream	45	205	0
Kidney, raw	375	1700	0
Lamb, raw			
With bone[2]	70	265	16
Without bone[2]	70	320	0
Lard and other animal fat	95	430	0
Liver, raw	300	1360	0
Lobster			
Whole[2]	200	235	74
Meat only[2]	200	900	0
Margarine			
All vegetable fat	0	0	0

From Watt, B.K., and Merrill, A.L.: Composition of foods — raw, processed, prepared, U.S. Department of Agriculture, Agriculture Handbook No. 8, Dec. 1963.

[1]Data apply to 100 g of edible portion of the item, although it may be purchased with the refuse indicated and described or implied in the first column.

[2]Items that have the same chemical composition for the edible portion but differ in the amount of refuse.

| Item | Amount of cholesterol in | | Refuse from item as purchased (%) |
	100 g edible portion[1] (mg)	Edible portion of 450 g (1 lb) as purchased (mg)	
Margarine — cont'd			
Two-thirds animal fat, one-third vegetable fat	65	295	0
Milk			
Fluid, whole	11	50	0
Dried, whole	85	385	0
Fluid, skim	3	15	0
Mutton			
With bone[2]	65	250	16
Without bone[2]	65	295	0
Oysters			
In shell[2]	>200	>90	90
Meat only[2]	>200	>900	0
Pork			
With bone[2]	70	260	18
Without bone[2]	70	320	0
Shrimp			
In shell[2]	125	390	31
Flesh only[2]	125	565	0
Sweetbreads (thymus)	250	1135	0
Veal			
With bone[2]	90	320	21
Without bone[2]	90	410	0

APPENDIX C
Dietary fiber in selected plant foods

Food	Amount	Weight (g)	Total dietary fiber (g)	Noncellulose polysaccharides (g)	Cellulose (g)	Lignin (g)
Apple	1 med					
Flesh		138	1.96	1.29	0.66	0.01
Skin		100	3.71	2.21	1.01	0.49
Banana	1 small	119	2.08	1.33	0.44	0.31
Beans						
Baked	1 cup	255	18.53	14.45	3.59	0.48
Green, cooked	1 cup	125	4.19	2.31	1.61	0.26
Bread						
White	1 slice	25	0.68	0.50	0.18	Trace
Whole meal	1 slice	25	2.13	1.49	0.33	0.31
Broccoli, cooked	1 cup	155	6.36	4.53	1.78	0.05
Brussels sprouts, cooked	1 cup	155	4.43	3.08	1.24	0.11
Cabbage, cooked	1 cup	145	4.10	2.55	1.00	0.55
Carrots, cooked	1 cup	155	5.74	3.44	2.29	Trace
Cauliflower, cooked	1 cup	125	2.25	0.84	1.41	Trace
Cereals						
All-Bran	1 oz	30	8.01	5.35	1.80	0.86
Corn Flakes	1 cup	25	2.75	1.82	0.61	0.33
Grapenuts	¼ cup	30	2.10	1.54	0.38	0.17
Puffed Wheat	1 cup	15	2.31	1.55	0.39	0.37
Rice Krispies	1 cup	30	1.34	1.04	0.23	0.07
Shredded Wheat	1 biscuit	25	3.07	2.20	0.66	0.21
Special K	1 cup	30	1.64	1.10	0.22	0.32
Cherries	10 cherries	68	0.84	0.63	0.17	0.05
Cookies						
Ginger	4 snaps	28	0.56	0.41	0.08	0.07
Oatmeal	4 cookies	52	2.08	1.64	0.21	0.22
Plain	4 cookies	48	0.80	0.68	0.05	0.06
Corn	1 cup	165	7.82	7.11	0.51	0.20
Canned	1 cup	165	9.39	8.20	1.06	0.13
Flour						
Bran	1 cup	100	44.00	32.70	8.05	3.23
White	1 cup	115	3.62	2.90	0.69	0.03
Whole meal	1 cup	120	11.41	7.50	2.95	0.96
Grapefruit	½ cup	100	0.44	0.34	0.04	0.06
Jam, strawberry	1 tbsp	20	0.22	0.17	0.02	0.03
Lettuce	⅙ head	100	1.53	0.47	1.06	Trace
Marmalade, orange	1 tbsp	20	0.14	0.13	0.01	Trace
Onions, raw, sliced	1 cup	100	2.10	1.55	0.55	Trace
Orange	1 cup	200	0.58	0.44	0.08	0.06

Adapted from Southgate, D.A.T., and others: A guide to calculating intakes of dietary fiber, J. Hum. Nutr. **30:**303, 1976. *Continued.*

Food	Amount	Weight (g)	Total dietary fiber (g)	Noncellulose polysaccharides (g)	Cellulose (g)	Lignin (g)
Parsnips, raw, diced	1 cup	100	4.90	3.77	1.13	Trace
Peanuts	1 oz	30	2.79	1.92	0.51	0.36
Peanut butter	1 tbsp	16	1.21	0.90	0.31	Trace
Peach, flesh and skin	1 med	100	2.28	1.46	0.20	0.62
Pear	1 med					
Flesh		164	4.00	2.16	1.10	0.74
Skin		100	8.59	3.72	2.18	2.67
Peas, canned	1 cup	170	13.35	8.84	3.91	0.60
Peas, raw or frozen	1 cup	100	7.75	5.48	2.09	0.18
Plums	1 plum	66	1.00	0.65	0.15	0.20
Potato, raw	1 med	135	4.73	3.36	1.38	Trace
Raisins	1 oz	30	1.32	0.72	0.25	0.35
Strawberries	1 cup	149	2.65	1.39	1.04	0.22
Tomato						
Raw	1 med	135	1.89	0.83	0.61	0.41
Canned, drained	1 cup	240	2.04	1.08	0.89	0.07
Turnips, raw	1 med	100	2.20	1.50	0.70	Trace

APPENDIX D
Sodium and potassium content of foods

Food and description	Sodium (mg)	Potassium (mg)
Almonds		
Dried	4	773
Roasted and salted	198	773
Apples		
Raw, pared	1	110
Frozen, sliced, sweetened	14	68
Apple juice, canned or bottled	1	101
Applesauce, canned, sweetened	2	65
Apricots		
Raw	1	281
Canned, syrup pack, light	1	239
Dried, sulfured, cooked, fruit, and liquid	8	318
Asparagus		
Cooked spears, boiled, drained	1	183
Canned spears, green		
Regular pack, solids and liquid	236[1]	166
Special dietary pack (low sodium), solids and liquid	3	166
Frozen		
Cuts and tips, cooked, boiled, drained	1	220
Spears, cooked, boiled, drained	1	238
Avocados, raw, all commercial varieties	4	604
Bacon, cured, cooked, broiled or fried, drained	1021	236
Bacon, Canadian, cooked, broiled or fried, drained	2555	432
Bananas, raw, common	1	370
Bass, black sea, raw	68	256
Beans, common, mature seeds, dry		
White		
Cooked	7	416
Canned, solids and liquid, with pork and tomato sauce	463	210
Red, cooked	3	340
Beans, lima		
Immature seeds		
Cooked, boiled, drained	1	422
Canned		
Regular pack, solids and liquid	236[1]	222
Special dietary pack (low sodium), solids and liquid	4	222
Frozen, thin-seeded types, commonly called baby limas, cooked, boiled, drained	129	394
Mature seeds, dry, cooked	2	612
Beans, mung, sprouted seeds, cooked, boiled, drained	4	156
Beans, snap		
Green		
Cooked, boiled, drained	4	151

Numbers in parentheses denote values inputed, usually from another form of the food or from a similar food. Dashes denote lack of reliable data for a constituent believed to be present in measurable amount. Values are selected from Watt, B.K., and Merrill, A.L.: Composition of foods — raw, processed, prepared, U.S. Department of Agriculture, Agriculture Handbook No. 8, Dec. 1963.

For notes, see end of table.

Food and description	Sodium (mg)	Potassium (mg)
Canned		
Regular pack, solids and liquid	236[1]	95
Special dietary pack (low sodium), solids and liquid	2	95
Frozen, cut, cooked, boiled, drained	1	152
Yellow or wax		
Cooked, boiled, drained	3	151
Canned		
Regular pack, solids and liquid	236[1]	95
Special dietary pack (low sodium), solids and liquid	2	95
Frozen, cut, cooked, boiled, drained	1	164
Beef		
Retail cuts, trimmed to retail level		
Round	60	370
Rump	60	370
Hamburger, regular ground, cooked	47	450
Beef, corned, boneless		
Cooked, medium fat	1740	150
Canned corned-beef hash (with potato)	540	200
Beef, dried, cooked, creamed	716	153
Beef potpie, commercial, frozen, unheated	366	93
Beets, common, red		
Canned		
Regular pack, solids and liquid	236[1]	167
Special dietary pack (low sodium), solids and liquid	46	167
Beet greens, common, cooked, boiled, drained	76	332
Biscuits, baking powder, made with enriched flour	626	117
Blackberries, including dewberries, boysenberries, and youngberries, raw	1	170
Blueberries		
Raw	1	81
Frozen, not thawed, sweetened	1	66
Bouillon cubes or powder	24,000	100
Bran, added sugar and malt extract	1060	1070
Bran flakes (40% bran), added thiamine	925	—
Bran flakes with raisins, added thiamine	800	—
Breads		
Cracked wheat	529	134
French or Vienna, enriched	580	90
Italian, enriched	585	74
Raisin	365	233
Rye, American (⅓ rye, ⅔ clear flour)	557	145
White, enriched, made with 3%-4% nonfat dry milk	507	105
Whole wheat, made with 2% nonfat dry milk	527	273
Bread stuffing mix and stuffings prepared from mix, dry form	1331	172
Broccoli		
Cooked spears, boiled, drained	10	267
Frozen, spears, cooked, boiled, drained	12	220
Brussels sprouts, frozen, cooked, boiled, drained	14	295

Continued.

Food and description	Sodium (mg)	Potassium (mg)
Buffalo fish, raw	52	293
Bulgur (parboiled wheat), canned, made from hard red winter wheat		
Unseasoned[2]	599	87
Seasoned[3]	460	112
Butter[4]	987	23
Buttermilk, fluid, cultured (made from skim milk)	130	140
Cabbage		
Common varieties (Danish, domestic, and pointed types)		
Raw	20	233
Cooked, boiled until tender, drained, shredded, cooked in small amount of water	14	163
Red, raw	26	268
Cakes		
Baked from home recipes		
Angel food	283	88
Fruit cake, made with enriched flour, dark	158	496
Gingerbread, made with enriched flour	237	454
Plain cake or cupcake, without icing	300	79
Pound, modified	178	78
Frozen, commercial, devil's food, with chocolate icing	420	119
Candy		
Caramels, plain or chocolate	226	192
Chocolate, sweet	33	269
Chocolate coated, chocolate fudge	228	193
Gum drops, starch jelly pieces	35	5
Hard	32	4
Marshmallows	39	6
Peanut bars	10	448
Carrots		
Raw	47	341
Canned		
Regular pack, solids and liquid	236[1]	120
Special dietary pack (low sodium), solids and liquid	39	120
Cashew nuts	15[5]	464
Cauliflower		
Cooked, boiled, drained	9	206
Frozen, cooked, boiled, drained	10	207
Celery, all, including green and yellow varieties		
Raw	126	341
Cooked, boiled, drained	88	239
Chard, Swiss, cooked, boiled, drained	86	321
Cheeses		
Natural cheeses		
Cheddar (domestic type, commonly called American)	700	82
Cottage (large or small curd)		
Creamed	229	85
Uncreamed	290	72
Cream	250	74

For notes, see end of table.

Food and description	Sodium (mg)	Potassium (mg)
Parmesan	734	149
Swiss (domestic)	710	104
Pasteurized process cheese, American	1136[6]	80
Pasteurized process cheese spread, American	1625[6]	240
Cherries		
Raw, sweet	2	191
Canned		
Sour, red, solids and liquid, water pack	2	130
Sweet, solids and liquid, syrup pack, light	1	128
Frozen, not thawed, sweetened	2	130
Chicken, all classes		
Light meat without skin, cooked, roasted	64	411
Dark meat without skin, cooked, roasted	86	321
Chicken potpie, commercial, frozen, unheated	411	153
Chili con carne, canned, with beans	531	233
Clams, raw		
Soft, meat only	36	235
Hard or round, meat only	205	311
Cocoa and chocolate-flavored beverage powders		
Cocoa powder with nonfat dry milk	525	800
Mix for hot chocolate	382	605
Cocoa, dry powder, high-fat or breakfast		
Plain	6	1522
Processed with alkali	717	651
Coconut meat, fresh	23	256
Cod		
Cooked, broiled	110	407
Dehydrated, lightly salted	8100	160
Coffee, instant, water-soluble solids		
Dry powder	72	3256
Beverage	1	36
Coleslaw, made with French dressing (commercial)	268	205
Collards, cooked, boiled, drained, leaves, including stems, cooked in small amount of water	25	234
Cookies		
Assorted, packaged, commercial	365	67
Butter, thin, rich	418	60
Gingersnaps	571	462
Molasses	386	138
Oatmeal with raisins	162	370
Sandwich type	483	38
Vanilla wafer	252	72
Corn, sweet		
Cooked, boiled, drained, white and yellow, kernels, cut off cob before cooking	Trace	165
Canned		
Regular pack, cream style, white and yellow, solids and liquid	236[1]	(97)
Special dietary pack (low sodium), cream style, white and yellow, solids and liquid	2	(97)

Continued.

Food and description	Sodium (mg)	Potassium (mg)
Frozen, kernels cut off cob, cooked, boiled, drained	1	184
Corn grits, degermed, enriched, dry form	1	80
Corn products used mainly as ready-to-eat breakfast cereals		
Corn flakes, added nutrients	1005	120
Corn, puffed, added nutrients	1060	—
Corn, rice, and wheat flakes, mixed, added nutrients	950	—
Corn bread, baked from home recipes, southern style, made with degermed cornmeal, enriched	591	157
Cornmeal, white or yellow, degermed, enriched, dry form	1	120
Cornstarch	Trace	Trace
Cowpeas, including blackeye peas		
Immature seeds, canned, solids and liquid	236[1]	352
Young pods, with seeds, cooked, boiled, drained	3	196
Crab, canned	1000	110
Crackers		
Butter	1092	113
Graham, plain	670	384
Saltines	(1100)	(120)
Sandwich type, peanut-cheese	992	226
Soda	1100	120
Cream, fluid, light, coffee, or table, 20% fat	43	122
Cream substitutes, dried, containing cream, skim milk (calcium reduced), and lactose	575	—
Cucumbers, raw, pared	6	160
Custard, baked	79	146
Doughnuts, cake type	501	90
Duck, domesticated, raw, flesh only	74	285
Eggs, chicken		
Raw		
Whole, fresh and frozen	122	129
Whites, fresh and frozen	146	139
Yolks, fresh	52	98
Eggplant, cooked, boiled, drained	1	150
Farina		
Enriched		
Regular		
Dry form	2	83
Cooked	144	9
Quick-cooking, cooked	165	10
Instant-cooking, cooked	188	13
Nonenriched, regular, dry form	2	83
Flatfishes (flounders, soles, sand dabs), raw	78	342
Fruit cocktail, canned, solids and liquid, water pack, with or without artificial sweetener	5	168
Garlic, cloves, raw	19	529
Grapefruit		
Raw, pulp, pink, red, white, all varieties	1	135
Canned, juice, sweetened	1	162

For notes, see end of table.

Food and description	Sodium (mg)	Potassium (mg)
Grapes, raw, American type (slip skin), such as Concord, Delaware, Niagara, Catawba, and Scuppernong	3	158
Haddock, cooked, fried	177	348
Halibut, Atlantic and Pacific, cooked, broiled	134	525
Ice cream and frozen custard, regular, approximately 10% fat	63[7]	181
Ice cream cones	232	244
Ice milk	68[7]	195
Jams and preserves	12	88
Kale, cooked, boiled, drained, leaves including stems	43	221
Lamb, retail cuts	70	290
Lettuce, raw crisphead varieties such as Iceberg, New York, and Great Lakes strains	9	175
Liver, beef, cooked, fried	184	380
Lobster, northern, canned or cooked	210	180
Macaroni, unenriched, dry form	2	197
Margarine[8]	987	23
Milk, cow		
Fluid (pasteurized and raw)		
Whole, 3.7% fat	50	144
Skim	52	145
Canned, evaporated (unsweetened)	118	303
Dry, skim (nonfat solids), regular	532	1745
Malted		
Dry powder	440	720
Beverage	91	200
Chocolate drink, fluid, commercial		
Made with skim milk	46	142
Made with whole (3.5% fat) milk	47	146
Molasses, cane		
First extraction or light	15	917
Third extraction or blackstrap	96	2927
Muskmelons, raw, cantaloupes, other netted varieties	12	251
Mustard greens, cooked, boiled, drained	18	220
Nectarines, raw	6	294
New Zealand spinach, cooked, boiled, drained	92	463
Noodles, egg noodles, enriched, cooked	2	44
Oat products used mainly as hot breakfast cereals, oatmeal or rolled oats		
Dry form	2	352
Cooked	218	61
Oat products used mainly as ready-to-eat breakfast cereals, with or without corn, puffed, added nutrients	1267	—
Okra		
Raw	3	249
Cooked, boiled, drained	2	174
Olives, pickled; canned or bottled		
Green	2400	55

Continued.

Food and description	Sodium (mg)	Potassium (mg)
Ripe, Ascolano (extra large, mammoth, giant jumbo)	813	34
Ripe, salt-cured, oil-coated, Greek style	3288	—
Onions, mature (dry), raw	10	157
Onions, young green (bunching varieties), raw, bulb and entire top	5	231
Oranges, raw, peeled fruit, all commercial varieties	1	200
Orange juice		
Raw, all commercial varieties	1	200
Canned, unsweetened	1	199
Frozen concentrate, unsweetened, diluted with 3 parts water, by volume	1	186
Oysters		
Raw, meat only, Eastern	73	121
Cooked, fried	206	203
Frozen, solids and liquid	380	210
Parsnips, cooked, boiled, drained	8	379
Peaches		
Raw	1	202
Canned, solids and liquid, water pack, with or without artificial sweetener	2	137
Frozen, sliced, sweetened, not thawed	2	124
Peanuts		
Roasted with skins	5	701
Roasted and salted	418	674
Peanut butters made with small amounts of added fat, salt	607	670
Pears		
Raw, including skin	2	130
Canned, solids and liquid, syrup pack, light	1	85
Peas, green, immature		
Cooked, boiled, drained	1	196
Canned, Alaska (early or June peas)		
Regular pack, solids and liquid	236[1]	96
Special dietary pack (low sodium), solids and liquid	3	96
Frozen, cooked, boiled, drained	115	135
Pecans	Trace	603
Peppers, sweet, garden varieties, immature, green, raw	13	213
Perch, yellow, raw	68	230
Pickles, cucumber, dill	1428	200
Piecrust or plain pastry, made with enriched flour, baked	611	50
Pineapple		
Raw	1	146
Frozen chunks, sweetened, not thawed	2	100
Pizza, with cheese, from home recipe, baked		
With cheese topping	702	130
With sausage topping	729	168
Plate dinners, frozen, commercial, unheated		
Beef pot roast, whole oven-browned potatoes, peas, corn	259	244
Chicken, fried; mashed potatoes; mixed vegetables (carrots, peas, corn, beans)	344	112
Meatloaf with tomato sauce, mashed potatoes, peas	393	115
Turkey, sliced; mashed potatoes; peas	400	176

For notes, see end of table.

Food and description	Sodium (mg)	Potassium (mg)
Plums		
Raw, Damson	2	299
Canned, solids and liquid, purple (Italian prunes), syrup packed, light	1	145
Popcorn, popped		
Plain	(3)	—
Oil and salt added	1940	—
Pork, fresh, retail cuts, trimmed to retail level, loin	65	390
Pork, cured, canned ham, contents of can	(1100)	(340)
Potatoes		
Cooked, boiled in skin	3[9]	407
Dehydrated mashed, flakes without milk		
Dry form	89	1600
Prepared, water, milk, table fat added	231	286
Pretzels	1680[10]	130
Prunes, dried, "softenized," cooked (fruit and liquid), with added sugar	3	262
Pudding mixes and puddings made from mixes, with starch base		
With milk, cooked	129	136
With milk, without cooking	124	129
Pumpkin, canned	2	240
Raspberries		
Canned, solids and liquid, water pack, with or without artificial sweetener, red	1	114
Frozen, red, sweetened, not thawed	1	100
Rice		
Brown		
Raw	9	214
Cooked	282	70
White (fully milled or polished), enriched, common commercial varieties, all types		
Raw	5	92
Cooked	374	28
Rice products used mainly as ready-to-eat breakfast cereals		
Rice flakes, added nutrients	987	180
Rice, puffed; added nutrients, without salt	2	100
Rice, puffed or open-popped, presweetened, honey and added nutrients	706	—
Roe, cooked, baked or broiled, cod and shad[11]	73	132
Rolls and buns, commercial, ready-to-serve		
Danish pastry	366	112
Hard rolls, enriched	625	97
Plain (pan rolls), enriched	506	95
Sweet rolls	389	124
Rusk	246	161
Rutabagas, cooked, boiled, drained	4	167
Rye, flour, medium	(1)	203
Rye wafers, whole grain	882	600

Continued.

Food and description	Sodium (mg)	Potassium (mg)
Salad dressings, commercial[12]		
Blue and Roquefort cheese		
Regular	1094	37
Special dietary (low calorie), low fat (approx. 5 kcal/tsp)	1108	34
French		
Regular	1370	79
Special dietary (low calorie), low fat (approx. 5 kcal/tsp)	787	79
Mayonnaise	597	34
Thousand Island		
Regular	700	113
Special dietary (low calorie, approx. 10 kcal/tsp)	700	113
Salmon, coho (silver)		
Raw	48[13]	421
Canned, solids and liquid	351[14]	339
Salt pork, raw	1212	42
Salt sticks, regular type	1674	92
Sandwich spread (with chopped pickle)		
Regular	626	92
Special dietary (low calorie, approx. 5 kcal/tsp)	626	92
Sardines, Atlantic, canned in oil, drained solids	823	590
Sardines, Pacific, in tomato sauce, solids and liquid	400	320
Sauerkraut, canned, solids and liquid	747[15]	140
Sausage, cold cuts, and luncheon meats		
Bologna, all samples	1300	230
Frankfurters, raw, all samples	1100	220
Luncheon meat, pork, cured ham or shoulder, chopped, spiced or unspiced, canned	1234	222
Pork sausage, links or bulk, cooked	958	269
Scallops, bay and sea, cooked, steamed	265	476
Soups, commercial, canned		
Beef broth, bouillon, and consomme, prepared with equal volume of water	326	54
Chicken noodle, prepared with equal volume of water	408	23
Tomato		
Prepared with equal volume of water	396	94
Prepared with equal volume of milk	422	167
Vegetable beef, prepared with equal volume of water	427	66
Soy sauce	7325	366
Spaghetti, enriched, cooked, tender stage	1	61
Spinach		
Cooked, boiled, drained	50	324
Canned		
Regular pack, drained solids	236[1]	250
Special dietary pack (low sodium), solids and liquid	34	250
Frozen, chopped, cooked, boiled, drained	52	333
Squash, summer, all varieties, cooked, boiled, drained	1	141

For notes, see end of table.

Food and description	Sodium (mg)	Potassium (mg)
Strawberries		
Raw	1	164
Frozen, sweetened, not thawed, sliced	1	112
Sweet potatoes		
Cooked, all, baked in skin	12	300
Canned, liquid pack, solids and liquid, regular pack in syrup	48	(120)
Dehydrated flakes, prepared with water	45	140
Tangerines, raw (Dancy variety)	2	126
Tea, instant (water-soluble solids), carbohydrate added		
Dry powder	—	4530
Beverage	—	25
Tomatoes, ripe		
Raw	3	244
Canned, solids and liquid, regular pack	130	217
Tomato catsup, bottled	1042[16]	363
Regular pack	200	227
Special dietary pack (low sodium)	3	227
Tomato puree, canned		
Regular pack	399	426
Special dietary pack (low sodium)	6	426
Tuna, canned		
In oil, solids and liquid	800	301
In water, solids and liquid	41[17]	279[17]
Turkey, all classes		
Light meat, cooked, roasted	82	411
Dark meat, cooked, roasted	99	398
Turkey potpie, commercial frozen, unheated	369	114
Turnips, cooked, boiled, drained	34	188
Turnip greens, leaves, including stems		
Canned, solids and liquid	236[1]	243
Frozen, cooked, boiled, drained	17	149
Veal, retail cuts, untrimmed	80	500
Waffles, frozen, made with enriched flour	644	158
Walnuts		
Black	3	460
Persian or English	2	450
Watermelon, raw	1	100
Wheat flours		
Whole (from hard wheats)	3	370
Patent		
All-purpose or family flour, enriched	2	95
Self-rising flour, enriched (anhydrous monocalcium phosphate used as a baking acid)[18]	1079	—[19]
Yogurt, made from whole milk	47	132

[1]Estimated average based on addition of salt in the amount of 0.6% of the finished product.
[2]Processed, partially debranned, whole-kernel wheat with salt added.

Continued.

[3]Processed, partially debranned, whole-kernel wheat with chicken fat, chicken stock base, dehydrated onion flakes, salt, monosodium glutamate, and herbs.

[4]Values apply to salted butter. Unsalted butter contains less than 10 mg of either sodium or potassium per 100 g. Value for vitamin A is the year-round average.

[5]Applies to unsalted nuts. For salted nuts, value is approximately 200 mg per 100 g.

[6]Values for phosphorus and sodium are based on use of 1.5% anhydrous disodium phosphate as the emulsifying agent. If emulsifying agent does not contain either phosphorus (P) or sodium (Na), the content of these two nutrients in milligrams per 100 g is as follows:

	P	Na
American process cheese	444	650
Swiss process cheese	540	681
American cheese food	427	—
American cheese spread	548	1139

[7]Value for product without added salt.

[8]Values apply to salted margarine. Unsalted margarine contains less than 10 mg/100 g of either sodium or potassium. Vitamin A value based on the minimum required to meet federal specifications for margarine with vitamin A added, 15,000 IUA/lb.

[9]Applies to product without added salt. If salt is added, an estimated average value for sodium is 236 mg/100 g.

[10]Sodium content is variable. For example, very thin pretzel sticks contain about twice the average amount listed.

[11]Prepared with butter or margarine, lemon juice or vinegar.

[12]Values apply to products containing salt. For those without salt, sodium content is low, ranging from less than 10 to 50 mg/100 g; the amount usually is indicated on the label.

[13]Sample dipped in brine contained 215 mg sodium/100 g.

[14]For product canned without added salt, value is approximately the same as for raw salmon.

[15]Values for sauerkraut and sauerkraut juice are based on salt content of 1.9% and 2.0%, respectively, in the finished products. The amounts in some samples may vary significantly from this estimate.

[16]Applies to regular pack. For special dietary pack (low sodium), values range from 5-35 mg/100 g.

[17]One sample with salt added contained 875 mg of sodium/100 g and 275 mg of potassium.

[18]The acid ingredient most commonly used in self-rising flour. When sodium acid pyrophosphate in combination with either anhydrous monocalcium phosphate or calcium carbonate is used, the value for calcium is approximately 120 mg/100 g; for phosphorus, 540 mg; for sodium, 1360 mg.

[19]90 mg of potassium/100 g contributed by flour. Small quantities of additional potassium may be provided by other ingredients.

APPENDIX E
Food Guide: Exchange Lists for Meal Planning (1986 revision)

The *exchange system of dietary control,* developed by two professional organizations—the American Dietetic Association and the American Diabetes Association—is based on a simple grouping of common foods according to generally equivalent nutritional values. This system may be used for any situation requiring caloric and food value control.

The foods are divided into six basic groups (with subgroups), called the "exchange lists." Each food item within a group or subgroup contains about the same food value as other food items in that group, allowing for exchange within groups, thus providing for variety in food choices as well as food value control. Therefore the term *food exchanges* is sometimes used to refer to food choices or servings. The total number of "exchanges" per day depends on individual nutritional needs, based on normal nutrition standards. Although there is some variation in the composition of foods within the exchange groups, for simplicity the following values for carbohydrate, protein, fat, and kcalories are used.

❖ *Exchange lists*

Food Groups	Carbohydrate (g)	Protein (g)	Fat (g)	Kcalories
Starch/Bread	15	3	trace	80
Meat				
Lean	—	7	3	55
Medium-fat	—	7	5	75
High-fat	—	7	8	100
Vegetable	5	2	—	25
Fruit	15	—	—	60
Milk				
Skim	12	8	trace	90
Low-fat	12	8	5	120
Whole	12	8	8	150
Fat	—	—	5	45

List 1: starch/bread list. (Whole grain foods have about 2 g fiber/serving. Foods containing 3 g fiber/serving or more are marked with the symbol *.)

Cereals/grains/pasta

* Bran cereals, concentrated	1/3 cup
* Bran cereals, flaked (such as Bran Buds, All Bran)	1/2 cup
Bulgur (cooked)	1/2 cup
Cooked cereals	1/2 cup
Cornmeal (dry)	2 1/2 Tbsp
Grapenuts	3 Tbsp
Grits (cooked)	1/2 cup
Other ready-to-eat unsweetened cereals	3/4 cup
Pasta (cooked)	1/2 cup
Puffed cereal	1 1/2 cup
Rice, white or brown (cooked)	1/3 cup
Shredded wheat	1/2 cup
* Wheat germ	3 Tbsp

Dried beans/peas/lentils

*Beans and peas (cooked; such as kidney, white, split, blackeye)	1/3 cup
*Lentils (cooked)	1/3 cup
*Baked beans	1/4 cup

Starchy vegetables

*Corn	1/2 cup
*Corn on cob, 6 in long	1
*Lima beans	1/2 cup
*Peas, green (fresh, frozen, or canned)	1/2 cup
*Plantain	1/2 cup
Potato, baked	1 small (3 oz)
Potato, mashed	1/2 cup
Squash, winter (acorn, butternut)	3/4 cup
Yam, sweet potato, plain	1/3 cup

Bread

Bagel	1/2 (1 oz)
Bread sticks, crisp (4 in long × 1/2 in)	2 (2/3 oz)
Croutons, low fat	1 cup
English muffin	1/2
Frankfurter bun or hamburger bun	1/2 (1 oz)
Pita (6 in across)	1/2
Plain roll, small	1 (1 oz)
Raisin, unfrosted	1 slice (1 oz)
*Rye, pumpernickel	1 slice (1 oz)
Tortilla, 6 in across	1
White (including French, Italian)	1 slice (1 oz)
Whole wheat	1 slice (1 oz)

Crackers/snacks

Animal crackers	8
Graham crackers (2½ in square)	3
Matzoth	3/4 oz
Melba toast	5 slices
Oyster crackers	2
Popcorn (popped, no fat added)	3 cups
Pretzels	3/4 oz
Rye crisp (2 in × 3½ in)	4
Saltine-type crackers	6
Whole wheat crackers, no fat added (crisp breads, such as Finn, Kavli, Wasa)	2-4 slices (3/4 oz)

Starch foods prepared with fat (count as 1 starch/bread serving + 1 fat)

Biscuit (2½ in across)	1
Chow mein noodles	1/2 cup
Corn bread (2 in cube)	1 (2 oz)
Cracker, round butter type	6
French fried potatoes (2 in to 3½ in long)	1 (1 1/2 oz)
Muffin, plain, small	1
Pancake (4 in across)	2
Stuffing, bread (prepared)	1/4 cup

Taco shell (6 in across)	2
Waffle (4½ in square)	1
Whole wheat crackers, fat added (such as Triscuits)	4-6 (1 oz)

List 2: meat and meat substitutes list. (To reduce fat intake, choose items mainly from the lean and medium-fat groups, using more fish and poultry [remove skin] as meat choices and trimming fat from all meats. Items having 400 mg sodium or more exchange are marked with the symbol **. None of the items on this list contributes fiber to the diet. One exchange is equal to the amount listed for each item. In the case of meat, for example, a serving may be 2-3 exchanges [2-3 oz].)

Lean meat and substitutes

Beef:	USDA Good or Choice grades of lean beef, such as round, sirloin, and flank steak; tenderloin; and chipped beef**	1 oz
Pork:	Lean port, such as fresh ham; canned, cured, or boiled ham**; Canadian bacon**; tenderloin	1 oz
Veal:	All cuts except for veal cutlets (ground or cubed)	1 oz
Poultry:	Chicken, turkey, Cornish hen (without skin)	1 oz
Fish:	All fresh and frozen fish	1 oz
	Crab, lobster, scallops, shrimp, clams (fresh or canned in water**)	2 oz
	Oysters	6 medium
	Tuna** (canned in water)	1/4 cup
	Herring (uncreamed or smoked)	1 oz
	Sardines (canned)	2 medium
Wild Game:	Venison, rabbit, squirrel	1 oz
	Pheasant, duck, goose (without skin)	1 oz
Cheese	Any cottage cheese	1/4 cup
	Grated parmesan	2 Tbsp
	Diet cheeses** (less than 55 kcal/oz)	1 oz
Other:	95% fat-free luncheon meat	1 oz slice
	Egg whites	3 whites
	Egg substitutes (less than 55 kcal/¼ cup)	1/4 cup

Medium-fat meat and substitutes

Beef:	Ground beef, roast (rib, chuck, rump), steak (cubed, Porterhouse, T-bone), and meatloaf (Most beef products are in this category.)	1 oz
Pork:	Chops, loan roast, Boston butt, cutlets (Most pork products fall into this category)	1 oz
Lamb:	Chops, leg, and roast (Most lamb products fall into this category)	1 oz
Veal:	Cutlet (ground or cubed, unbreaded)	1 oz
Poultry:	Chicken (with skin), domestic duck or goose (well drained of fat), ground turkey	1 oz
Fish:	Tuna** (canned in oil and drained)	1/4 cup
	Salmon** (canned)	1/4 cup
Cheese:	Skim or part-skim cheeses, such as:	
	Ricotta	1/4 cup
	Mozzarella	1 oz
	Diet cheeses** (56-80 kcal/oz)	1 oz

Other:	86% fat-free luncheon meat**	1 oz
	Egg (high in cholesterol, limit to 3/week)	1
	Egg substitutes (56-80 kcal per ¼ cup)	1/4 cup
	Tofu (2 1/2 in × 2 3/4 in × 1 in)	4 oz
	Liver, heart, kidney, sweetbreads (high in cholesterol, limit use)	1 oz

High-fat meat and substitutes. (These items are high in saturated fat, cholesterol, and kcalories; limit to occasional use, not more than 3 times/week.)

Beef:	USDA Prime cuts, ribs; corned beef**	1 oz
Pork:	Spareribs, ground pork, pork sausage**	1 oz
Lamb:	Ground lamb patties	1 oz
Fish:	Any fried fish product	1 oz
Cheese:	Regular cheeses**, such as American, Blue, Monterey Jack, Swiss	1 oz
Other:	Luncheon meat,** such as bologna, salami, pimento loaf	1 oz slice
	Sausage**, such as Polish, Italian	1 oz
	Knockwurst, smoked	1 oz
	Bratwurst**	1 oz
	Frankfurter** (turkey or chicken)	1 frank (10/lb)
	Frankfurter** (beef, pork, or combination) (count as 1 high-fat meat + 1 fat)	1 frank (10/lb)
	Peanut butter	1 Tbsp

List 3: vegetable list. (Unless otherwise noted, one vegetable exchange is 1 cup raw vegetable or 1/2 cup cooked vegetable or vegetable juice. Vegetables containing 400 mg sodium or more/serving are marked with the symbol †. Fresh and frozen vegetables have less added salt. Canned vegetables contain more salt, but rinsing will help remove much of it. In general, vegetables contain 2-3 g dietary fiber/serving. Starchy vegetables are found in the Starch/Bread List. Other free vegetables are in the Free Food List.)

Artichoke (½ medium)	Mushrooms, cooked
Asparagus	Okra
Bean sprouts	Onions
Beans (green, wax, Italian)	Pea pods
Beets	Peppers (green)
Broccoli	Rutabaga
Brussels sprouts	Sauerkraut†
Cabbage	Spinach
Carrots	Summer squash (crookneck)
Cauliflower	Tomato (1 large)
Eggplant	Tomato/vegetable juice
Greens (collard, mustard, turnip)	Turnips
Kohlrabi	Water chestnuts
Leeks	Zucchini

List 4: fruit list. (Fruits containing 3 g dietary fiber or more/serving are marked with the symbol *. Portions are usual serving sizes of commonly eaten fruits.)

Fresh, unsweetened frozen, and unsweetened canned fruit

Apple (raw, 2 in across)	1 apple
Applesauce (unsweetened)	1/2 cup
Apricots (medium, raw)	4 apricots
Apricots (canned)	1/2 cup or 4 halves
Banana (9 in long)	1/2 banana
* Blackberries (raw)	3/4 cup
* Blueberries (raw)	3/4 cup
Canteloupe (5 in across)	1/3 melon
Canteloupe (cubes)	1 cup
Cherries (large, raw)	12 cherries
Cherries (canned)	1/2 cup
Figs (raw, 2 in across)	2 figs
Fruit cocktail (canned)	1/2 cup
Grapefruit (medium)	1/2 grapefruit
Grapefruit (segments)	3/4 cup
Grapes (small)	15 grapes
Honeydew melon (medium)	1/8 melon
Honeydew melon (cubes)	1 cup
Kiwi fruit (large)	1 kiwi fruit
Mandarin oranges (segments)	3/4 cup
Mango (small)	1/2 mango
* Nectarine (1½ in across)	1 nectarine
Orange (2½ in across)	1 orange
Papaya (small cubes or balls)	1 cup
Peach (2¾ in across)	1 peach
Peach (slices)	3/4 cup
Peaches (canned)	1/2 cup or 2 halves
Pear	1/2 large pear or 1 small
Pears (canned)	1/2 cup or 2 halves
Persimmon (medium, native)	2 persimmons
Pineapple (raw, cubes)	3/4 cup
Plum (raw, 2 in across)	2 plums
* Pomegranate	1/2 pomegranate
* Raspberries (raw)	1 cup
* Strawberries (raw, whole)	1 1/4 cups
Tangerine (2½ in across)	2 tangerines
Watermelon (cubes or balls)	1 1/4 cup

Dried Fruit

* Apples	4 rings
* Apricots	7 halves
Dates	2½ medium
* Figs	1½
* Prunes	3 medium
Raisins	2 Tbsp

Fruit Juice

Apple juice or cider	1/2 cup
Cranberry juice cocktail	1/3 cup
Grape juice	1/3 cup

Grapefruit juice	1/3 cup
Orange juice	1/2 cup
Pineapple juice	1/2 cup
Prune juice	1/3 cup

List 5: milk list. (Milk may be used alone or in combination with other foods. See the Combination Foods List.)

Skim and very lowfat milk

Skim or nonfat milk	1 cup
½% milk	1 cup
1% milk	1 cup
Lowfat buttermilk	1 cup
Evaporated skim milk	1/2 cup
Dry nonfat milk	1/3 cup
Plain nonfat yogurt	8 oz

Lowfat milk

2% milk	1 cup
Plain lowfat yogurt (with added nonfat milk solids)	8 oz

Whole milk (more than 3¼% butterfat; limit use)

Whole milk	1 cup
Evaporated whole milk	1/2 cup
Whole plain yogurt	8 oz

List 6: fat list. (Measure carefully; use mainly unsaturated fats. Sodium content varies widely, so check labels.)

Unsaturated fats

Avocado	1/8 medium
Margarine	1 tsp
Margarine, diet	1 Tbsp
Mayonnaise	1 tsp
Mayonnaise, reduced kcalories	1 Tbsp
Nuts and seeds:	
Almonds, dry roasted	6 whole
Cashews, dry roasted	1 Tbsp
Peanuts	20 small or 10 large
Pecans	2 whole
Walnuts	2 whole
Other nuts	1 Tbsp
Seeds, pine nuts, sunflower (shelled)	1 Tbsp
Pumpkin seeds	2 tsp
Oil (corn, cottonseed, safflower, soybean, sunflower, olive, peanut)	1 tsp
Olives	10 small or 5 large
Salad dressing (all varieties)	1 Tbsp
Salad dressing, mayonnaise type	2 tsp
Salad dressing, mayonnaise type, low kcal	1 Tbsp
* Salad dressing, low kcal	2 Tbsp
(2 Tbsp low-caloric salad dressing is a free food)	

Saturated fats

Butter	1 tsp
Bacon	1 slice
Chitterlings	1/2 oz
Coconut, shredded	2 Tbsp
Coffee whitener, liquid	2 Tbsp
Coffee whitener, powder	4 tsp
Cream (light, coffee, table)	2 Tbsp
Cream (heavy, whipping)	1 Tbsp
Cream, sour	2 Tbsp
Cream cheese	1 Tbsp
Salt pork	1/4 oz

Free foods. (Any food or drink containing less than 20 kcal/serving is "free." If a serving size is given, 2-3 servings/day are sufficient. Higher fiber* and sodium** foods are indicated. Use **nonstick pan spray** for cooking as desired.)

Drinks

Bouillon** or broth, fat-free	
Bouillon, low sodium	
Carbonated drinks, sugar-free	
Carbonated water	
Club soda	
Cocoa powder, unsweetened	1 Tbsp
Coffee/tea	
Drink mixes, sugar-free	
Tonic water, suger-free	

Condiments

Catsup	1 Tbsp
Horseradish	
Mustard	
Pickles**, dill, unsweetened	
Salad dressing, low kcal	2 Tbsp
Taco sauce	1 Tbsp
Vinegar	

Seasonings

Basil (fresh); other herbs
Celery seeds
Cinnamon; other spices
Chili powder
Chives
Curry
Dill
Flavoring extracts (vanilla, almond, walnut, butter)
Garlic, fresh and powder
Hot pepper sauce and flakes
Lemon, juice and zest (outer skin)
Lemon pepper
Lime, juice and zest
Mint, fresh leaves

Onion powder
Oregano
Paprika
Parsley
Pepper
Pimento

Soy sauce**	
Soy sauce, low sodium— "lite"	
Wine, used in cooking	1/4 cup
Worchestershire sauce	

Fruits

Cranberries, unsweetened	1/2 cup
Rhubarb, unsweetened	1/2 cup

Vegetables

Cabbage
Celery
Chinese cabbage*
Cucumber
Green onion
Hot peppers
Mushrooms
Radishes
Zucchini*

Salad greens

Endive
Escarole
Lettuce
Romaine
Spinach

Sweet substitutes

Candy, hard, sugar-free
Gelatin dessert, sugar-free

Gum, sugar-free		Sugar substitutes (saccharin,	
Jam/jelly, sugar-free	2 tsp	Aspartame)	
Pancake syrup, sugar-free	1-2 Tbsp	Whipped topping	2 Tbsp

Combination foods. (Check the *American Dietetic Association/American Diabetes Association Family Cookbooks* and the *American Diabetes Association Holiday Cookbook* for many recipes and much information, including combination foods.)

Food	Amount	Exchanges
Casseroles, homemade	1 cup (8 oz)	2 starch, 2 med-fat meat, 1 fat
Cheese pizza**, thin crust	1/4 of 10 in	2 starch, 1 med-fat meat, 1 fat
Chili beans*, **	1 cup (8 oz)	2 starch, 2 med-fat meat, 2 fat
Chow mein*, ** (without noodles or rice)	2 cups	1 starch, 2 vegetables, 2 lean meat
Macaroni and cheese**	1 cup	2 starch, 1 med-fat meat, 2 fat
Soup		
Bean*, **	1 cup	1 starch, 1 vegetable, 1 lean meat
Chunky, all varieties**	10 3/4 oz can	1 starch, 1 vegetable, 1 med-fat meat
Cream** (made with water)	1 cup	1 starch, 1 fat
Vegetable** or broth**	1 cup	1 starch
Spaghetti and meatballs (canned)	1 cup	2 starch, 1 med-fat meat, 1 fat
Sugar-free pudding (made with skim milk)	1/2 cup	1 starch

Beans used as a meat substitute:

Dried beans*, peas*, lentils* (cooked)	1 cup	2 starch, 1 lean meat

Foods for occasional use

Food	Amount	Exchanges
Angel food cake	1/12 cake	2 starch
Cake, plain no icing	1/12 cake or 3 in square	2 starch, 2 fat
Cookies	2 small (3/4 in across)	1 starch, 1 fat
Frozen fruit yogurt	1/3 cup	1 starch
Gingersnaps	3	1 starch
Granola	1/4 cup	1 starch, 1 fat
Granola bars	1 small	1 starch, 1 fat
Ice cream, any flavor	1/2 cup	1 starch, 2 fat
Ice milk, any flavor	1/2 cup	1 starch, 1 fat
Sherbet, any flavor	1/4 cup	1 starch
Snack chips**, all varieties	1 oz	1 starch, 2 fat
Vanilla wafers	6 small	1 starch, 1 fat

APPENDIX F
Nutrient Recommendations for Canadians

❖ *Summary of examples of recommended nutrients based on energy expressed as daily rates*

Age	Sex	Energy (kcal)	Thiamin (mg)	Riboflavin (mg)	Niacin (NE[b])	n-3 PUFA[a] (g)	n-6 PUFA (g)
Months							
0–4	Both	600	0.3	0.3	4	0.5	3
5–12	Both	900	0.4	0.5	7	0.5	3
Years							
1	Both	1100	0.5	0.6	8	0.6	4
2–3	Both	1300	0.6	0.7	9	0.7	4
4–6	Both	1800	0.7	0.9	13	1.0	6
7–9	M	2200	0.9	1.1	16	1.2	7
	F	1900	0.8	1.0	14	1.0	6
10–12	M	2500	1.0	1.3	18	1.4	8
	F	2200	0.9	1.1	16	1.2	7
13–15	M	2800	1.1	1.4	20	1.5	9
	F	2200	0.9	1.1	16	1.2	7
16–18	M	3200	1.3	1.6	23	1.8	11
	F	2100	0.8	1.1	15	1.2	7
19–24	M	3000	1.2	1.5	22	1.6	10
	F	2100	0.8	1.1	15	1.2	7
25–49	M	2700	1.1	1.4	19	1.5	9
	F	1900	0.8	1.0	14	1.1	7

Continued.

From Scientific Review Committee: *Nutrition recommendation*, Ottawa, Canada, 1990, Health and Welfare.
[a] PUFA, polyunsaturated fatty acids
[b] Niacin Equivalents
[c] Level below which intake should not fall
[d] Assumes moderate physical activity

❖ *Summary of examples of recommended nutrients based on energy expressed as daily rates—cont'd*

Age	Sex	Energy (kcal)	Thiamin (mg)	Riboflavin (mg)	Niacin (NE[b])	n-3 PUFA[a] (g)	n-6 PUFA (g)
Years—cont'd							
50–74	M	2300	0.9	1.2	16	1.3	8
	F	1800	0.8[c]	1.0[c]	14[c]	1.1[c]	7[c]
75+	M	2000	0.8	1.0	14	1.1	7
	F[d]	1700	0.8[c]	1.0[c]	14[c]	1.1[c]	7[c]
Pregnancy (additional)							
1st trimester		100	0.1	0.1	1	0.05	0.3
2nd trimester		300	0.1	0.3	2	0.16	0.9
3rd trimester		300	0.1	0.3	2	0.16	0.9
Lactation (additional)		450	0.2	0.4	3	0.25	1.5

❖ *Summary of examples of recommended nutrients based on energy expressed as daily rates—cont'd*

Age	Sex	Weight (kg)	Protein (g)	Vit A (RE[a])	Vit D (µg)	Vit E (mg)	Vit C (mg)	Folate (µg)	Vit B$_{12}$ (µg)	Calcium (mg)	Phosphorus (mg)	Magnesium (mg)	Iron (mg)	Iodine (µg)	Zinc (mg)
Months															
0–4	Both	6.0	12[b]	400	10	3	20	25	0.3	250[c]	150	20	0.3[d]	30	2[d]
5–12	Both	9.0	12	400	10	3	20	40	0.4	400	200	32	7	40	3
Years															
1	Both	11	13	400	10	3	20	40	0.5	500	300	40	6	55	4
2–3	Both	14	16	400	5	4	20	50	0.6	550	350	50	6	65	4
4–6	Both	18	19	500	5	5	25	70	0.8	600	400	65	8	85	5
7–9	M	25	26	700	2.5	7	25	90	1.0	700	500	100	8	110	7
	F	25	26	700	2.5	6	25	90	1.0	700	500	100	8	95	7

10–12	M	34	34	800	2.5	8	25	120	1.0	900	700	130	8	125	9
	F	36	36	800	2.5	7	25	130	1.0	1100	800	135	8	110	9
13–15	M	50	49	900	2.5	9	30	175	1.0	1100	900	185	10	160	12
	F	48	46	800	2.5	7	30	170	1.0	1000	850	180	13	160	9
16–18	M	62	58	1000	2.5	10	40[e]	220	1.0	900	1000	230	10	160	12
	F	53	47	800	2.5	7	30[e]	190	1.0	700	850	200	12	160	9
19–24	M	71	61	1000	2.5	10	40[e]	220	1.0	800	1000	240	9	160	12
	F	58	50	800	2.5	7	30[e]	180	1.0	700	850	200	13	160	9
25–49	M	74	64	1000	2.5	9	40[e]	230	1.0	800	1000	250	9	160	12
	F	59	51	800	2.5	6	30[e]	185	1.0	700	850	200	13	160	9
50–74	M	73	63	1000	5	7	40[e]	230	1.0	800	1000	250	9	160	12
	F	63	54	800	5	6	30[e]	195	1.0	800	850	210	8	160	9
75+	M	69	59	1000	5	6	40[e]	215	1.0	800	1000	230	9	160	12
	F	64	55	800	5	5	30[e]	200	1.0	800	850	210	8	160	9
Pregnancy (additional)															
1st Trimester		5		0	2.5	2	0	200	0.2	500	200	15	0	25	6
2nd Trimester		20		0	2.5	2	10	200	0.2	500	200	45	5	25	6
3rd Trimester		24		0	2.5	2	10	200	0.2	500	200	45	10	25	6
Lactation (additional)		20		400	2.5	3	25	100	0.2	500	200	65	0	50	6

a Retinal Equivalents
b Protein is assumed to be from breast milk and must be adjusted for infant formula.
c Infant formula with high phosphorus should contain 375 mg calcium.
d Breast milk is assumed to be the source of the mineral.
e Smokers should increase vitamin C by 50%.

Glossary

absorption (L. *ab*, away; *sorbere*, to suck in) Process by which digested food materials pass through the mucosal epithelial cells lining the gastrointestinal tract, mainly in the small intestine, into the blood or lymph.

acid (L. *acidus*, sour) Substance that buffers or neutralizes base substances by donating hydrogen ions. Acids are essentially ionized hydrogen donors—in solution they provide hydrogen ions.

adipose (L. *adeps*, fat; *adiposus*, fatty) Fat present in cells of adipose (fatty) tissue.

adynamic ileus (Gr. *a-*, prefix: want, absence; *dynamis*, might; *ilein*, to roll up) Obstruction of the intestines caused by lack of normal bowel motility.

aerobic capacity (Gr., L., *aer*, air or gas) Ability to perform activity that requires oxygen to proceed.

albumin (L. *albus*, white) A major protein in many animal and some plant tissues; specialized plasma protein maintaining normal blood volume.

aldosterone Main hormone of the cortex (outer layer) of the adrenal glands; acts on the distal nephron tubules in the kidney to reabsorb sodium and water, the *aldosterone mechanism*.

alkaline (L. *alkalinus*, alkali) Chemical nature of substances having the reactions of an alkali; generally having basic or nonacidic qualities.

amino acids Nitrogen-bearing compounds that form the structural units of protein. The various food proteins, when digested, yield their specific constituent amino acids, which are then available for use by the cells to synthesize specific tissue proteins.

amino peptidase Specific protein-splitting enzyme secreted by glands in the walls of the small intestine that breaks off the nitrogen-containing amino ($-NH_2$) end of the peptide chains that form proteins, producing smaller short-chained peptides and free amino acids.

anabolism (Gr. *anabole*, building up) Constructive metabolic processes that build up the body substances and tissues; opposite of *catabolism*, processes that break down body substances and tissues.

analog (or analogue) (Gr. *analogos*, due ratio, proportionate) A chemical compound having a similar structure to that of another compound but differing in a particular component.

anemia (Gr. *an-* negative prefix; *haima* blood) Blood condition characterized by decreased number of circulating red blood cells, hemoglobin, or both.

angina pectoris (Gr. *angeion*, vessel; L. *pectus*, breast) Chest pain, usually radiating down the arm, with a feeling of suffocation; caused most often by lack of oxygen to the heart muscle, sometimes precipitated by effort or excitement.

antibodies Specific protein substances circulating in the blood designed to interact with and destroy their specific disease agents—*antigens*.

antidiuretic hormone (ADH) Hormone secreted by the posterior pituitary gland in response to body stress; acts on the distal tubules of the kidney's nephrons to cause water reabsorption and thus protect vital body water. It is also called *vasopressin*.

antigens (*antibody* + Gr. *gennan*, to produce) Any disease agents, such as toxins, bacteria, viruses, or other foreign substances, that stimulate the production of specific *antibodies* to combat them.

anuria Complete lack of urine secretion by the kidneys.

apoprotein (Gr. *apo-*, from) Protein part of a lipoprotein compound.

ascites (Gr. *askites*, from; *askos*, bag) Outflow and accumulation of fluid in the abdominal cavity.

atherosclerosis (Gr. *athers*, gruel; *sklerosis*, hardness) Condition in which yellowish fatty plaques *(atheromas)* form within the medium and large arteries, eventually filling in the vessel at that point and blocking blood circulation.

atrophy (Gr. *atrophia*) Wasting away; reduced size of a cell, tissue, or organ.

basal metabolism (Gr. *basis*, base; *metabole*, change) The amount of energy needed by the body for maintenance of life when the person is at digestive, physical, and emotional rest. This basal metabolic rate (BMR) is reported as the percent of variation in the person above or below the normal number of kilocalories required for a person of like height, weight, and sex.

blood urea nitrogen (BUN) Blood test used to identify any disorder in kidney function.

botulism (L. *botulus*, sausage) A type of food poisoning caused by a neurotoxin, botulin, produced by the growth of the bacteria *Clostridium botulinum* in improperly preserved or canned foods.

cachexia (Gr. *kakos*, bad; *hexis*, habit) A specific profound effect caused by a disturbance in glucose metabolism, usually seen in patients with advanced cancer; general poor health and malnutrition usually indicated by an emaciated appearance.

callus (L. *kalus*, hard) Unorganized meshwork of newly grown, woven bone developed on pattern of original fibrin clot (formed after fracture) and normally replaced by hard adult bone.

caloric density Concentration of energy (kilocalories) in a given quantity of food.

carbonic acid–base bicarbonate buffer system The body's main buffer system, a combination of carbonic acid and base (sodium) bicarbonate designed to protect the body fluids against entry of either acid or base substances and maintain an internal environment compatible with life.

carcinogens (Gr. *karkinos*, a crab; *gennan*, to produce) Agents capable of producing cancer.

carotene (L. *carot*, carrot) Any of three (alpha, beta, and gamma) yellow or orange pigments found in many plants, especially carrots, that are provitamin substances converted to vitamin A in the body. Beta-carotene is the one of greatest significance in human nutrition.

catabolism (Gr. *katabole*, a throwing down) The breaking-down phase of metabolism in which complex substances in tissues are progressively broken down into simpler ones; process of tissue breakdown.

cell metabolism Sum of complex interrelated chemical reactions in cells by which life of the body is maintained; sometimes called intermediary metabolism.

cellulitis (L. *cella*, compartment; suffix *-itis*, inflammation) Diffuse inflammation of the soft or connective tissue from infection producing a watery exudate, sometimes leading to an ulcer or abscess.

cerebrovascular accident (CVA) Stroke; brain tissue damage caused by reduced blood flow from arterial blockage or breakage.

cholecalciferol Chemical name for activated form of vitamin D most important in human nutrition; activated 7-dehydrocholesterol, vitamin D_3.

cholesterol (Gr. *chole*, bile; *stereos*, solid) A fat-related compound, a sterol, found only in animal tissue; a normal constituent of bile and a principal constituent of gallstones. In the body, cholesterol is synthesized mainly by the liver. In the diet, it is found only in animal food sources. In human body metabolism, cholesterol is important as a precursor of various steroid hormones such as sex hormones and adrenal corticoids. However, in disordered lipid metabolism, it is a major factor in atherosclerosis, the underlying disease process leading to heart disease.

chyme (Gr. *chymos*, juice) Semifluid food mass in the gastrointestinal tract following gastric digestion.

chymotrypsin A protein-splitting enzyme produced by the pancreas that acts in the small intestine. Together with trypsin, it breaks down proteins to shorter chain polypeptides and dipeptides.

collagen disease Connective tissue diseases such as rheumatoid arthritis, scleroderma, lupus erythematosus, and others.

complex carbohydrate Larger, more complex molecules of carbohydrates. Complex forms of dietary carbohydrates are starch, which is digestible and provides a major energy source, and fiber, which is nondigestible and provides important bulk to the diet.

continuous ambulatory peritoneal dialysis (CAPD) A form of kidney dialysis that does not require a kidney dialysis machine and can be used at home.

coronary heart disease General term used for heart disease involving the coronary arteries, usually caused by the underlying vascular disease process atherosclerosis.

cystinuria (*cystine* + *uria*, from Gr. *ouron*, urine) Condition caused by a rare hereditary defect in metabolism of the amino acid cystine, characterized by excessive urinary excretion of cystine (a sulfur-containing amino acid). Cystine crystals often accumulate and form small, smooth, yellow kidney stones (cystine renal calculi).

deamination (L., *de-*, from; Gr. *amino*, nitrogen-containing chemical group—NH_2) Chemical reaction that splits off the amino group from its carrier compound.

dehiscence (L. dehiscere, *to gape*) Splitting open, separation of the layers of a surgical wound.

dialysis (Gr. *dia*, through; *lysis*, separate) Separating substances in solution by taking advantage of the different rates at which they pass through a semipermeable membrane; filtering process done outside the body by special machines in cases of advanced renal failure when the damaged kidneys no longer function.

dietetics Management of diet and the use of food; the science concerned with the nutritional planning and preparation of foods.

diffusion (L. *diffundere*, to spread or pour forth) Processes by which particles in solution spread throughout the solution and across separating membranes from the place of highest solute concentration to all surrounding spaces of lesser solute concentration.

digestion (L. *dis*, apart; *genere*, to carry; *digerere*, to separate, arrange, dissolve, digest) Process by which food is broken down chemically in the gastrointestinal tract through the action of secretions containing specific enzymes. Digestion separates complex food structures into their simpler parts, which are the chemicals the body needs to sustain life.

dipeptidase A protein-splitting enzyme produced by glands in the walls of the small intestine, which breaks the final dipeptides into free amino acids.

disaccharide (L. *di-*, two; *saccharum*, sugar) Class of compound or "double" sugars composed of two molecules of "single" sugars or monosaccharides. The three common members of this class are sucrose (table sugar), lactose (milk sugar), and maltose (grain sugar).

diuresis (Gr. *diourein*, to urinate) Increased urination.

edema (Gr. *oidema*, swelling) Large abnormal amounts of fluid filling the intercellular tissue spaces; may be either localized or systemic.

elemental formula A formula whose components cannot be broken down into simpler parts, so it requires no further digestion and is ready for immediate absorption.

enteral (Gr. *enteron*, intestine) Within, or by way of, the intestines; feeding by way of the gastrointestinal tract, either regular oral feedings or tube feedings.

essential hypertension High blood pressure of unknown cause; usually related to a strong family history of hypertension.

exudate (L. *exsudare*, to sweat out) Material that escapes from blood vessels and is deposited in tissues or on tissue surfaces; has a high content of protein, cells, or other cellular solid matter.

fatty acid The structural components of fats.

gastric lipase Fat-splitting enzyme secreted by the stomach; ributyrinase.

gastrostomy A surgical opening into the stomach for special tube feeding.

gene (Gr. *gennan*, to produce) The biologic unit of heredity; located at specific sites on particular threads of chromosomes in the cell nucleus.

glyceride Chemical group name for fats; formed from glycerol base with one, two, or three fatty acids attached. Glycerides are the principal constituents of adipose tissue and are found in animal and vegetable fats and oils.

glycogen (Gr. *glykys*, sweet; *gennan*, to produce) A polysaccharide, the main storage form of carbohydrate, largely stored in the liver and to a lesser extent in muscle tissue.

glycosuria (Gr. *glykys*, sweet; *ouron*, urine) Sugar in the urine, an abnormal condition.

health A state of optimal well-being—physical, mental, and social; relative freedom from disease or disability.

health promotion (A.S. *hal*, hale, sound; L. *promovere*, to move forward) Active involvement in behaviors or programs that advance positive well-being.

hematuria (Gr. *haima*, blood; *ouron*, urine) Blood in the urine.

hemoglobin (Gr. *haima*, blood; L. *globus*, globe) A conjugated protein in red blood cells; composed of a compact rounded mass of polypeptide chains forming *globin*, the protein portion, attached to an iron-containing red pigment called *heme*. Carries oxygen in the blood to cells.

homeostasis (Gr. *homoios*, like, unchanging; *stasis*, standing) State of relative dynamic equilibrium within the body's internal environment; a balance achieved through the operation of various interrelated physiologic mechanisms.

hyperglycemia (Gr. *hyper*, above; *glykys*, sweet) An abnormal increase in the level of blood glucose.

hypertension Medical term for chronic condition of high blood pressure.

hypoglycemia (Gr. *hypo*, under; *glykys*, sweet) An abnormal decrease in the level of blood glucose.

immunocompetence (L. *immunis*, free, exempt; *competere*, to be fitting or suffice) To be immune; ability to produce antibodies in response to antigens.

insulin (L. *insula*, island) Hormone formed in the B cells of the pancreas; secreted when blood glucose levels rise and assists its entry into cells for cell metabolism and ultimate energy production. Commercial insulin used by persons with diabetes who lack available internal insulin.

intestinal lipase Fat-splitting enzyme produced by glands in the walls of the small intestine; secretion triggered by the presence of fat.

isotonicity (Gr. *isos*, equal; *tonos*, tone, tension) State of having the same tension or pressure. Two given solutions are isotonic if they have the same concentration of particles in solution and thus the same osmotic pressure; as such they balance one another. For example, the law of isotonicity governs the movement of water and electrolytes between the gastrointestinal tract and the surrounding extracellular fluid.

ketoacidosis Abnormally high concentration of ketone bodies (ketones) in body tissues and fluids; a complication of diabetes mellitus and starvation.

ketones Intermediate products of fat metabolism; acids such as acetone.

ketosis General synonymous term for ketoacidosis.

kilocalorie (Fr. *chilioi*, thousand; L. *calor*, heat) The general term *calorie* refers to a unit of heat measure and is used alone to designate the *small calorie*. The calorie used in nutritional science and the study of metabolism is the *large calorie*, 1000 calories, or kilocalorie, to be more accurate and avoid the use of very large numbers in calculations.

lactated Ringer's solution A sterile water solution of sodium chloride, potassium chloride, calcium chloride, and sodium lactate given to replenish fluid and electrolytes; named for Sydney Ringer (1835-1910), an English physiologist.

lipectomy (Gr. *lipos*, fat; *ektome*, excision) The removal of fat from adipose tissue by a suction process, commonly called *liposuction*.

lipid (Gr. *lipos*, fat) The chemical group name for organic substances of fatty nature. The lipids include fats, oils, waxes, and related compounds such as cholesterol.

lipoprotein Chemical complexes of fat with protein. The lipoproteins serve as the major carriers of lipids in the plasma, since most of the plasma fat is associated with them. They vary in density according to the size of the fat load being carried; the lower the density, the higher the fat load. The combination package with water-soluble protein makes possible the transport of nonwater-soluble fatty substances in the water-based blood circulation.

lymphocytes (L. *lympha*, water; *kytos*, hollow vessel, anything that contains or covers) Special white blood cells that function as components of the body's immune system.

major minerals The name given those minerals that occur in the body in larger amounts than the trace elements. The term has no meaning of greater importance; *all* minerals have specific vital roles in body metabolism.

metabolism (Gr. *metaballein*, to turn about, change, alter) The sum of all chemical changes that take place in the body by which it maintains itself and produces energy for its functioning. Products of these various reactions are called *metabolites*.

microvilli (Gr. *mikros*, small; L. *villus*, tuft of hair) Minute hairlike projections from the surface of cells, especially cells of the intestinal mucosa, which greatly increase the absorbing surface area.

mutation (L. *mutare*, to change) A change in form or quality; in genetics, a permanent change in a specific gene that can then be transmitted to offspring.

myocardial infarction (Gr. *mys*, muscle; *kardia*, heart; L. *infarctus*, dead tissue) Heart attack; an area of dead tissue in the heart muscle caused by local lack of oxygen resulting from obstruction in the artery serving that tissue. The obstruction is caused by atherosclerosis, fatty buildup within the blood vessel, or a blood clot cutting off the circulation.

neoplasm (Gr. *neo*, new; *plasma*, a formation or growth) Any new or abnormal growth; uncontrolled or progressive growth. Also called a tumor.

nephrosis (Gr. *nephros*, kidney) General term for disease of the kidney characterized by degenerative lesions in the nephron tubules and marked by gross edema; nephrotic syndrome.

nutrient density Concentration of nutrients in a portion of food.

nutrition (L. *nutritic*, nourishment) The sum of the processes involved in taking in nutrients, assimilating and using them to maintain body tissue and provide energy; a foundation for life and health.

nutritional science The body of science, developed through controlled research, that relates to the processes involved in nutrition—international, community, and clinical.

oliguria (Gr. *oligos*, little; *ouron*, urine) Reduced amount of urine in comparison to fluid intake.

osmosis (Gr. *osmos*, a thrusting) Passage of a solvent such as water through a membrane that separates solutions of differing concentrations. Water molecules pass through the membrane from the area of lower concentration of solute particles to that of higher concentration of particles, in order to equalize the concentrations of the two solutions.

pancreatic amylase (Gr. *amylon*, starch) Starch-splitting enzyme produced by the pancreas and acting in the small intestine.

pancreatic lipase (Gr. *lipos*, fat) Fat-splitting enzyme produced by the pancreas and acting in the small intestine.

parenteral (Gr. *para*, alongside, beyond; *enteron*, intestine) Shot through the intestine; feeding of nutrient solutions into veins, peripheral or central, when the gastrointestinal tract cannot be used or a greater concentration of nutrients is necessary.

pepsin (Gr. *pepsis*, digestion) The main gastric enzyme specific for proteins. Pepsin begins breaking large protein molecules into shorter chain polypeptides. Gastric hydrochloric acid is necessary to activate pepsin.

pinocytosis (Gr. *pinein*, to drink; *kytos*, cell) Engulfing of nutrient solutions by cells as a means of absorption; "cell drinking."

plasma protein Any of a number of protein substances carried in the circulating blood. A major one of these plasma proteins is *albumin*, which maintains the fluid volume of the blood through its colloidal osmotic pressure.

precursor (L. *praecursor*, a forerunner) A substance from which another substance is made. For example, beta-carotene is a precursor of vitamin A.

proteinuria Abnormal loss of protein in the urine; also called *albuminuria*.

purine Chemical compound found in various animal and plant foods, of which uric acid is a metabolic end product.

Recommended Dietary Allowances (RDAs) Recommended daily allowances of nutrients and energy intake for population groups according to age and sex, with defined weight and height. Established and reviewed periodically by a representative group of nutritional scientists, in relation to current research. These standards vary very little among the developed countries.

Registered Dietitian (RD)   A professional dietitian, accredited by academic degree course of university and graduate study and having passed required registration examinations administered by the American Dietetic Association.

retinol   (L. *ret*, net; *retina*, eye part; *-ol*, alcohol) Vitamin A; the form of vitamin A found in mammals. Its chemical structure is that of a 20-carbon higher alcohol. Its major functions relate to the light-dark vision cycle in the eye and to the health of epithelial tissue. In the eye, a lack of vitamin A can cause blindness because of deterioration of epithelial tissue with formation of nonfunctioning scar tissue.

saccharide   (L. *saccharum*, sugar) Chemical name for sugar molecules. May occur as single molecules in monosaccharides (glucose, fructose, galactose), as two molecules in disaccharides (lactose, sucrose, maltose), or as multiple molecules in polysaccharides (starch, fiber, glycogen).

salivary amylase   Starch-splitting enzyme secreted by the salivary glands and acting in the mouth; ptyalin. This action is small because food is usually not held in the mouth long enough for continued action, which is good reason for chewing food more thoroughly.

saturated   (L. *saturare*, to fill) State of being filled; state of fatty acid components of fat being filled in all of their available carbon bonds with hydrogen, making the fat harder and more solid. Such solid food fats are from animal sources.

simple carbohydrate   Simple sugars, mono- and disaccharides.

steroids   Group of synthetic derivatives of the male sex hormone testosterone that have pronounced anabolic effects.

stoma   (Gr. *stoma*, mouth) Surgical opening through abdominal wall to the large intestine for elimination of fecal material from the body; a colostomy or an ileostomy.

tocopherol   (Gr. *tokos*, childbirth; *pherein*, to carry) Vitamin E; named at time of early discovery through experiments with rats and observed necessity of the vitamin for reproduction in rats. However, in continued study with humans this function did not prove true, but the early name remained.

total parenteral nutrition (TPN)   Process of feeding concentrated nutrient solutions through large central subclavian vein directly into superior vena cava, providing complete nutrition. Used in cases when gastrointestinal tract is not available and increased nutritional support is required for an extended period of time.

trace element   Minerals occurring in very small amounts in the body, but having essential functions.

triglyceride   Chemical name for fats in the body or in foods. Compound of three fatty acids attached to a glycerol base.

trypsin   A protein-splitting enzyme secreted by the pancreas and acting in the small intestine; reduces proteins to shorter chain polypeptides and dipeptides.

vegan   Person following a strict vegetarian diet containing no complete animal protein (milk, cheese, egg, meat), who must carefully plan a good mixture of complementary combinations of incomplete plant proteins to obtain a balanced diet and not suffer deficiencies of protein and other nutrients, such as vitamin B_{12}, contained in animal proteins.

villi   Fingerlike projections on the mucosal surface of the small intestine, each of which is covered with still smaller hairlike microvilli called the *brush border*. Together these structures greatly increase the intestinal absorbing surface area.

Answers to self-test questions

Chapter 1
True-False
1. T
2. F
3. F
Multiple Choice
1. a
2. d
3. a

Chapter 2
True-False
1. F
2. T
3. F
4. T
5. F
6. T
Multiple Choice
1. d
2. b

Chapter 3
True-False
1. F
2. T
3. F
4. F
5. T
Multiple Choice
1. a
2. c
3. b

Chapter 4
True-False
1. F
2. T
3. F
4. F
5. F
6. F
7. T
8. T
9. T
10. F
11. T
Multiple Choice
1. a
2. d
3. c

Chapter 5
True-False
1. F
2. F
3. T
4. F
5. F
6. F
Multiple Choice
1. b
2. c
3. c
4. c
5. d
6. c

Chapter 6
True-False
1. F
2. F
3. T
4. F
5. T
6. T
Multiple Choice
1. b
2. c
3. d

Chapter 7
True-False
1. F
2. T
3. F
4. T
5. F
6. F
7. F
8. T
Multiple Choice
1. c
2. a
3. b

Chapter 8
Matching
1. k
2. g
3. n
4. a
5. l
6. b
7. f
8. h
9. i
10. p
11. d
12. o
13. j
14. c
15. e
16. m

Chapter 9
True-False
1. F
2. T
3. F
4. T
5. F
6. F
7. T

Multiple Choice
1. d
2. c
3. c
4. b
5. d
6. a

Chapter 10
True-False
1. T
2. F
3. F
4. T
5. F
6. F
7. T
8. T
9. T
10. T
Multiple Choice
1. a
2. b
3. b
4. d

Chapter 11
True-False
1. F
2. F
3. F
4. F
5. F
Multiple Choice
1. a
2. c
3. b

Chapter 12
True-False
1. F
2. F
3. F
4. F
5. T
6. F
7. F
Multiple Choice
1. d
2. a
3. a
4. d

Chapter 13
True-False
1. F
2. F
3. F
4. T
5. F

6. T
7. F
8. T
Multiple Choice
1. d
2. c

Chapter 14
True-False
1. F
2. T
3. T
4. T
5. F
6. F
Multiple Choice
1. d
2. b
3. c
4. b
5. c

Chapter 15
True-False
1. F
2. F
3. F
4. T
5. F
Multiple Choice
1. d
2. b
3. b

Chapter 16
True-False
1. F
2. F
3. T
4. F
5. F
6. T
7. T
8. F
9. T
Multiple Choice
1. b
2. d
3. d
4. a
5. c

Chapter 17
True-False
1. T
2. F
3. T
4. F
5. F
6. T
7. F
8. T
9. F
10. F
Multiple Choice
1. d
2. c
3. b
4. d
5. b

Chapter 18
True-False
1. F
2. F
3. T
4. F
5. F
6. T
7. T
8. T
9. T
Multiple Choice
1. d
2. b
3. c
4. b

Chapter 19
True-False
1. T
2. F
3. F
4. F
5. T
6. T
7. T
8. F
9. F
10. F
Multiple Choice
1. b
2. a
3. a

Chapter 20
True-False
1. F
2. F
3. F
4. T
5. T
6. T
7. T
8. F
9. F
10. F
Multiple Choice
1. c
2. a
3. d

Chapter 21
True-False
1. T
2. F
3. F
4. T
5. T
6. F
7. T
8. F
9. T
10. T
Multiple Choice
1. b
2. a
3. a

Chapter 22
True-False
1. T
2. T
3. F
4. T
5. F
6. F
7. F
8. F
9. F
10. T
Multiple Choice
1. a
2. b
3. a
4. c
5. b

Chapter 23
True-False
1. F
2. T

3. T
4. F
5. T
6. F

7. F
8. T
Multiple Choice
1. b

2. c
3. b
4. a
5. d

Index

Median Heights and Weights and Recommended Energy Intake

Category	Age (years) or Condition	Weight (kg)	Weight (lb)	Height (cm)	Height (in)	FEE[a] (kcal/day)	Average Energy Allowance (kcal)[b] Multiples of REE	Average Energy Allowance (kcal)[b] Per kg	Average Energy Allowance (kcal)[b] Per day[c]
Infants	0.0–0.5	6	13	60	24	320		108	650
	0.5–1.0	9	20	71	28	500		98	850
Children	1–3	13	29	90	35	740		102	1,300
	4–6	20	44	112	44	950		90	1,800
	7–10	28	62	132	52	1,130		70	2,000
Males	11–14	45	99	157	62	1,440	1.70	55	2,500
	15–18	66	145	176	69	1,760	1.67	45	3,000
	19–24	72	160	177	70	1,780	1.67	40	2,900
	25–50	79	174	176	70	1,800	1.60	37	2,900
	51 +	77	170	173	68	1,530	1.50	30	2,300
Females	11–14	46	101	157	62	1,310	1.67	47	2,200
	15–18	55	120	163	64	1,370	1.60	40	2,200
	19–24	58	128	164	65	1,350	1.60	38	2,200
	25–50	63	138	163	64	1,380	1.55	36	2,200
	51 +	65	143	160	63	1,280	1.50	30	1,900
Pregnant	1st Trimester								+ 0
	2nd Trimester								+ 300
	3rd Trimester								+ 300
Lactating	1st 6 months								+ 500
	2nd 6 months								+ 500

[a] Resting energy expenditure (REE); calculation based on FAO equations, then rounded.

[b] In the range of light to moderate activity, the coefficient of variation is ±20%.

[c] Figure is rounded.